Fourth Edition

VOLUME 2

Family Nurse Practitioner Review

EDITED BY

Elizabeth Blunt, PhD, RN, FNP-BC, and
Courtney Reinisch, DNP, MSN, FNP-BC, DCC

ANCC

CREDENTIALING KNOWLEDGE CENTER | Conferences.
Consultation.
Education.

Library of Congress Cataloging-in-Publication Data

Family nurse practitioner (2009).
Family nurse practitioner review manual / edited by Elizabeth Blunt and Courtney
Reinisch.—4th edition.
      p. ;   cm.
   Preceded by Family nurse practitioner : nursing review and resource manual / edited by
Elizabeth Blunt. 3rd ed. 2009.
   Includes bibliographical references.
   ISBN 978-1-935213-41-3
   I. Blunt, Elizabeth, editor of compilation. II. Reinisch, Courtney, editor of compilation.
III. Title.
   [DNLM: 1. Family Nursing—Examination Questions. 2. Nurse Practitioners. WY 18.2]
RT73
610.7306'92076—dc23
                              2013037137

The American Nurses Credentialing Center (ANCC), a subsidiary of the American
Nurses Association (ANA), provides individuals and organizations throughout the
nursing profession with the resources they need to achieve practice excellence. ANCC's
internationally renowned credentialing programs certify nurses in specialty practice areas;
recognize healthcare organizations for promoting safe, positive work environments through
the Magnet Recognition Program® and the Pathway to Excellence® Program; and accredit
providers of continuing nursing education. In addition, the ANCC Credentialing Knowledge
Center™ provides leading-edge information and education services and products to
support its core credentialing programs.

Volume 2: ISBN 13: 978-1-935213-45-1

© 2013 American Nurses Credentialing Center.
8515 Georgia Ave., Suite 400
Silver Spring, MD 20910
All rights reserved.

Contents

VOLUME 2

Mood Disorders
Depressive Disorders
Substance Use Disorders
Domestic Violence and Abuse
Sexual Assault and Abuse
Eating Disorders
Other Disorders

FEMALE REPRODUCTIVE SYSTEM DISORDERS

Barbara Seibert, DNP, CRNP, FNP-BC, CNE

GENERAL APPROACH

Description

▶ Because of the high number of women who seek health care, the primary care clinician must be prepared to handle a broad variety of women's health concerns.

▶ The clinician may view women's health concerns in terms of common groupings: menstrual cycle, normal changes (menopause), variations (PMS), abnormalities of that cycle (abnormal bleeding), and fertility issues.

RED FLAGS

Ovarian Cancer

▶ High-risk women: Familial cancer syndromes; history of breast, colon, or uterine cancer; 2 first-degree relatives with ovarian cancer; smokers

▶ Presentation with ovarian cancer is vague: Mild, nonspecific gastrointestinal symptoms; dyspareunia; abdominal pain; bloating; urinary symptoms; dyspepsia; abdominal fullness; increasing abdominal girth; cramping; irregular vaginal bleeding; fatigue; or pelvic pressure; 60%–75% present with advanced disease

▶ In a recent study, predominance of the following symptoms differentiated cases of ovarian cancer vs. controls: unusual bloating (71%); unusual abdominal or lower back pain (52%); and fullness, abdominal pressure, and lack of energy (43%).

▶ Weight loss and anorexia are poor prognostic signs.

▶ Physical exam findings occur late in disease: palpable adnexal mass; ascites (poor prognostic sign)

▶ If suspicious, get transvaginal ultrasound. Consider getting CA-125 as you refer to GYN oncology specialist.

▶ Refer women in high-risk groups — premenarchal or postmenopausal females with a palpable ovary, reproductive-age women with persistent ovarian cyst ≥ 5 cm (beyond 6 weeks) — to GYN oncologist.

Endometrial Cancer

▶ Risks include any condition leading to unopposed estrogen, including prolonged anovulation, oligomenorrhea nulliparity, obesity, diabetes, early menarche or late menopause, endometrial hyperplasia, hormone replacement therapy with estrogen alone, smokers, polycystic ovary syndrome (PCOS), tamoxifen therapy; if diagnosed in early stages, 5-year survival is 85%–95%.

▶ 80%–90% present with painless abnormal bleeding pattern as cardinal sign, but may also present with watery vaginal discharge.

▶ Pelvic pain, pressure, or mass present late in disease (entire uterus may be boggy, enlarged)

▶ Refer if Pap smear reports atypical glandular cells of undetermined significance (AGCUS) or if transvaginal ultrasound reports endometrial stripe ≥ 10 mm among postmenopausal women.

▶ Any postmenopausal vaginal bleeding merits a referral to gynecology for further work-up; women over 35 or with risk factors should have a pelvic ultrasound, an endometrial biopsy, or both, as should younger women with vaginal bleeding unresponsive to therapies.

Vulvar Cancer

▶ Pruritus most common symptom, followed by burning or dysuria, bleeding, pain, or discharge

▶ Common areas for lesions include labia majora, clitoris, and periurethral areas, but may occur anywhere on vulva

▶ Suspicious findings include changes in pigmentation or tissue that is thickened, reddened, ulcerated, nodular, fissured, or with abnormal raised areas.

▶ Refer any lesions that fail to spontaneously resolve in several weeks or with therapy; promptly refer new lesions among women ≥ 60 years of age.

Vaginal Cancer

▶ Frequently secondary to cervical or endometrial cancer, diethylstilbestrol (DES) exposure

▶ Signs and symptoms include bleeding from vaginal wall, chronic pruritus, vaginal or pelvic pain.

▶ Usually found in proximal one-third of posterior vagina; most lesions raised, granular, friable; lesions may be palpable, but not visible

▶ Refer all lesions for biopsy.

Ectopic Pregnancy

▶ Represents 1%–2% of pregnancies but accounts for 13% of maternal deaths

   » Majority of ectopics implant in fallopian tubes (97%).

   » Most common time for rupture is during the first 8–12 weeks

▶ Risk factors include history of sexually transmitted infections (STIs; especially multiple episodes), pelvic inflammatory disease (PID), adhesions, intra-uterine device (IUD) use, tubal ligation failure, pelvic or abdominal surgery, prior ectopic gestation, inconsistent or nonuse of birth control methods, infertility therapy

▶ Classic symptoms: Amenorrhea, abdominal pain, abnormal bleeding

▶ Commonly see late menses that is lighter than normal *or* amenorrhea of 4–6 weeks' duration followed by erratic vaginal bleeding (75%)

▶ Abdominal tenderness (95%); adnexal tenderness (87%–99%); adnexal mass (33%–53%); cervical motion tenderness in almost all cases

▶ Peritoneal signs: Involuntary guarding, rigidity (75%)

▶ Late and more ominous signs indicating potential rupture: Syncope or orthostatic blood pressure changes (shock, 2%–17%), shoulder pain similar to cholecystitis (10%), increase in vaginal bleeding (dark red or bright red), and significant worsening of abdominal pain

▶ If urine hCG or serum β-hCG is positive, get series of quantitative serum hCG (low and not doubling every 24–48 hours indicates ectopic); if urine hCG is negative, get serum β-hCG. A negative serum β-hCG rules out pregnancy and thus presence of an ectopic pregnancy.

▶ Transvaginal ultrasound may be done to rule out intrauterine pregnancy more than 6 weeks from last menstrual period (LMP).

▶ If condition is stable, refer to gynecologist for possible medical treatment with methotrexate, laparoscopy, or laparotomy.

▶ Transfer to emergency facility immediately for signs of rupture.

▶ RhoGAM 300 mcg will also need to be given to an Rh-negative woman.

Toxic Shock Syndrome

▶ Caused by strain of *Staphylococcus aureus*; risk factors include menstruation (especially with tampon use), skin and respiratory infections, post-surgery, postpartum

▶ Signs and symptoms: 2–3 day prodrome including but not limited to malaise, myalgias, fever (> 102° F), erythematous rash (particularly palms and soles), vomiting, watery diarrhea, or abdominal pain followed by signs of shock and organ failure

▶ Consult with physician promptly for hospitalization or immediate transfer to emergency facility.

CONTRACEPTION

Description

▶ Voluntary control of childbearing

▶ In the United States, more than 3.5 million women unintentionally become pregnant each year because of birth control failures and nonuse of method.

▶ Most popular methods in the U.S. are oral contraceptives, female sterilization, condoms, and male sterilization. Many forms of contraception do not decrease risk of STIs.

▶ Abstinence is the only method with 100% safety and efficacy for preventing pregnancy and STIs.

▶ Surgical sterilization via tubal ligation has efficacy > 99%; should be considered irreversible.

▶ Choice of contraceptive method is based on lifestyle, developmental level, efficacy, safety, and characteristics of sexual relationships. Adolescents are typically sexually active 6 months before seeking counseling and information regarding contraception; contraception failure rates are highest among adolescents.

▶ By high school graduation, approximately 65% of all adolescents are sexually active and 15.3% of adolescents surveyed have had multiple (> 4) sexual partners (Centers for Disease Control and Prevention, 2012)

▶ Providers must know state regulations regarding adolescent confidentiality when seeking contraception.

Spermicides

▶ Spermicides (gels, creams, suppositories; vaginal film, foam) usually contain Nonoxynol-9 (N-9), are sold over the counter with specific instructions for each type, and are hormone-free. Nonoxnol-9 (N-9) or octoxynol-9, the active ingredients, are detergents that damage membranes and inhibit or kill sperm. They must be present in the vagina before intercourse to be effective.

▶ Spermicidal products sold separately in the U.S. are intended for use alone, with condoms, or with vaginal or cervical barrier devices.

▶ Products intended for use alone or with condoms contain 4% N-9 and are free of petroleum products.

▶ Products designed for use with cervico-vaginal barriers contain 2% N-9 or octoxynol-9.

▶ For optimal effectiveness, spermicides must be placed in the vagina before each coital act (5–15 minutes up to 1 hour, or according to package labeling) and retained for 6 hours afterward. If spermicide is used alone, it should be reapplied before each ejaculation.

▶ Spermicides may be combined with periodic abstinence or withdrawal to improve efficacy.

▶ Avoid douching after placement of spermicide until 6 hours after the last ejaculation.

▶ Can be effective if used consistently, but first-year failure rate of typical users is 21%

▶ More effective when combined with barrier method

▶ Spermicides with a petroleum base should not be used with latex condoms; they may damage or weaken the latex.

▶ May irritate vagina or urinary tract; alters normal vaginal flora or may alter normal vaginal barriers (mucus, flora, pH) that protect from infection

▶ No major contraindications except women with allergy to N-9, octoxynol-9, or the additives commonly found in N-9 should avoid exposure; common product additives are methylparaben, sorbic acid, cellulose gum, lactic acid, povidone, propylene glycol, and sorbitol.

▶ No systemic side effects; safe in postpartum or breastfeeding women

▶ Appropriate for women with infrequent coitus or those using contraceptives to space their children and who accept a moderate risk of contraceptive failure

▶ *Warning:* The Centers for Disease Control and Prevention (CDC) have indicated that vaginal spermicides that contain N-9 are not effective in the prevention of STIs and HIV. Furthermore, frequent use of spermicides containing N-9 has been associated with disruption of the genital epithelium, which might be associated with an increased risk for HIV transmission if exposed to the virus. Therefore, N-9 is not recommended for STI or HIV prevention or use in the rectum.

▶ If contraception is used improperly or not used at all, emergency contraception as a backup method is available OTC for those age15 and above and should be recommended to decrease the risk of unplanned pregnancy.

Nonprescription Barrier Methods

▶ Female or male condoms prevent sperm from physically entering woman

▶ Female condom: Single-use, polyurethane sheath with 8 hours of maximal wear time

   ▹ Up to 97% effective if perfect use (99% if combined with spermicide)

▶ Latex condoms are good choice for protection from STIs and HIV when used appropriately; require partner cooperation

   ▹ Screen for latex allergy (nonlatex products may offer less STI and HIV protection)

▶ Contraceptive sponge

   ▹ Nonprescription barrier method of reversible birth control; inserted deep into the vagina before intercourse; made of solid polyurethane foam containing 1 gram N-9 spermicide; soft, round, pillow-shaped, and about 2 inches in diameter; has a nylon loop attached to the bottom for removal

   ▹ Covers the cervix and blocks sperm from entering the uterus; continuously releases spermicide that immobilizes sperm; cannot reduce the risk of STIs

   ▹ *Advantages*

      ▷ No prescription or fitting needed

      ▷ Can be used during breastfeeding

      ▷ Portable

      ▷ Does not affect a woman's natural hormones

      ▷ Does not interrupt sex play

   ▹ Method of use: Before inserting the sponge, wet it with at least two tablespoons of clean water. Gently squeeze the sponge. The spermicide will become active when the sponge is thoroughly wet. Fold the sides of the sponge upward and away from the loop on the bottom to make it look long and narrow. Slide the sponge as far back into vagina as fingers will reach. The sponge will unfold and cover the cervix once released. To make sure the cervix is covered, slide a finger around the edge of the sponge and check its position. The nylon loop on the bottom of the sponge should also be felt.

» Can be inserted up to 24 hours before intercourse; must be left in place for at least 6 hours after the last act of intercourse; during that time, intercourse may be repeated without additional preparation during the first 24 hours. It should not be worn for more than 30 hours in a row. Use sponge only once, then discard.

» To remove the sponge, insert a finger inside the vagina and through the loop. Pull the sponge out slowly and gently.

» *Contraindications for use:* Allergy to polyurethane, spermicide, or sulfa drugs; current menstruation; current reproductive tract infection; difficulty with insertion; discomfort with touching one's genitals; history of toxic shock syndrome; recent abortion, childbirth, or miscarriage; vaginal obstructions; during any kind of vaginal bleeding, including menstruation.

» *Disadvantages:* Few side effects reported. Sponge may be difficult to remove. If the sponge cannot be removed, or if it breaks into pieces that cannot be completely removed, instruct patient to be seen by her healthcare provider immediately. Some women may notice vaginal irritation. Sponge users may be at slightly increased risk of toxic shock syndrome, which is also associated with the prolonged use of highly absorbent tampons.

Emergency Contraception (EC)

▶ Emergency contraception (EC) is used within short interval after coital event to reduce chance of pregnancy.

▶ May be used within 72 hours and up to 120 hours after unprotected vaginal intercourse to prevent pregnancy; however, is most effective when used as soon as possible after having unprotected sex

▶ Available OTC in the U.S. to men and women age 15 and older

▶ Mechanism of action: Depends on where woman is in her menstrual cycle; inhibition or delay in ovarian follicular development or maturation; typically prevents luteinizing hormone (LH) surge and thus ovulation; alters endometrium to prevent implantation; promotes thickening of cervical mucous, impeding sperm transport; or alteration of fallopian tube transport of sperm, egg, or fertilized ovum. The Copper T IUD prevents fertilization of the ovum and may prevent implantation of a fertilized egg.

▶ Use of EC could prevent as many as 1.5 million unintended pregnancies annually; 90% of pregnancies following rape could be prevented if all women had access to EC after a sexual assault; an estimated 51,000 abortions were avoided due to EC use in 2000; most women seeking EC use a regular form of contraception, usually condoms; up to 50% of patients request EC after condom failure.

▶ Options for EC in the U.S. are ulipristal acetate progesterone agonist/antagonist (prescription only); combined estrogen and progestin; progestin-only (Plan B One-Step, Next Choice One Dose, Next Choice, or levonorgestrel tablets); and Copper T IUD.

▶ Combined estrogen and progestin pills (Yuzpe Method): Take 2 doses of pills p.o. 12 hours apart as soon as possible up to 120 hours after unprotected intercourse; each dosage contains 100–120 mg ethinyl estradiol and 0.50–0.60 mg levonorgestrel; the regimen is one dose followed by a second dose 12 hours later, where each dose consists of 1, 2, 4, 5, or 6 pills, depending on brand used; approximately 75% effective, may cause nausea and vomiting.

▶ Plan B One-Step (this has replaced the 2-pill predecessor Plan B) and Next Choice One Dose (a generic form of Plan B One-Step) 1-pill system: Take 1 tablet p.o. single dose as soon as possible up to 120 hours after unprotected intercourse; the dosage contains 1.5 mg levonorgestrel; much less nausea and vomiting reported than seen with combined estrogen and progestin pills use; 89% effective

▶ Next Choice and levonorgestrel tablets (generic forms of the original 2-pill version of Plan B): Take 2 tablets p.o. together or 1 tablet p.o. 12 hours apart as soon as possible up to 120 hours after unprotected intercourse; each dosage contains 0.75 mg levonorgestrel.

▶ Ulipristal acetate progesterone agonist/antagonist antiprogestin pill (prescription only): Brandname Ella—take one pill p.o. single dose as soon as possible up to 120 hours after unprotected intercourse; the dosage contains 30 mg ulipristal acetate; ulipristal binds to the human progesterone receptor, thereby preventing the binding of progesterone; contraindicated in pregnancy; unlike other hormonal ECs, existing pregnancy must be ruled out before prescribing ulipristal, because of the risk of fetal loss if used in the first trimester of pregnancy; obtain urine hCG (or serum β-hCG if indicated) before administering; patient must return if menses does not occur after taking ulipristal to assess for pregnancy and to rule out ectopic pregnancy if severe abdominal pain occurs 3–5 weeks after the dose.

▶ Copper T IUD: May be inserted within 5 days (120 hours) after unprotected intercourse to reduce the risk of pregnancy by 99.9%; prevents fertilization of ovum and may prevent implantation of a fertilized egg

▶ Educate regarding correct use of emergency contraceptive regimen selected.

▶ Emergency contraception needs to be initiated within 120 hours of need, preferably as soon as possible after unprotected intercourse.

▶ Nausea (30%–50%) and vomiting (15%–20%) are the most common complaints associated with emergency contraception with combination pills; take pills with food, not on an empty stomach.

▶ Advise the patient to return for a pregnancy test if no menses in next 3–4 weeks.

▶ Medications that reduce the efficacy of EC are rifampin, griseofulvin, phenytoin, St. John's wort, and some antiretroviral agents.

▶ Emergency follow-up is recommended if patient experiences severe abdominal pain or other severe side effects possibly related to the treatment, ectopic gestation, or miscarriage.

▶ Obtain date of LMP and if it was normal; determine date and time of first episode and most recent episode of unprotected intercourse.

▶ Physical exam is not necessary before EC use when otherwise asymptomatic; before IUD insertion, perform a pelvic exam to assess uterine size and position and rule out pelvic infection.

▶ Plan for future use of a reliable contraceptive method.

▶ Note: EC is not the same as mifepristone (RU-486) and does not cause an abortion. EC is not effective if a woman is already pregnant and, other than ulipristal as described above, will not adversely affect an established pregnancy.

Natural Family Planning

▶ Efficacy is variable, but can be high if couple is very dedicated.

▶ Several visits or specialized classes are recommended to provide instructions for using one or more of the natural family planning methods, practicing the record-keeping, and learning to observe the signs correctly; instructor should be specially trained.

▶ *The calendar rhythm method* uses calendar charting to calculate a woman's fertile period, averaging longest and shortest cycles, and identifying times of likely ovulation.

▶ Basal body temperature (BBT) method: Daily a.m. basal body temperatures are monitored for a sustained rise (0.4° F–0.8° F degrees) at ovulation that continues until next menses.

▶ *Ovulation or "Billings" method:* Daily cervical mucus changes are observed for characteristics at ovulation (sticky and pasty precedes ovulation, silky and stretchy occurs at ovulation).

▶ A variety of factors may interfere with the cervical mucus characteristics: Douching, spermicides, vaginal infections, lubricants, semen, vaginal medications, and normal lubrication of sexual arousal.

▶ *Symptothermal method:* Combines mucus and cervical changes and recognition of ovulation symptoms with BBT; charted daily and used to assess fertile times

▶ Cooperation between partners and agreement about any backup methods are needed. Typically, the ovum is viable for 24 hours and sperm up to 72 hours; however, ova can survive up to 72 hours and sperm can survive 72 or more hours, so this must factor into fertile interval planning; needs regular cycles to be most successful. Studies have shown that conception can occur up to 6 days before ovulation and 1 day after.

Prescription Barrier Methods

▶ Diaphragms, caps, and shields are soft latex or silicone barrier devices that cover the entire cervix, blocking the opening to the uterus to prevent sperm from physically entering the cervix; used with spermicidal jelly or cream to enhance contraceptive effect.

▶ *A diaphragm* is a shallow, dome-shaped cup with a flexible spring rim. There are several types of diaphragms as determined by the spring rim: coil, flat, or arcing. Coil-spring and flat-spring diaphragms become a flat oval when compressed for insertion. Arcing diaphragms form an arc or half-moon when compressed and are the easiest to insert. Efficacy may reach 96% if used properly; use with 1 teaspoon of spermicidal jelly; insert to back of vagina and tuck behind the pubic bone, ensuring the cervix is covered; must stay in place 6 hours after last act of intercourse; if intercourse is repeated or occurs more than 6 hours after insertion, leave the diaphragm in place and apply more spermicide; do not leave the diaphragm in place for more than 24 hours.

▶ *FemCap* is a silicone rubber cup-shaped device that fits securely in the vagina to cover the cervix; efficacy may reach 94% if used properly. Cap must stay in place for 8 hours after intercourse; do not leave cap in place for more than 48 hours; cannot use cervical cap if have short or irregular cervix, post-cervical conization, or abnormal Pap smear. Use with spermicidal jelly; insert cap into the vagina and onto the cervix, ensuring the cervix is completely covered; with each act of intercourse, check that cap is still covering the cervix; apply more spermicide if needed.

▶ *Lea's Shield* is a medical-grade silicone rubber cup that covers the cervix with an air valve and a loop to aid in removal. Use with spermicidal jelly placed in dome, coating the inside of the bowl around the hole, the front of the rim, and outer part of the valve with spermicide; insert the shield into the vagina with the valve facing down and the thickest end inserted first; push the shield up as far in the vagina as is possible; be sure that the loop is not sticking out of vagina; the air between the cervix and shield will be vented out through the valve to create a proper fit; the valve may be pressed a few times after insertion to be sure that the air is removed; with each act of intercourse, check that the shield is still covering the cervix; additional spermicide may be added to the vagina for subsequent acts of intercourse if needed; the shield must stay in place 8 hours after the last intercourse; do not leave in place for more than 48 hours.

▶ Fitting or sizing done by a clinician to determine the correct size for diaphragm and cap

▶ No major contraindications, no systemic side effects; may be increased urinary tract infections (UTIs) in some women; ask about allergy to latex and N-9, or history of toxic shock syndrome

▶ Protection may be increased by ensuring cervix is covered before each act of intercourse; spermicide is used as recommended; or using a latex condom.

▶ Diaphragms, caps, and shields offer no protection against sexually transmitted infection. Use a latex condom to reduce the risk of infection.

▶ Diaphragms are available in many sizes and designs. A new size may be needed after any of the following: full-term pregnancy; abdominal or pelvic surgery; miscarriage; abortion after 14 weeks of pregnancy; or 20% change in weight.

▶ FemCap is available in three sizes: small, for women who have never been pregnant; medium, for women who have had an abortion or a cesarean delivery; large, for women who have given birth vaginally.

▶ The shield only comes in one size.

Warning Signs

▶ Toxic shock syndrome: Rare cases of toxic shock syndrome (TSS) have been reported with diaphragm, sponge, and other cervical barrier method use. Symptoms include a sunburn-type rash; diarrhea; dizziness, faintness, weakness; sore throat; aching muscles and joints; sudden high fever; and vomiting.

Contraindications

▶ Allergy to latex, silicone, or spermicide; childbirth in the last 6 weeks (10 weeks for FemCap); difficulty with insertion; discomfort with touching one's genitals; history of toxic shock syndrome; recent cervical surgery; recent abortion after the first trimester (after any recent abortion for FemCap); uterine prolapse; vaginal obstructions

▶ Inability to use a diaphragm if woman has frequent urinary tract infections or poor vaginal muscle tone

▶ Inability to use FemCap if patient has breaks in the vaginal or cervical tissue; cancer of the uterus, vagina, or vulva; reproductive tract infection; poor vaginal muscle tone

▶ Inability to use a shield if patient has breaks in the vaginal or cervical tissue; frequent urinary tract infections; reproductive tract infection

▶ Diaphragm, cap, or shield should never be used during any kind of vaginal bleeding, including menstruation.

Advantages

▶ Can be used during breastfeeding; portable; generally cannot be felt by either partner; immediately effective and reversible; no effect on a woman's natural hormones; no interruption of sex play; can be inserted hours ahead of time

Disadvantages

▶ Cannot be used during menstruation; may be difficult for some women to insert; may be pushed out of place by some sexual positions; must be in place every time a woman has vaginal intercourse; diaphragms and caps may require refitting

▶ Use of spermicide N-9 many times a day by people at risk for HIV may irritate tissue and increase risk of HIV and other sexually transmitted infections.

Care of Diaphragms, Caps, and Shields

▶ Diaphragm and cap may last 2 years and the shield may last 6 months; wash with warm soapy water and air dry; do not use powders; never use oil-based lubricants such as petroleum jelly (Vaseline), creams, or lotions, which will damage latex; examine devices for small holes or fill the cup of the diaphragm or cap with water and look for leaks; diaphragms, caps, and shields can still be used if the rubber becomes discolored. However, if the rubber puckers, especially near the rim, it has become too thin.

Intra-Uterine Contraceptives (IUCs)

▶ IUCs are small, T-shaped contraceptive devices made of flexible plastic; can be embedded with progestin or wrapped with copper; sit in uterine cavity and prevent implantation of fertilized ovum; > 99% effective, no user error or inconsistency

▶ Two types are now available in the U.S.: ParaGard (Copper T 380A) contains copper and can be left in place for 10 years, but effective for 12 years; Mirena LNG-releasing IUC continuously releases a small amount of the hormone progestin and is approved for 5-year use, but effective for 7 years.

▶ Both contain barium sulfate for detection by radiograph.

▶ Hormonal IUC thickens cervical mucus, disrupts the pattern of ovulation, and impairs uterine and tubal motility.

▶ Levonorgesterol intra-uterine system: Mirena approved December 2000; T-shaped polyethylene device; reservoir contains levonorgesterol 52 mg; delivers 20 mcg/day of the progestin; approved for 5 years of use; decreases bleeding and cramping; 20% become amenorrheic; must be inserted by a trained clinician; irregular bleeding or spotting first 3 months; abdominal pain, back pain, breast pain, mood changes, acne, headaches, and nausea may occur; patient must be comfortable checking string monthly

▶ Copper-based IUC: ParaGard (Copper T 380A) contains copper and can be left in place for 10 years; causes increased copper in ions, enzymes, and prostaglandins that enhance inflammatory response and impede sperm transport, fertilization, and implantation

▶ Choose candidates based on careful assessment of risk factors (PID risk related to multiple partners; history of heavy menses; dysmenorrhea); need special training for insertion

▶ Nulliparous women can safely use IUCs.

▶ IUCs are not abortifacients.

▶ May be inserted any time in woman's cycle if negative hCG, midcycle, and no unprotected coitus since LMP; may insert immediately after an uncomplicated abortion or delivery

▶ Common complaints

  » Dysmenorrhea and increased blood flow

  » Should consider IUC removal in addition to antibiotic therapy when treating endometritis, STI, PID; IUC should be removed at time pregnancy is diagnosed if strings are visible, regardless of patient's plan for the pregnancy; 40%–50% risk of spontaneous abortion if IUC is left in place and 30% risk of spontaneous abortion after IUC is removed

▶ ParaGard is effective immediately after insertion.

▶ Mirena is effective immediately if inserted within 7 days of LMP. If Mirena is inserted at any other time of the menstrual cycle, patient will need to use another method of birth control if vaginal intercourse occurs during the first week after insertion. Protection will begin after 7 days.

Risk Factors

▶ Highest risk of perforation is at time of insertion; early warning signs are:

  » **P:** Period late, abnormal spotting, bleeding

  » **A:** Abdominal pain, or pain with intercourse

  » **I:** Infection exposure (sexually transmitted infections [STIs]), abnormal discharge, itching, pain

  » **N:** Not feeling well, fever, chills, fatigue

  » **S:** String missing, shorter, or longer (check monthly)

Hormonal Contraception

▶ The first question to be decided is whether the presence of estrogen is medically acceptable and not contraindicated for the woman.

Oral, Transdermal, Vaginal, Injectable Progestin, and Progestin Implants

▶ Hormonal methods interfere with negative feedback loop with steady hormonal doses, which inhibit ovulation, decrease endometrial lining (less flow, less area to implant in), and alter cervical mucus.

▶ Estrogen effects: Follicle-stimulating hormones (FSH) and luteinizing hormone (LH) are suppressed, ovary is not stimulated, and secretions and cellular structure of endometrium are altered.

▶ Progestin effects: Inhibits FSH and LH, which suppresses ovulation, thickens cervical mucus so sperm transport is inhibited; decidualized endometrial bed inhibits implantation

▶ Contraindications

  » Thrombophlebitis; thromboembolic disease; cerebrovascular accident (CVA); coagulopathies; uncontrolled hypertension (may use progestin-only pills); vascular disease (coronary artery disease (CAD), peripheral vascular disease (PVD); breast cancer; estrogen-dependent neoplasia; hepatic adenoma or cancer; pregnancy; impaired renal function or hepatitis; diabetes with nephropathy, neuropathy, retinopathy, or other vascular disease; lactation, < 6 weeks postpartum; major surgery with immobilization; hypertension (160+/100+); smoking (age > 35 smoking > 20 cigarettes/day); migraines with focal neurologic symptoms that worsen with any hormonal contraceptive use; usually not given to smokers

> » Relative contraindications, exercise caution: Undiagnosed vaginal bleeding, active gallbladder disease, family history of hyperlipidemia or myocardial infarction (MI) < age 50, smoking (age > 35 smoking > 15 cigarettes/day)

> » No significant adverse fetal effects have been documented regarding exposure before and early in pregnancy.

▶ Highly effective (> 98%) when used correctly; reversible, widely studied for years, menstrual benefits (especially with endometriosis)

▶ No STI protection is provided.

▶ Side effects

> » Acne (with high androgenic activity pills), light or no menses (rule out pregnancy), breakthrough bleeding or spotting between periods, breast pain (mastalgia), depression, headaches, libido changes, nausea, weight changes

> » Serious: Stroke, pulmonary embolus, thrombophlebitis, hepatitis; stroke risk increased in smokers

> » Some drugs reduce oral contraceptive levels (carbamazepine [Tegretol], phenytoin [Dilantin], rifampin [Refadin])

▶ Antibiotics that *do not* decrease steroid levels in women using oral contraceptives: Ampicillin, clarithromycin (Biaxin), metronidazole (Flagyl), quinolone antibiotics (ciprofloxacin, ofloxacin), doxycycline, tetracycline, fluconazole (Diflucan)

Oral Contraceptives (OCs)

▶ Multiple dosage arrangements are available combining estrogens and progestins in fixed amounts during 21 days of the cycle, or varying amounts of progestin and sometimes estrogen. Side effects (breakthrough bleeding) and beneficial effects (acne reduction) based on the estrogenic, progestational, androgenic, endometrial, and lipid biological activity of each type.

▶ Acts on pituitary and hypothalamus to inhibit gonadotropin secretion, thereby preventing ovulation; progestin suppresses LH secretion, eliminating the LH surge; estrogen suppresses FSH secretion, decreasing follicular maturation

▶ Progestational agent also thickens cervical mucus, decreases peristalsis in fallopian tube, and makes endometrium unreceptive to implantation; estrogen stabilizes the endometrium to prevent irregular bleeding.

▶ Perfect use failure rate is 0.1%; typical use failure rate is 7.6%

▶ Menstrual suppression: OCs taken for 91 days (84/7 regimen) resulting in 4 periods/year; 84 days of hormonal pills, followed by 7 days of placebo pills or 7 days of pills containing 10 mcg ethinyl estradiol (EE).

▶ Low-dose estrogen OCs (20–25 mcg) decrease estrogen side effects; possible increased breakthrough bleeding; decreased suppression of cyst formation or reduction; decreased margin of error for noncompliance, late or missed dosing; variety of cycle regimens are available: 21/7 (hormonally active/placebo), 21/2/5 (hormonally active/placebo/EE), 24/4 (hormonally active/placebo); monophasic pills contain the same dose of EE and progestin for all hormonally active days; multiphasic preparations use varying levels of EE or progestin.

▶ Progestin-only OCs "mini-pill": Contains only progestin, not estrogen; norethindrone 0.35 mg is available in the U.S.; 28 pills per month, all pills contain active hormone dose, no placebos; failure rate is 5 times that of combined OCs; taken continuously with no placebos; breakthrough bleeding more common especially if pills are missed or taken late; need backup method for missed or late pills

Warning Signs

▶ Abdominal pain (severe)

▶ Chest pain (severe, cough, short of breath, sharp pain on breathing in)

▶ Headache (severe), dizziness, weakness, numbness, especially if one-sided

▶ Eye (visual blurring, visual loss), speech problem

▶ Severe leg pain (calf or thigh)

OC Initiation

▶ Screen patient for personal or family history of venous thromboembolism, complicated valvular heart disease, history of an estrogen-dependent tumor, or known or suspected breast cancer.

▶ Use pill with the fewest bleeding side effects, better lipid profiles, less estrogenic effects

▶ Can be initiated on any day of the menstrual cycle; pregnancy test is not necessary for first cycle since the pill is easily withdrawn and has excellent safety record in early pregnancy over past 40 years

▶ "Quick start" method: Initiation of the pill on the day patient is given the prescription improves compliance and does not increase breakthrough bleeding; use a backup method for 7–10 days

▶ Use alternative contraception in addition to OCs during first 7–10 days of starting pill, unless started on first day of menses; also use alternative contraception if missed pills, late pills, certain drugs used with pills

▶ With combined form OCs: If one pill is missed, take it immediately or 2 pills together the next day; if 2 days of pills are missed, take 2 pills immediately and 2 pills the following day, avoid intercourse on days when pills are missed or use condoms for 7 days. If more than 2 days of pills are missed in a row, discard the pack, use another form of birth control such as condoms, and start a new pack within 7 days of the onset of the next menses.

▶ With progestin-only forms: If minipill is even 2–3 hours late, use backup method. Report severe headache, or severe lower abdominal pain that may indicate pregnancy or ruptured cyst.

▶ In the first 6 weeks postpartum, avoid combination OCs due to clotting risk; progestin-only pill may be used; OCs pose no apparent harm to the neonate but lactation may be impaired.

▶ Thorough history and physical exam with attention to the breasts, blood pressure, abdomen, pelvic organs, and cervical cytology should be done on initiation of the pill and at least yearly.

Transdermal Patch

▶ Ortho Evra transdermal contraceptive patch releases norelgestromin 150 mcg and ethinyl estradiol 20 mcg per 24 hours. The patch is applied to abdomen, buttock, upper outer arm, or upper torso (except breasts) weekly × 3, followed by a patch-free week causing withdrawal bleeding or menses to occur. A backup method should be used the first week after starting the patch.

▶ Start first patch cycle on day 1 of menses or the first Sunday after first day of menses.

▶ Same indications, risk factors, mechanisms, and side effects as OCs

▶ May be less effective in women who weigh more than 198 pounds

▶ About 2%–4.7% of patches have to be replaced due to detachment.

▶ No powder, lotion, or other products should be applied around the site of the patch.

▶ May bathe, exercise, and swim

▶ 3% discontinuation rate due to application-site reaction

▶ Increased breakthrough bleeding in first 1–2 cycles

▶ Most antibiotics do not affect contraceptive efficacy of the patch; rifampin is the exception.

Vaginal Ring Contraceptive

▶ NuvaRing: Etonogestrel 120 mcg and ethinyl estradiol 15 mcg, both amounts released each day; 21 days on/7 days off; flexible donut-shaped ring (2 inches); ethylene vinylacetate copolymer (not latex)

▶ Insert 1 ring vaginally on day 1–5 of menstrual cycle. Leave in place for 3 weeks, then remove and discard for 1 week, allowing menses to occur; insert new ring following menses and repeat 3-weeks-in/1-week-out pattern; backup method recommended during initial week.

▶ If ring falls out for < 3 hours, it may be reinserted.

▶ Same indications, risk factors, mechanisms, and side effects as OCs; may cause some irregular bleeding, leukorrhea, vaginitis, foreign body sensation, coital problems, and expulsion

Warning Signs

▶ Cautious use in women with vaginal abnormalities (rectoceles, stenosis, cervical prolapse)

Depo Medroxyprogesterone Acetate (DMPA; Depo-Provera)

▶ Depo-Provera: Progesterone only, 150 mg IM injection every 12–13 weeks (not later than 14 weeks), may use deltoid or gluteal muscles, do not rub site after injection; given within first 5 days of menses; cannot be immediately reversed, may take 6–18 months for return of fertility; recommend a urine hCG before administering first two DMPA injections to rule out pregnancy

▶ Amenorrhea, spotting, irregular bleeding are most common in first 3 months

▶ Start Depo-Provera at 30 days postpartum.

▶ *Note:* Lunelle is no longer available in the U.S.

Complications

▶ Frequently causes weight gain, headaches, mood changes, menstrual irregularities (amenorrhea in 60%–70%), hair loss or thinning, lowering of high-density lipoprotein (HDL), decreased bone density

Contraindications

▶ Absolute: Pregnancy and unexplained vaginal bleeding

▶ Relative: Weight gain issues, headaches, and liver or gallbladder disease

▶ May take as long as 18–22 months for fertility to return after stopping DMPA; therefore, another contraceptive method may be more appropriate for women considering a pregnancy within the next year.

▶ Bone mineral density (BMD) fully recovers in teens and adult women following DMPA discontinuation; it should not be withheld due to skeletal health concerns.

Nexplanon and Implanon

▶ Single rod, progestin-only subdermal implant; effective for up to 3 years; packaged as a sterile, disposable, preloaded applicator; rod is 4 cm × 2 cm; solid core imbedded containing etonogestrel 68 mg; initial release is 60–70 mcg/day; after a few weeks, 40–50 mcg/day; end of the third year 25–30 mcg/day; after third year, not enough of hormone is produced to prevent pregnancy; may cause irregular bleeding

▶ The difference between the newly developed Nexplanon and older Implanon is that Implanon is not radiopaque and Nexplanon is radiopaque containing barium sulfate. This enables Nexplanon to be identified by X-ray, CT scan, ultrasound, or MRI to confirm placement. The insertion applicator device for Nexplanon is also different than Implanon. The new preloaded applicator prevents insertion errors from occurring, such as the device being inserted too deeply into the arm.

▶ Inserted subdermally in the grove between the bicep and tricep muscles; clinician may insert or remove device after completing a sponsored training program

▶ Inhibits ovulation, increases viscosity of cervical mucus; drug below detectable levels within 1 week of removal, > 90% women ovulated well within 3 months post-removal

▶ *Contraindications*

▷ Pregnancy, current or past history of thrombotic disease, undiagnosed vaginal bleeding, history of breast cancer, hypersensitivity to any of the components; not recommended with hepatic enzyme inducer drugs, women desiring to use implantable birth control advised to quit such drugs before beginning this form of birth control

▶ Immediately after insertion, the clinician and patient have to check the rod for placement in the arm. If the rod cannot be felt, a nonhormonal backup birth control method such as condoms should be used until placement is confirmed.

▶ No STI protection is provided.

Essure Permanent Birth Control System

▶ Essure micro-insert is placed in proximal portion of each fallopian tube lumen; micro-insert expands upon release and anchors itself in the tube; subsequent benign local tissue in-growth over a 3-month period; scarring blocks fallopian tube, device permanently anchored in occluded fallopian tube, resulting in permanent contraception; provider must be experienced hysteroscopist

▶ Candidates: Women who prefer this approach to laparoscopy; especially for women with obesity (BMI of ≥ 45), abdominal mesh that prevents laparoscopy, permanent colostomy, multiple abdominal or pelvic surgeries (adhesions), use of anticoagulation medications, medical problems that contraindicate general anesthesia

▶ Menstrual function: Some transient or recurrent menstrual changes that may or may not be related to Essure; women reported both heavier and lighter than normal menstrual flow; few persistent changes in menstrual function

▶ Essure confirmaton test and postplacement follow-up: Low-pressure hysterosalpingogram (HSG) is recommended 3 months after Essure; if tubal occlusion is confirmed, the woman can rely on Essure for pregnancy protection; if tubal occlusion is not demonstrated, repeat HSG 3 months later.

▶ Benefits: No incisions or general anesthesia required; micro-insert contains no hormones; can be used in patients not eligible for incisional surgery (morbid obesity, prior abdominal or pelvic surgery)

CONDITIONS OF THE MENSTRUAL CYCLE

NORMAL MENSTRUAL CYCLE

Description

▶ Complex rhythmical, hormonal interchange among the hypothalamus, pituitary gland (the hypothalamic-pituitary axis), ovaries, and uterine endometrium

▶ Cycle requires intact hormonal feedback, functional organs, and open cervical and vaginal orifices

▶ Cycle divided into 2 phases: Follicular starts with day 1 of menses and ends with luteinizing hormone (LH) surge; luteal begins with pre-ovulatory LH surge and ends with menses

▶ Low estrogen level causes the hypothalamus to produce pulsatile waves of gonadotropin-releasing hormone (GnRH).

▶ GnRH causes anterior pituitary to produce follicle-stimulating hormone (FSH) and LH.

▶ Ovary responds to FSH production and higher level of estrogen (estradiol) with follicle stimulation to prepare the ovum. Estrogen also produces proliferation of the endometrial lining.

▶ Rising estrogen provides feedback to the pituitary; LH surges, stimulates release of the egg follicular material (ovulation).

▶ Estradiol continues to rise and progesterone starts increasing.

▶ Progesterone thickens and stabilizes the endometrial lining (if the zygote needs to implant, the endometrium is ready). From LH surge to endometrial shed (menses) is approximately 14 days for most women.

▶ A negative feedback cycle occurs as rising estrogen and progesterone levels "switch off" the stimulating hormones from the pituitary and hypothalamus.

▶ Corpus luteum begins to shut down, estrogen and progesterone production falls, and the endometrial tissue loses hormonal support.

▶ Ischemia and vasoconstriction ensues 4–24 hours before menstruation and causes degeneration of the endometrium, which eventually sloughs away.

▶ Average age of menarche 12 years; range 10–16 years

▶ Average duration of menses is 2–7 days and average interval between menstrual periods is 28 days ± 7 days. The normal amount of blood loss per menstrual period is approximately 30 mL.

▶ If a conceptus implants in the endometrial lining, the β-hCG produced will help the ovary maintain the corpus luteum, which helps maintain the progesterone levels, which maintains the protective endometrial lining and supports the developing gestation. This short-circuits the "negative feedback loop."

PREMENSTRUAL SYNDROMES (PMS)

Description

▶ Clusters of mood and behavioral symptoms (somatic, affective, or both) occurring or worsening cyclically during the luteal phase (between ovulation and onset of menstruation), followed by resolution after menses

▶ Has some negative impact on one or more aspects of patient's life (work, social, lifestyle, interpersonal relationships)

▶ Premenstrual symptom clusters occur within a continuum

  ▸ Premenstrual syndrome (PMS), a mild to moderate form

  ▸ Premenstrual dysphoric disorder (PMDD), a subset of PMS; more severe with major impairment

▶ Diagnosis of exclusion (see differential list)

Etiology

▶ Precise pathogenesis unknown; presumed to relate to hormonal fluctuations preceding menses

▶ Psychophysiologic disorder tied to menses by unknown biological link

▶ May be increased sensitivity of one or more neurotransmitters the cyclic fluctuation of ovarian hormones, particularly for PMDD; theorized to be due to neurotransmitter dysregulation

▶ Deficit of serotonin may play role

Incidence and Demographics

▶ 90% of all women report at least one premenstrual symptom.

▶ 10% of these women report adverse lifestyle impact of symptoms and have severe PMS or PMDD.

▶ These syndromes most frequently affect 25- to 45-year-old parous women.

▶ Symptom onset often occurs in adolescence; affects approximately ⅓ of premenopausal women.

Risk Factors

▶ Strongly associated with a past personal or family history of mood disorders (including depression and anxiety) and psychiatric disorders; history of sexual abuse or domestic violence; stress may precipitate condition

▶ Familial trend in female relatives

Prevention and Screening

▶ Balanced diet; regular exercise; decreased alcohol intake; elimination of caffeine, sodium to reduce symptoms; smoking cessation; adequate sleep

Assessment

History

▶ PMS and PMDD are diagnoses of exclusion.

▶ Begin 7–10 days before menses, after ovulation.

  » Fatigue, lack of energy, sleep changes

  » Depression, affective lability, panic attacks, anxiety, lethargy, persistent marked anger or irritability, changes in libido, difficulty concentrating, feelings of being overwhelmed or out of control

  » Breast tenderness

  » Abdominal bloating, thirst, and appetite changes

  » Other: Headaches, edema, joint or muscle pain, weight gain

▶ Anxiety may peak 1–2 days before menses.

  » Severe emotional symptoms predominate for PMDD; symptoms also tend to become more severe and of greater duration with time. In mild or moderate PMS, symptoms do not cause functional impairment; neither the affective nor somatic symptoms predominate.

Physical Exam

▶ Affect, speech, mood, mental status, depression scale to evaluate for other mood disorder

▶ General appearance, skin, thyroid exam to look for signs of adrenal or thyroid disorder

▶ Cardiac exam for changes with thyroid disorder, substance abuse

▶ Musculoskeletal exam for trigger points of fibromyalgia

▶ Complete pelvic examination screening for focal pain, masses

▶ Complete neurologic exam to evaluate headache, mood changes

Diagnostic Studies

▶ Thyroid-stimulating hormone (TSH) cortisol level as indicated to rule out thyroid adrenal disorders; prolactin if headache severe

▶ Consider CBC, glucose and serum chemistries, liver function tests, renal function to evaluate lethargy

▶ If perimenopausal or premature menopause is suspected: FSH, estradiol, progesterone, testosterone, and dehydroepiandrosterone sulfate (DHEA-S) hormone testing may be indicated.

▶ Can do Self-Rating Scale for PMS (Steiner, Haskett, & Carroll, 1980) or calendar of symptoms; must have a minimum of 2 months of charting of symptoms

▶ To differentiate PMDD from PMS, see Table 11–1.

TABLE 11–1
DSM-IV CRITERIA FOR PREMENSTRUAL DYSPHORIA DISEASE (PMDD)

Patients must have 5 or more of the following symptoms, and 1 of them must be from column 1. None of the symptoms can be an exacerbation of another disorder.

COLUMN 1	COLUMN 2
Feeling sad, hopeless, or self-deprecating	Decreased interest in usual activities, which may be associated with withdrawal from social relationships
Feeling tense, anxious, or "on edge"	Difficulty concentrating
Marked lability of mood interspersed with frequent fearfulness	Feeling fatigue, lethargic, or lacking in energy
Persistent irritability, anger, and increased interpersonal conflicts	Marked changes in appetite, which may be associated with binge eating or craving certain foods
	Hypersomnia or insomnia
	A subjective feeling of being overwhelmed or out of control
	Physical symptoms such as breast tenderness or swelling; headaches, joint, or muscle pain; sensations of bloating or weight gain with tightness of fit of clothing, shoes, or rings
	Symptoms interfere with work or usual activities or relationships

Differential Diagnosis

- ▶ Thyroid disorders
- ▶ Substance abuse
- ▶ Adrenal disorders (Cushing's)
- ▶ Depression (often with suicide ideation)
- ▶ Dysthymia
- ▶ Anxiety disorders
- ▶ Fibromyalgia
- ▶ Chronic fatigue syndrome

- ▶ Irritable bowel syndrome
- ▶ Personality disorders
- ▶ PCOS
- ▶ Sleep disorders
- ▶ Chronic pelvic pain syndromes; endometriosis
- ▶ Perimenopause
- ▶ Menopause
- ▶ Drug & alcohol abuse

Management

- ▶ Focus therapeutic management on self-care approaches and lifestyle modification. No treatment of PMS has been validated by evidence-based studies. However, the following lifestyle changes are reported effective for some patients with PMS.

Nonpharmacologic Treatment

- ▶ During evaluation, consider discontinuing all self-remedies such as vitamins and supplements.
- ▶ Menstrual charting for symptom assessment during management
- ▶ Aerobic exercise 3–4× weekly, especially during luteal phase
- ▶ Stress reduction
- ▶ Reduction of alcohol, caffeine, sugar, sodium during most-symptomatic times
- ▶ Balanced diet; increase consumption of dairy and complex carbohydrates
- ▶ Adequate sleep
- ▶ Smoking cessation

Pharmacologic Treatment

- ▶ Calcium carbonate 1,200 mg daily
- ▶ Dietary supplements: Vitamin B_6 100 mg/day, vitamin E 400 IU/day, and magnesium 200–400 mg/day
- ▶ SSRIs, tricyclic antidepressants, benzodiazepines helpful in clinical trials; SSRIs are the drug of choice for PMDD
- ▶ NSAIDs taken with food are effective for pain and cramping components
- ▶ Evening primrose oil, oral contraceptives (OC), progesterone, MAO inhibitors, bromocriptine, vitamins, lithium, spironolactone not demonstrated in clinical trials to reduce PMS symptoms
- ▶ Use of monophasic OCs continuously (tricycling is taking 3 or 4 months of 21-day packets without placebo interval) or with first-day start (begin new packet with first day of menses)

may improve PMS but recurrence is common with discontinuation of OC. Continuous-use OCs for menstrual suppression may also be helpful in reducing symptoms.

▶ Psychological support is helpful for severe manifestations affecting functioning.

How Long to Treat

▶ Therapy is based on patient response; expect long intervals of treatment.

Special Considerations

▶ Accurate identification of premenstrual syndromes requires ruling out other disorders and careful evaluation of menstrual charts and symptom diaries for at least 3 months.

▶ Placebo effect very potent; confidence in clinician, improved understanding of condition, eliminates some fears, provides some hope, improves self-control

▶ Complementary therapies may offer variable efficacy, although clinical trials are lacking to support these modalities.

When to Consult, Refer, Hospitalize

▶ Psychological counseling may be indicated.

Follow-up

▶ After charting symptoms for 2–3 cycles; follow-up every 3–4 months to assess or evaluate effectiveness of therapy.

Expected Course

▶ In the absence of treatment, signs and symptoms expected to persist as long as the woman has ovulatory menstrual cycles; spontaneous remission occurs with menopause and otherwise anovulatory cycles

Complications

▶ None

AMENORRHEA

Description

▶ Absence of menses

   ▸ *Physiologic amenorrhea* occurs with pregnancy, lactation, and menopause.

   ▸ *Primary amenorrhea* is lack of menarche by 14 years of age with absence of secondary sex characteristics, or lack of menarche by age 16 regardless of presence of secondary sex characteristics, or absence of menses > 5 years after thelarche.

   ▸ *Secondary amenorrhea* is the absence of menses for a minimum of 90 days or 3 missed cycles to 6 months' cessation of menses after menarche has been previously established.

Etiology

For Primary Amenorrhea

► Constitutional delay of puberty

- » Müllerian agenesis (2nd most common cause of primary amenorrhea) includes:

   ▷ 46,XX-Rokitansky-Kuster-Hauser syndrome: Absent vagina and uterus, but ovaries and sexual hair normal

   ▷ 46,XY-androgen sensitivity syndrome (testicular feminization): X-linked recessive defect; uterus and adnexa absent with testes and blind-pouched vagina; breasts well-developed but scant sexual hair; elevated testosterone

- » Müllerian fusion anomalies: Müllerian duct fails to fuse with urogenital sinus, resulting in transverse septum of vagina, usually located in middle or upper vagina; normal uterine development

- » 45,XO-Turner syndrome: Ovarian dysgenesis, most common chromosomal abnormality causing gonadal failure and primary amenorrhea

- » Gonadal dysgenesis: Lack of mature breast and pubic hair development, but some initial stages of development may be present

- » Approximately 30% of patients with primary amenorrhea have associated genetic abnormality

- » Congenital defects in steroid synthesis

- » Late-onset congenital adrenal hyperplasia

   ▷ Depending on onset, some disorders classified under secondary amenorrhea may present as primary amenorrhea.

For Secondary Amenorrhea

► Pregnancy is most common cause of secondary amenorrhea. The next five most common causes are polycystic ovary syndrome (PCOS), hypothalamic amenorrhea, thyroid dysfunction, hyperprolactinemia, and ovarian failure.

► Hormonal contraception such as depot medroxyprogesterone (Depo-Provera), combined oral contraceptives

► Hypothalamic dysfunction, including excessive exercise, severe drop in body fat (< 22%) as in anorexia nervosa, severe malnutrition, severe systemic illness, and stress

► Pituitary dysfunction (adenoma, idiopathic hyperprolactinemia)

► Other endocrine causes: Severe hypo- or hyperthyroidism, adrenal disorders, diabetes

► Ovarian dysfunction: Premature ovarian failure; polycystic ovary disease (characterized by amenorrhea, obesity, infertility, and hirsutism)

► Other medications: Phenothiazines, antidepressants, antihypertensives, complication of chemotherapy or radiation therapy, systemic steroids, GnRH agonists

► Surgical: Oophorectomy, hysterectomy

► Outflow tract obstruction: Severe cervical stenosis, severe endometrial scarring and obliteration of endometrium, vaginal scarring, labial fusion

Incidence and Demographics

▶ Incidence for primary amenorrhea = 0.3%

▶ Incidence for secondary amenorrhea = 3.3%

Risk Factors

▶ Varies according to underlying etiology

▶ Endocrine disorders, stressful life events, and a variety of medications (phenothiazines, antidepressants, antihypertensives, chemotherapy, systemic steroids, GnRH agonists) may produce amenorrhea.

▶ Obesity, weight loss, excessive exercise, chronic disease

Assessment

History

▶ Assess first for pregnancy, then galactorrhea (in addition to amenorrhea).

  ▹ Gynecologic history: Infertility, PID, STIs, surgical procedures such as dilation and curettage (D&C), cryotherapy, ovarian wedge resection (for polycystic ovary disease), myomectomy, hysterectomy

  ▹ Pubertal development history

  ▹ Menstrual history with attention to past episodes of erratic bleeding or absence of bleeding

  ▹ Update obstetrical history; update contraceptive history

  ▹ Endocrine: Thyroid, diabetes signs and symptoms

  ▹ Headaches, visual changes

  ▹ Acne, hirsutism (include adolescent as well as family history)

  ▹ Emotional stress: Recent major life events such as divorce, death

  ▹ Depression or other psychological symptoms

  ▹ Nutritional patterns, weight changes, history of eating disorder

  ▹ Family history of genetic anomalies

  ▹ Athletes who exercise excessively

Physical Exam

▶ Weight changes since last visit, body habitus and height

▶ Observe for common anomalies associated with gonadal dysgenesis such as neck folds and low-set ears

▶ Secondary sexual characteristics and Tanner staging: Pubic and axillary hair patterns, breast development, genital appearance

▶ Eyes: Impaired visual fields, ptosis, nystagmus, papilledema

▶ Skin: Hirsutism, acne, hyperpigmentation, vitiligo, fat distribution

▶ Thyroid: Tenderness, nodules, enlargement

▶ Breasts: Galactorrhea, engorgement

▶ Pelvic: Assess for presence or absence of normal structures; clitoromegaly, vulvar or vaginal atrophy, imperforate hymen, uterine enlargement (pregnancy), cervical stenosis, tenderness, adnexal masses, ovary greater than 5 cm, masses.

Diagnostic Studies

▶ First rule out pregnancy with a urine hCG or serum β-hCG test.

▶ Work-up for primary amenorrhea

   » If secondary sex characteristics absent or poorly developed, obtain karyotype to rule out genetic etiology

   » If breast tissue absent or poorly developed and uterus present, obtain serum FSH

      ▷ If elevated, suggests ovarian failure; obtain karyotype to rule out ovarian dysgenesis

      ▷ If low, suggests pituitary or hypothalamic dysfunction

   » If breast development present but absent uterus, obtain serum testosterone

   » If results appropriate for males, obtain karyotype to rule out testicular feminization

   » If breast tissue and uterus present, obtain serum prolactin

      ▷ If elevated, include pituitary tumor in differential diagnosis

      ▷ If normal, begin progesterone challenge test (see below)

   » If work-up negative, proceed to work-up for secondary amenorrhea

   » Work-up for secondary amenorrhea (obtain serum prolactin at start of challenge): CBC, erythrocyte sedimentation rate (ESR), TSH levels, bone age, FSH and LH levels, estradiol level, liver function tests, BUN, creatinine levels, urinalysis (UA), urine hCG, karyotyping, DHEA-S levels, rostenedione levels, testosterone levels, adrenal suppression test for 17-hydroxyprogesterone, MRI of brain to rule out pituitary tumor (prolactinoma)

   » Progesterone challenge: Prescribe oral Provera (medroxyprogesterone acetate [MPA]) 10 mg daily for 5 days.

   » Positive: Withdrawal bleeding (or spotting) within 7 days of last MPA pill suggests adequate endogenous estrogen present to prime endometrium; suggests anovulation meaning presence of intact outflow tract; intact functioning of endometrium, ovary, pituitary, central nervous system (CNS). If prolactin is normal and there is no galactorrhea, no further work-up is needed.

   » Negative: No withdrawal bleeding or spotting suggests either inadequate estrogen levels to prime uterus or absent endometrial cavity (in case of primary amenorrhea). If negative progesterone challenge, wait 2 weeks, then prescribe conjugated estrogen 1.25 mg daily for 21 days *or* 2 mg estradiol p.o. q.d. for 21 days, with Provera (MPA) 10 mg p.o. for the last 5 days of the estrogen, or combination oral contraceptives (monophasic) 1 tab p.o. for 21 days.

      ▷ Positive: Withdrawal bleeding or spotting within 14 days; no outflow tract problem (uterus, cervix, or vagina) but estrogen deficiency

▷ Negative: No withdrawal bleeding suggests end-organ failure possibly due to congenital malformation or distortion (e.g., intrauterine adhesions) of the uterus, vagina; need to repeat estrogen/MPA trial to confirm.

▷ If negative, obtain serum TSH/thyroid panel, FSH, LH, and LH/FSH ratio

▷ If TSH elevated, suggests hypothyroidism

▷ If TSH low or undetectable, suggests hyperthyroidism

▷ If LH elevated or LH/FSH ratio > 3 (especially with signs of androgen excess), include polycystic ovary syndrome in differential

▷ If LH normal or low, include hypothalamic or pituitary regulation defect in differential

▷ If low LH, low FSH, suggests hypothalamic etiology, e.g., stress, excessive exercise, anorexia, or pituitary malfunction

▷ If high LH, high FSH, suggests ovarian failure or menopause secondary to radiation, chemotherapy, autoimmune disease, chromosomal abnormalities

▶ If Cushing's suspected, check ACTH (adrenocorticotrophic hormone), DHEA-S, urinary free cortisol

▶ Transvaginal and pelvic ultrasounds if any abnormality found on physical exam (masses, absent organs, enlarged organs) or if PCOS suspected

▶ If galactorrhea or elevated prolactin, must get an MRI of the sella turcica to assess for adenoma, necrosis, or ischemia (Sheehan syndrome); coned down X-ray of sella turcica is also appropriate

Differential Diagnosis

▶ Pregnancy

▶ Chromosomal abnormality

▶ Secondary causes

Management

▶ Treat any underlying conditions or abnormality identified and assess in 3–6 months for spontaneous return of menses

Nonpharmacologic Treatment

▶ Pituitary adenoma: May need surgical treatment

▶ Increase caloric intake if underweight, encourage adequate calcium intake, reduce exercise if excessive, help patient cope with stress, refer to eating disorder center as needed, and maintain appropriate body weight.

Pharmacologic Treatment

▶ If positive MPA challenge, give MPA monthly 10 mg q.d. for a minimum of 10 days or progesterone (Prometrium) 100–200 mg p.o. q.d. (day 14–16 until menses onset) for 3–6 cycles *or* can treat with combined OCs for minimum of 3–6 cycles.

▹ Start hormonal therapy with oral contraceptives *or* hormone replacement therapy (HRT) regimen if no menstruation present for more than 6 months (or sooner if estradiol levels < 20, FSH levels > 20).

▹ Suggest *not* using progestin-only contraception until regular cycles recur.

▶ If no withdrawal bleed occurs, further exploration is needed.

▶ For pituitary adenoma, referral to an endocrinologist for bromocriptine (Parlodel) treatment.

Special Considerations

▶ Endometrial biopsy is recommended for a long duration of unopposed estrogen (e.g., erratic, variable episodes of bleeding without premenstrual prodrome), amenorrhea for more than 12 months, or more than 3-month history of undiagnosed abnormal vaginal bleeding.

When to Consult, Refer, Hospitalize

▶ Consult with an endocrinologist for pituitary adenoma or PCOS.

▶ Refer to a gynecologist if no withdrawal bleeding occurs, for patients who do not respond to therapy, if prolonged amenorrhea recurs, or for infertility management or HRT.

Follow-up

▶ As appropriate for cause

Complications

▶ Endometrial cancer is a complication of unopposed estrogen.

▶ Reduced bone mass with prolonged amenorrhea

DYSMENORRHEA

Description

▶ Painful menstruation may be primary (absence of pelvic pathology) or secondary (organic cause of pain may be identified)

Etiology

▶ Typically worst in early years of menses and lessens after early 20s

▶ Not common in the first 2–3 years after menarche, when most menstrual cycles are anovulatory

▶ Incidence of primary dysmenorrhea decreases with age, parity, and the use of hormonal contraceptives.

▶ Considered to be chiefly prostaglandin-mediated (PGE and PGF), produced within the endometrial tissue by influence of progesterone and secretory phase of cycle

▶ Diagnosed by history and ruling out other causes, especially pregnancy and PID

▶ Presents as crampy middle to lower abdominal pain, occurs with menses, worst the first 1–2 days; may radiate to the lower back, thighs

▶ Secondary dysmenorrhea is painful menstruation due to an identifiable organic cause.

» Occurs chiefly in women years after menarche and into fourth decade; incidence increases with age

» Associated with pain frequently but not limited to the menstrual phase; the pattern of pain may become more severe over time

» Symptoms suggest a specific etiology, such as endometriosis, tumors, adhesions, adenomyosis, leiomyomas, polyps, or infection.

Incidence and Demographics

▶ Affects 50%–75% of menstruating women; approximately 10% suffer from severe symptoms

▶ High incidence in adolescents, 60%–92%

Risk Factors

▶ Primary dysmenorrhea: Adolescent age, nulliparity, heavy menstrual flow, cigarette smoking, low fish intake, depression/anxiety/sexual abuse and poor school/work performance are weaker factors

▶ Secondary dysmenorrhea: Varies with etiology, usually > 30 years, PID/STIs, endometriosis, family history of endometriosis, unmedicated IUD use, uterine fibroids

Assessment

History

▶ History should direct the clinician to a likely etiology; emphasis on menstrual history, descriptors of pain relative to menses

▶ Low midline pain, cramping in character, occurs in waves, may radiate to back or thighs, lasts 1 or more days with headache, diarrhea, vasomotor flushing, nausea

▶ Associated symptoms indicating underlying problem include fever, unilateral pain, dizziness, unusual bleeding, increased pain with coitus

▶ Symptoms associated with primary dysmenorrhea include fatigue, nervousness, irritability dizziness, syncope, bloating, headache, mood changes, nausea, vomiting, constipation, diarrhea.

▶ Primary dysmenorrhea is menstrual pain occurring a few years after menarche in the absence of pathology.

▶ Review past medical history, surgeries, complications of pregnancy (infection), fibroids, STIs, bowel disorders

Physical Exam

▶ Assess for fever or signs of shock (i.e., low blood pressure, rapid pulse)

▶ Abdominal masses; abdominal tenderness, guarding, or rebounding; focal abdominal pain, can identify source (e.g., LLQ suggests bowel, ureter, fallopian tube, ovary)

▶ Vaginal discharge, odor

▶ Cervical erythema, purulent mucus, friability, cervical motion tenderness

▶ Uterine enlargement or tenderness, masses, immobility, firmness

▶ Adnexal or ovarian masses, or adnexal tenderness

▶ Exam and diagnostic studies will be normal in primary dysmenorrhea.

Diagnostic Studies

▶ Vaginal and cervical smear and wet mount to rule out STI; increased WBCs indicating STIs or PID

▶ Chlamydia and gonorrhea testing

▶ Pregnancy test

▶ Pap screen may be deferred if obvious vaginal or cervical infection exists; obtain later

▶ Ultrasound if ectopic or intrauterine pregnancy, ovarian masses, or fibroids suspected

Differential Diagnosis

▶ Pregnancy

▶ Ectopic gestation

▶ Endometriosis

▶ STIs

▶ PID

▶ Leiomyoma (fibroids)

▶ Chronic pelvic pain syndromes

▶ Irritable bowel syndrome (IBS) or other bowel disorder

▶ Fibroids

▶ Urinary tract disorder (calculi, UTI)

▶ Must always consider carcinoma

Management

Nonpharmacologic Treatment

▶ Treat causes of secondary dysmenorrhea as indicated.

▶ For primary dysmenorrhea, evidence of interference in activities of daily living and severity of complaints determines management protocols.

» Grade 1 (mild dysmenorrhea): Little or no interference in activities of daily living, mild somatic complaints

» Grade 2 (moderate–severe dysmenorrhea): Complaints of significant interference in daily living, positive systemic somatic complaints

» Grade 3 (severe dysmenorrhea): Severely restricted activities, large degree of systemic somatic complaints

▶ Supportive treatment of primary dysmenorrhea: Eat regularly, use dry or moist heat to abdomen to hasten pain relief; high intake of fish rich in omega-3 fatty acids and aerobic exercise are helpful for some women.

▶ Transcutaneous electrical nerve stimulator (TENS) appliance may be helpful.

Pharmacologic Treatment

▶ NSAIDs are the treatment of choice for primary dysmenorrhea; work most effectively when taken before pain becomes severe. Take with food.

» Take NSAIDs 2 days or more (up to 1 week) before onset of menses, at regular intervals around the clock; take with food to avoid GI upset.

» If inadequate response, increase dosage or switch to other product; allow minimum of 2–3 cycles to evaluate before switching

» Ibuprofen (Motrin), 400–800 mg p.o. t.i.d.–q.i.d. p.r.n.

» Mefenamic acid (Ponstel) 500 mg p.o. loading dose, then 250–500 mg p.o. q6h p.r.n.

» Naproxen (Anaprox, Naprosyn), 500 mg p.o. loading dose, then 250 mg p.o. q6–8h p.r.n. (maximum 24 hour dose = 1,250 mg)

» Naproxen sodium extended release (Anaprox DS) 550 mg tablet p.o. b.i.d. p.r.n. (single dose) or (Naprelan) 500 mg, 2 tablets p.o. once daily (single dose)

» Ketoprofen extended release (Oruvail) 200 mg caplet p.o. daily (single dose)

» Another class of NSAIDs has been proven to work for treatment of primary dysmenorrheal as well as first-generation NSAIDs: cyclooxygenase-2 (COX-2) specific inhibitor; drugs approved: celecoxib (Celebrex)

» See Table 11–2.

▶ Controlling menses with oral contraception can also be beneficial; options include:

» Combined OCs may be considered for first-line of therapy in a sexually active female with 21/7 or extended cycling.

» Tricycling (take active contraceptive pills for 3 cycles without allowing withdrawal bleeding) is especially beneficial.

» Use the first-day start system.

» After 2–6 cycles, some patients can discontinue OCs and will respond to NSAIDs.

» Consider DMPA or levonorgestrel intrauterine system (Mirena).

▶ Vitamin B_1 100 mg p.o. daily

▶ Magnesium (limited evidence, optimal regimen unknown)

TABLE 11–2
PROSTAGLANDIN INHIBITORS

DRUG	INITIAL DOSE	SUBSEQUENT DOSING
Acetic acid/Salicylic acids		
Indomethacin (Indocin)	50 mg	25 mg b.i.d.
Diflunisal (Dolobid)	500 mg	500 mg q12h
Diclofenac Potassium (Voltaran)	50 mg	50 mg b.i.d.
Propionic acids		
Ibuprofen (Motrin)	400–800 mg	400–800 mg q4–6h
Naproxen (Naprasyn)	500 mg	250 mg q6–8h
Naproxen sodium (Naproxen)	550 mg	275 mg q6–8h
Fenamates		
Mefenamic Acid (Polsen)	500 mg	250 mg q6h

Adapted from *Pharmacology for the Primary Care Provider* (3rd. ed.) by M. W. Edmunds & M. S. Mayhew, 2009, St. Louis, MO: Mosby.

Special Considerations

▶ Aspirin, a mild prostaglandin inhibitor, tends to increase menstrual flow while ibuprofen, a potent prostaglandin inhibitor, lessens flow and controls cramping more effectively.

When to Consult, Refer, Hospitalize

▶ Refer to gynecologist if poor response to NSAID therapy or need evaluation and management of secondary dysmenorrheal.

Follow-up

▶ Every 2–3 months as necessary to evaluate efficacy of therapy or as appropriate for underlying cause

Expected Course

▶ Primary dysmenorrhea tends to improve with age and pregnancy.

▶ Symptoms resolve with NSAIDs or OCs within 3 cycles.

▶ For Grade 1, use medication for 24–72 hours; Grade 2, treat with NSAIDs for 3–4 cycles or continuous NSAIDs for 3–4 months; Grade 3, try NSAIDs, then use OC for 2–6 months then stop; retry NSAIDs.

▶ Secondary dysmenorrhea: Depends on cause

Complications

▶ Primary dysmenorrhea: None

▶ Secondary dysmenorrhea: Depends on cause

ABNORMAL UTERINE BLEEDING (AUB)

Description

▶ Any vaginal bleeding that is not attributed to normal menstrual flow. It is classified as premenopausal or postmenopausal; bleeding at inappropriate times, amount, or duration. It is a symptom, not a diagnosis.

▶ DUB (dysfunctional uterine bleeding) is a diagnosis of exclusion defined as painless, irregular bleeding due to anovulation.

▶ AUB can be classified as:

  ▹ Blood loss during normal menses averages 60 cc over a maximum of 7 days

    ▷ Menorrhagia: Menstrual periods occurring at regular intervals but of excessive duration and flow; total blood loss of > 80 cc and duration > 7 days

    ▷ Metrorrhagia: Menstrual periods occurring at irregular intervals of varying flow and duration

    ▷ Oligomenorrhea: Menstrual periods occurring irregularly at intervals of greater than 40 days, but less than 6 months

▷ Hypomenorrhea: Regular menstrual periods but with reduced amount or duration, < 60 cc

▷ Menometrorrhagia: Irregular menstrual periods of increased amount or duration

▷ Polymenorrhea: Regular menstrual periods but at intervals of less than 21 days

▷ A single spot of blood with ovulation is common and benign.

Etiology

▶ Women < 20 years: Anovulation due to immature pituitary-hypothalamic-ovarian axis

» Over 90% of AUB is anovulatory in this age range.

» Estimates suggest 55% of teens have anovulatory cycles the first year after menarche.

» Less frequent cycles and erratic ovulation may lead to AUB (mostly anovulatory), intervals of amenorrhea, and reduced fertility.

▶ Women age 20–40 years

» Usually ovulatory (less than 20% of cases are due to anovulatory problems)

» Pregnancy, PID, OCs, DMPA, other drugs, IUCs, severe stress, thyroid disease, endometriosis, polyps, fibroids, and neoplasm

▶ Women > 40 years

» Anovulation due to perimenopause, aging, polyps, fibroids, uterine atrophy or thickening (hyperplasia), uterine cancer

» 40% of all DUB cases occur in women over age 40 — more likely to have disruptions in ovarian function

» Perimenopausal women have menstrual changes, including altered intermenstrual intervals (shorter, longer, or variable) and altered menstrual flow (heavier, lighter, longer, or shorter patterns).

Incidence and Demographics

▶ 25% of all AUB is from pregnancy-related complications.

Risk Factors

▶ Adolescents and perimenopausal women; copper IUD, disorders of systemic hemostasis

Assessment

History

▶ Complete menstrual history and patterns; STI; nipple or vaginal discharge; contraceptive patterns; abdominal pain; dyspareunia; heat or cold intolerance; bleeding or bruising; weight changes; headaches; visual problems; male pattern hair growth; drugs and medication, including oral and long-acting contraceptive use

▶ Abnormal bleeding is primary symptom

Physical Exam

▶ Perform a thorough pelvic exam to rule out structural abnormality of the uterus and pelvic organs.

▶ Thyroid nodules, enlargement, tenderness

▶ Visual field defects

▶ Galactorrhea: Often present with hyperprolactinemia

▶ Abdominal pain, guarding, rebound

▶ Pelvic: Polyps, lesions, cervical motion tenderness, cervicitis, cervical discharge or blood, enlarged uterus, adnexal pain or masses, infection, pregnancy

▶ Moon facies, truncal obesity, abdominal striae, elevated blood pressure (BP); include Cushing's disease in differential

▶ Check for hirsutism.

Diagnostic Studies

▶ Urine or serum hCG, CBC, TSH, Pap test, prolactin, chlamydia *and* gonorrhea testing

▶ If indicated by history or physical exam:

  ▹ Glucose, renal function, hepatic function, bleeding studies (platelet count, PT, PTT, bleeding time); adolescents with heavy menstrual bleeding should be evaluated for underlying systemic disorder such as von Willebrand factor or other inherited disorders of hemostasis

  ▹ Endometrial biopsy or hysteroscopy: Need determined by history but generally more than 3–6 months of unexplained AVB despite therapies

  ▹ Pelvic or transvaginal ultrasound: Rule out pregnancy or its related complications, assess endometrial stripe to rule out endometrial hyperplasia, other masses (e.g., fibroids)

  ▹ Dexamethasone test, ACTH, serum cortisol, and urine cortisol

  ▹ FSH, LH, LH/FSH ratio

  ▹ MRI of sella turcica

Differential Diagnosis

▶ Pregnancy

▶ Spontaneous abortion

▶ Ectopic pregnancy

▶ Polyps

▶ Hyper- or hypothyroidism

▶ PCOS

▶ Infection

▶ Gynecologic cancer (usually endometrial)

▶ Salpingitis (especially chronic)

▶ Endometritis

▶ Fibroids

▶ Adenomyosis

▶ Copper IUD

▶ Thrombocytopenia

▶ Coagulopathy

▶ Blood dyscrasia

▶ Hyperprolactinemia (r/o pituitary adenoma, medications)

Management

- ▶ Main goal of management is to determine who requires intervention and who can just be monitored

- ▶ In adolescents, advise that the problem is often self-limiting and should resolve within a year or two of menarche.

- ▶ Treat any causes identified as indicated.

- ▶ DUB is the working diagnosis if other causes are ruled out.

Pharmacologic Treatment

- ▶ Oral contraceptives or hormone replacement therapy for several cycles

- ▶ Monophasic combination OC with 30–35 mcg estrogen may be given 1 tab p.o. b.i.d.–q.i.d. for 7–10 days until bleeding is controlled.

- ▶ If bleeding stops within the treatment period, advise one OC q.d., uninterrupted without a withdrawal bleed, for another 21 days.

- ▶ Delayed withdrawal bleeding after 6–12 weeks allows gradual thinning of the endometrium, results in a lighter bleed than if withdrawal bleeding occurs within the 10 days

- ▶ Another treatment is 1.25 mg conjugated estrogens p.o. or 2 mg estradiol p.o. q4h for 24 hours, then a daily dose for 7–10 days

- ▶ Follow with progestin coverage allowing withdrawal bleed; treatment after this is OC cycles × 3.

- ▶ Consider continuous or extended OC cycle therapy.

- ▶ Medroxyprogesterone acetate (MPA or Provera)
  - » May be given 10 mg p.o. for 10–14 days every month
  - » The first withdrawal bleed will be heavy but the woman should cycle after that.
  - » MPA may be used monthly.

- ▶ Depot medroxyprogesterone acetate (DMPA, Depo-Provera)
  - » Give Depo-Provera 150 mg IM every 12 weeks

- ▶ Levonorgestrel- IUS: Progestin-impregnated IUD
  - » Reduces blood loss by up to 94% in first 3 months of use.
  - » Amenorrhea in 20%–40% at 1 year

- ▶ Supportive therapy
  - » Iron replacement therapy if needed for anemia
  - » NSAIDs (prostaglandin synthetase inhibitors): 20%–30% reduction in bleeding may occur. Start NSAIDs the first day of menses and continue through the heavy flow days.
    - ▷ Mefenamic acid (Ponstel) 500 mg p.o. t.i.d. for 3 days
    - ▷ Naproxen (Naprosyn) 500 mg p.o. b.i.d.
    - ▷ Ibuprofen (Motrin) 400 mg q6h

Surgical Treatment

▶ Surgical interventions for idiopathic heavy menstrual bleeding are usually reserved for those patients who have failed or are intolerant of medical therapy and who are willing to forego fertility; surgical interventions may include but are not limited to endometrial ablation and hysterectomy.

Special Considerations

▶ With postmenopausal women, any bleeding or spotting is presumed to be of malignant origin until proven otherwise.

When to Consult, Refer, Hospitalize

▶ Refer to gynecologist for acute menorrhagia if the bleeding is severe enough to cause volume depletion, shortness of breath, fatigue, palpitations, and other related symptoms. This level of anemia necessitates hospitalization for intravenous fluids and possible transfusion, intravenous estrogen therapy, or both. Patients who do not respond to medical therapy may require surgical intervention to control the menorrhagia.

Follow-up

▶ Varies according to etiology

Expected Course

▶ Varies with etiology

Complications

▶ Varies with etiology

ENDOMETRIOSIS

Description

▶ Endometrial glands and stroma outside of uterine endometrial cavity, sometimes well outside of pelvic cavity

▶ Common cause of secondary dysmenorrhea, abnormal bleeding patterns, altered fertility, dyspareunia

▶ Staging: Based on the site(s) and severity of involvement at the time of surgery

  » Stage I (minimal): Isolated implants, no significant adhesions

  » Stage II (mild): Superficial implants with < 5 cm of total disease, no significant adhesions

  » Stage III (moderate): Multiple superficial and deep implants, with or without peritubal and periovarian adhesions

  » Stage IV (severe): Multiple superficial and deep implants, large ovarian endometrioma(s), with presence of adhesions

Etiology

▶ Pathogenesis poorly understood; theories include retrograde menstruation, abnormal cellular process from embryogenesis, lymphatic or vascular transplantation, autoimmune disorders

Incidence and Demographics

▶ 3%–10% prevalence in fertile women and 25%–35% in infertile women

▶ Commonly diagnosed in mid-20s

Risk Factors

▶ Increased risk with affected first-degree female relatives

▶ History of uninterrupted, prolonged menstrual cycles

▶ Delayed childbearing or parity

▶ Increased incidence in women with uterine anomalies leading to outflow obstruction, such as transverse vaginal septum

Assessment

History

▶ Gradual onset of constant, achy pain starting at or near menses, with increasing severity for few days and relenting only when menses starts to abate

▶ History of pain-free cycles then gradual pain, with recurrences for months or years with increasing intensity over time will help rule out most acute abdominal conditions.

▶ History of large doses of NSAID analgesics with or without narcotics can be a tip toward assessing pain severity.

▶ Severity of symptoms may not correlate with extent of disease.

▶ Symptoms include pain, infertility, dysmenorrhea, nonmenstrual pelvic pain, dyspareunia, low back pain, bladder pain, frequency and dysuria, irregular vaginal bleeding, partial bowel obstruction, IBS, perimenstrual chest and shoulder pain, abdominal wall pain, and nonpelvic pain.

Physical Exam

▶ Physical examination at time of menses may identify typical patches of enlarged tissue palpable at points of pain (some only identifiable at time of laparoscopic examination).

▶ There may be fixed uterine position, adnexal enlargement, cervical motion tenderness, or tenderness in vaginal cul-de-sac.

Diagnostic Studies

▶ Diagnosis is suggested by history and physical, and tests to exclude other sources.

▶ Lab test to rule out other causes of pain: STIs screens, urinalysis, Hemoccult testing, Pap testing

► Vaginal or abdominal ultrasound may show complex fluid-filled masses or diagnose endometrioma.

► Abdominal CT or MRI may show masses but not small implants; may help in mapping extent of disease.

► Confirmation of diagnosis via direct visualization can only be made by laparoscopy or surgical exploration with biopsy.

Differential Diagnosis

► Leiomyomas

► STIs or PID

► Irritable bowel other GI disorders

► Adenomyosis

► Ectopic pregnancy

► Urinary tract disorders

► Chronic pelvic pain

► Nerve pain syndromes

► Musculoskeletal pain disorders

► Ruptured ovarian cyst

► Neoplasms

► Pelvic adhesions

Management

Nonpharmacologic Treatment

► Laparoscopy with destruction of identifiable lesions via excision, laser vaporization, electrocautery, or endocoagulation

► Surgical management may also involve excision of implants, lysis of adhesions, reduction of ovarian tissue, or hysterectomy with bilateral salpingo-oophorectomy (TAH-BSO).

Pharmacologic Treatment

► Treatment goals are pain relief, control of endometrial patch growth, preservation of fertility

► These first-line therapies should be combined with NSAIDs; additional analgesics may be necessary when menses occur:

  » Hormonal contraception may be used (omitting the withdrawal bleed interval) for 6–12 months (continuous use OCs daily without placebo pills or break, Depo-Provera injections on accelerated schedule). Continuous OCs may be associated with breakthrough bleeding (BTB) if taken for more than 3 months continuously. Patient must be informed about this possibility.

  » Provera tablets p.o. 30 mg daily (side effects: change in lipid profile, depression, BTB common)

  » Danazol 600–800 mg/day for a course of 6 months

  » LNG-IUS: Limited data suggest improvement in dysmenorrhea and menorrhagia with use.

How Long to Treat

► Until pain relief, pregnancy, or menopause (biologic or surgical)

Special Considerations

▶ Calcium supplementation is advised during therapy.

▶ Needs HRT (both estrogen progesterone, to reduce endometrial cancer risk from residual implants) and calcium supplementation after TAH-BSO

When to Consult, Refer, Hospitalize

▶ Refer to gynecologist if poor response to medical therapy or if fertility assistance is desired.

▶ Refer for other hormonal suppression with GnRH analogs such as leuprolide (Lupron), or androgens such as danazol (Danocrine); significant side effect profile and expense

Follow-up

▶ Gynecologist should be managing any follow-up required if receiving GnRH agonists or danazol, to assess side effects and evaluate efficacy.

Expected Course

▶ After surgery or suppressive drug therapies (e.g., GnRH agonists or danazol), women may have 18–24 months of pain relief.

Complications

▶ Infertility

PERIMENOPAUSE AND MENOPAUSE

Description

▶ Age-related biologic reduction in ovarian function with end of fertility and menstrual cycle

▶ Biological menopause is natural failure of ovaries after age 40–45, resulting in absence of fertility and > 12 months without menses

Etiology

▶ The actual cause of natural menopause is unknown.

▶ Ovary is less responsive to FSH (so pituitary increases production). Contrary to past understanding, estrogen levels remain normal or slightly elevated until cessation of menses, but there is inconsistent ovulation each cycle.

▶ Fluctuation in estrogen level (controversial) creates menstrual cycle changes, hot flashes and sweats (vasomotor instability), sleep disturbances, fatigue, irritability, PMS, mood changes, vaginal dryness, and urinary complaints.

▶ Perimenopause is suggested when FSH levels are greater than 20 IU/mL despite continued menstrual bleeding.

▶ Adverse postmenopausal body changes include:

  ▹ Increased bone reabsorption and decreased bone formation, leading to decreased bone density (osteoporosis)

> » Rise in total cholesterol, low-density lipoprotein (LDL), and very low density lipoprotein (VLDL); high-density lipoprotein (HDL) declines and triglycerides show no change
>
> » Diminished bladder control (may occur months to years later)
>
> » Infertility (depending on the woman's reproductive desire)

► Positive postmenopausal changes include:

> » FSH levels greater than 30 IU/mL
>
> » Reduction in myomas, endometriosis, adenomyosis
>
> » Gradual decrease in PMS-type symptoms is common: less mastodynia, bloating, edema, headache, and cyclical mood swings.
>
> » Infertility (again, depending on the woman's reproductive desire)

Incidence and Demographics

► Average age at perimenopause is 47.5 years, with a duration of approximately 4 years.

► Approximately 95% reach menopause at 45–55 years.

► Average age of biological menopause is 51.4 years

► About 10% of women have abrupt cessation of menses and 90% of women have menstrual changes before menstrual cessation.

► About 0.9% of women experience menopause before age 40 (premature menopause).

► Artificial menopause can occur at any time the ovaries are removed or irradiated before biologic failure occurs.

Risk Factors (for premature menopause)

► Turner syndrome (mosaic variant)

► Autoimmune endocrinopathy

► Severe systemic illness

► Chemotherapy and radiation

► Possible familial component

Prevention and Screening

► All women should be asked about menstrual history and onset of menopausal symptoms after age 40.

► Assess risk for coronary heart disease (CHD), osteoporosis, breast and endometrial cancer

Assessment

History

► Obtain complete medical, GYN, and menstrual history, contraceptive use, and medication use, and family history of menopause.

► Associated symptoms: Mood, sleep, hot flashes, vaginal dryness, and vaginal bleeding not related to menses

Physical Exam

▶ Complete physical exam, including breast and pelvic exam; uterus and ovaries become smaller

▶ Leiomyomata or adenomyosis reduced

▶ Rectovaginal exam, stool for occult blood in women > 50 years

Diagnostic Studies

▶ Some experts suggest diagnosis should be based on clinical, not laboratory, criteria (cessation of menses, age, vasomotor symptomatology), but pregnancy test (must be done if there is any possibility), TSH, and FSH if suspect thyroid problems.

▶ Fluctuation of FSH, LH, and estradiol levels is common until menopause.

▶ Within 1 year after cessation of menses, there is a 3–4-fold increase in FSH and a 3-fold increase in LH (confirm ovarian failure) with estradiol levels below 20 pg/mL.

▶ Predominance of immature epithelial cells on vaginal wet mount (simple, inexpensive)

▶ CBC, TFTs, Pap testing, mammogram, DEXA Scan, STI testing if indicated, FOB or sigmoidoscopy. Follow Periodic Health Screening and Evaluation for Adults as recommended by the U.S. Preventive Services Task Force (USPSTF, 2010).

Differential Diagnosis

▶ Pregnancy

▶ Depression

▶ Thyroid or other endocrine disorders

▶ PMS

▶ Hot flashes

▶ Pheochromocytoma

▶ Cancer

▶ Leukemia

▶ Thyroid tumors

▶ Pancreatic tumors

Management

Nonpharmacologic Treatment

▶ Exercise and weight management

▶ Smoking cessation reduces heart disease and osteoporosis risk, may relieve hot flashes, may avoid early menopause.

▶ Healthy nutritional and dietary practices, including well-balanced diet consisting of fresh fruits and vegetables, whole grains, lean proteins, low saturated fats; daily multivitamin, daily recommended dosage of calcium (1,500 mg/day), vitamin D (800 IU per day for women at risk of deficiency). See Chapter 14 for osteoporosis prevention; avoid hot flash triggers such as spicy foods, face heat, hot baths, tanning booths, etc.

   ▸ Limit alcohol to 1 drink per day or less; limit caffeine.

   ▸ Kegel exercises for coitus and urinary incontinence; weight-bearing exercise

   ▸ Vaginal lubricants for coitus

   ▸ In a meticulously conducted yearlong clinical trial funded by the National Institutes of Health (NIH) and published in late 2006, black cohosh, soy products, red clover, and vitamin E were found to be no better than placebos for relieving hot flashes. The women given these products reported the same number of daily hot flashes as did the women given a placebo.

Pharmacologic Treatment

▶ Women's Health Initiative study has changed what the medical profession thought about HRT:

  » Data suggest long-term estrogen plus progestin (combination HRT) increase risk of breast cancer

  » HRT has no beneficial effect on coronary heart disease (CHD).

  » HRT may increase the risk of CHD among generally healthy postmenopausal women, especially during the first year after the initiation of hormone use.

  » HRT increases the risk of thromboembolic events and stroke.

▶ Other research suggests long-term combination HRT may increase chance of dementia and breast cancer.

▶ Some women will still require hormone replacement therapy; regimen should be individualized and based on the specific diagnosis.

  » Relieves vasomotor flushing and may prevent osteoporosis; available in oral forms or transdermal patch; progestin alone for those who cannot take estrogen; progestin *must* be included for women with intact uterus to protect against endometrial hyperplasia or cancer.

  » Absolute contraindications: Pregnancy, thromboembolus, unexplained genital bleeding, endometrial cancer, undiagnosed breast mass, active liver disease

  » Relative contraindications: Seizure disorder, hypertension, familial hyperlipidemia, migraines, gallbladder disease, past history of thrombosis

▶ Vaginal creams for atrophic vaginitis (stop after 3–6 months; reassess)

  » Estradiol 0.01% cream (Estrace) 1 g twice weekly for 3 weeks, off for 1 week

  » Estropipate 1.5 mg/g cream (Ogen) 2–4 g daily for 3 weeks, off for 1 week

  » Conjugated estrogens 0.625 mg/g cream (Premarin) 0.5–2 g daily for 3 weeks, off for 1 week

▶ Vaginal ring

  » Estring vaginal ring releases estradiol 7.5 mcg/24 hours; inserted deeply into upper ⅓ of vaginal vault by patient; remove and replace after 90 days. Reassess at 3–6 month intervals.

▶ Preparation for hot flashes

  » Hormone therapy: Gold standard for relief of hot flashes; contraindicated in women with hormonally mediated cancers, undiagnosed vaginal bleeding, active liver disease, increased risk of clotting, and CAD

  » Estrogen therapy (ET) for women without uteri and estrogen plus progesterone therapy (EPT) for women with uteri; unopposed estrogen increases risk of endometrial cancer; progestin therapy reduces risk back to baseline

  » Goal is to use lowest dose for shortest amount of time

    ▷ MPA 10–20 mg q.d. or depo MPA (Depo-Provera) 150 mg IM q 3 months

    ▷ Megestrol acetate (Megace) 20 mg b.i.d.

    ▷ Progesterone (Prometrium) 100 mg q.d. (or 200 mg 12 days a month)

▶ The Food and Drug Administration has approved the following drugs specifically to treat hot flashes; however, they are approved for treating other conditions as well. Information is available on the FDA website at www.fda.gov.

  ▹ **Antidepressants:** Low doses of certain antidepressants may decrease hot flashes. Antidepressants from classes of medications known as selective serotonin reuptake inhibitors (SSRIs) and serotonin and norepinephrine reuptake inhibitors (SNRIs)— including venlafaxine (Effexor), paroxetine (Paxil), fluoxetine (Prozac), citalopram (Celexa), and others—have been found to relieve hot flashes in some clinical trials. Many clinicians now consider these antidepressants the treatment of choice for moderate to severe hot flashes for patients who refuse or are not candidates for HRT. However, these medications are not as effective as hormone therapy for severe hot flashes and may cause unwanted side effects, such as nausea, dizziness, weight gain, or sexual dysfunction.

  ▹ **Gabapentin (Neurontin):** Some studies have found that gabapentin, approved for treating seizures or pain associated with shingles, is moderately effective in reducing hot flashes. Side effects can include drowsiness, dizziness, nausea, imbalance when walking, and swelling.

  ▹ **Clonidine:** Typically used to treat high blood pressure, clonidine in pill or patch form may provide some relief from hot flashes. Side effects such as dizziness, drowsiness, dry mouth, and constipation are common, sometimes limiting the medication's usefulness for treating hot flashes.

    ▷ Transdermal clonidine 0.1 mg/d applied weekly (side effects: hypotension, dizziness, nausea, mood swings)

    ▷ Clonidine 0.1 mg daily orally or transdermally is another option to treat vasomotor flushing

▶ Prevention and treatment of osteoporosis

  ▹ Oral bisphosphonates (alendronate, risedronate, ibandronate) for prevention and treatment; raloxifene

How Long to Treat

▶ Until symptoms resolve or, with HRT use, for no more than 10 years (controversial)

Special Considerations

▶ Do not start HRT in a woman who is being treated for ovarian or breast cancer or who has a history of either; consult with the oncologist or surgeon.

▶ Do not use HRT as a birth control method.

▶ All undiagnosed vaginal bleeding in postmenopausal women is cancer until proven otherwise.

When to Consult, Refer, Hospitalize

▶ Consult or refer for all relative contraindications and questionable uses for HRT.

▶ Consult or refer for endometrial biopsy for episodes of vaginal spotting or bleeding, even though this side effect of HRT is common.

Follow-up

▶ 3 months after initiating HRT or as often as necessary to evaluate efficacy and side effects

▶ Review danger signs of HRT: Vaginal bleeding not associated with HRT use, calf pain, chest pain, shortness of breath, hemoptysis, severe headache, vision problems, breast changes, abdominal pain, and jaundice

▶ After HRT regimen established, annual exams

Complications

▶ Postmenopausal problems: Cardiovascular problems, osteoporosis, vasomotor symptoms, urogenital atrophy and incontinence, atrophic vaginitis, diminished libido

BREAST CONDITIONS

BREAST CANCER, BREAST MASSES

Description

▶ Malignancy of the breast

Etiology

▶ Precise etiology unknown

▶ Noninvasive: Intraductal tumors, including ductal carcinoma in situ (DCIS) or lobular carcinoma in situ (LCIS)

▶ Invasive: Tumor no longer contained within basement membrane

▶ Invasive ductal carcinoma is most common; originates from epithelial cells lining mammary ducts; subtypes include medullary, papillary, tubular, colloid

▶ Invasive lobular carcinoma arises from mammary lobules

Incidence and Demographics

▶ 1 in 8 women (lifetime risk)

▶ Second leading cause of cancer death in women ages 30–70

▶ Rare in women under 25; 48% of new breast cancer cases and 56% of breast cancer deaths occur in women > 65 years

▶ Peak age at diagnosis is age 45–65, with > 75% occurring over age 50

▶ About 70% are invasive; invasive ductal more common than lobular (96%–97% vs. 3%–4%)

▶ Most common site is upper outer quadrant (49%)

Risk Factors

▶ Female gender; living in North America, northern Europe; older age; early menarche (before age 11) or late menarche (after age 14); late menopause (after age 55 or more than 35 years' duration of menses); nulliparity; first pregnancy after age 35 (1.5× risk); prior breast cancer (5–10× risk); obesity (may be linked to hyperinsulinemia or fat cell production of androgens converted to estrogens); android fat distribution; excess alcohol use; tobacco use; never any breastfeeding; use of combined estrogen plus progestin use for > 4 years.

▶ 20% family history (autosomal dominant with maternal linkage) relative risk (RR) 2.2 with first-degree relatives, with bilateral disease in premenopausal relatives (10.5 RR), bilateral disease in postmenopausal relatives (5.5 RR)

▶ 90% of women with breast cancer have *no* family history.

▶ BRCA (breast cancer recessive autosomal) carriers have substantially higher risks for breast and ovarian cancers, usually early onset.

  ▹ BRCA 1 have 57% breast cancer risk and 40% ovarian cancer risk with estrogen receptor negative

  ▹ BRCA 2 have 45% breast cancer risk with estrogen receptor positive and 11% ovarian cancer risk

Prevention and Screening

Protection

▶ Protection may be conferred by exercise, weight control, especially in postmenopausal years.

▶ Tamoxifen as prophylaxis in high-risk women (watch for endometrial abnormalities)

▶ In a huge multicenter study, raloxifene (Evista), a common osteoporosis drug, was shown to be as effective as tamoxifen (Nolvadex) in preventing invasive breast cancer, but had fewer side effects as reported by the data accrued from the "Study of Tamoxifen and Raloxifene," a project of the National Surgical Adjuvant Breast and Bowel Project and National Cancer Institute (NCI).

  ▹ Further studies comparing raloxifene and an aromatase inhibitor have already been submitted to the NCI for approval. Aromatase inhibitors have been shown to be more effective than tamoxifen in preventing second breast cancers.

▶ Breastfeeding may reduce the risk by about 4% per year; is cumulative per child.

  ▹ Women with BRCA1 mutations who breastfed for more than 1 year are less likely to have breast cancer than those who never breastfed.

▶ Avoid methylxanthines.

Screening

▶ While some controversy surrounds the breast self-exam (BSE), it is still recommended by many clinicians.

▶ Age 20–39: Monthly BSE and clinical breast examination q 1–3 years

▶ For women with family history of breast cancer, baseline digital mammogram 10 years earlier than age of onset of a first-degree relative with history of breast cancer

▶ 40–49: Monthly BSE, annual clinical breast examination, digital mammography every 2 years per patient's history and risk factors

▶ Age 50–74: Monthly BSE, annual clinical breast examination, digital mammography every 1–2 years (reduces cancer mortality by 30%–50% in women ages 50–69; over age 70, data are conflicting; no evidence of benefit to women over age 75)

▶ False negative rate of 10%–15%, false positive rate of 15%–20% for screening digital mammogram

▶ Clinical breast examination to find changes that may indicate a malignancy soon enough for timely intervention, and to teach or to reinforce BSE

▶ Yearly digital mammogram for women who have had breast cancer; MRI for women with history of breast cancer for close surveillance

Assessment

History

▶ Assess for risk factors

▶ Obtain detailed medical and GYN history; history of breast mass development; document all prior mammogram dates and results, contraceptive and HRT use, prior breast biopsies and breast surgery

▶ Painless or tender persistent breast mass; unilateral nipple inversion, discharge, itching; breast cellulitis that fails to respond or resolve; symptoms of systemic disease: bone pain, cough, or shortness of breath, epigastric discomfort or nausea; family history of breast and ovary cancers; ethnicity: Ashkenazi Jewish or Scandinavian

Physical Exam

▶ Persistent nipple itching or burning suggests Paget's disease; may present with minimal skin changes, no mass palpable, may have erosion or ulceration

▶ Exam shows solitary, nontender, firm to hard mass without well-defined margins, often fixed position

▶ Ominous signs are enlarged or tender lymphs, skin color changes, skin erosion, peau d'orange (edema), dimpling, nipple retraction, pain, breast enlargement

▶ Assess for nipple discharge, thickening, scaling, or inversion.

▶ Lymphadenopathy noted in axilla, neck, or suraclavicular regions

Diagnostic Studies

▶ Negative test results are not necessarily diagnostic in the presence of a palpable breast mass.

▶ Diagnostic mammography

▶ Ultrasound (US)

▶ CBC, liver function tests (LFT), chest X-ray (CXR), estrogen and progesterone receptor determination (usually ordered once biopsy done), bone scan, CT or US to assess lymph node involvement and metastasis

▶ Sentinel node biopsy is accurate tool for assessment of axilla in early breast cancer

▶ Breast MRI if exam suspicious and mammogram is not definitive

▶ Cystologic tests of nipple discharge

Differential Diagnosis

- ▶ Fibrocystic changes
- ▶ Fibroadenoma
- ▶ Intraductal papilloma
- ▶ Lipoma
- ▶ Fat necrosis

Management

- ▶ Mastectomy (radical and modified radical) or lumpectomy combined with radiation appear to have similar cure rates.
- ▶ In addition to surgical excision:
  - ▹ Premenopausal women with positive lymph nodes often receive cytoxic chemotherapy, followed by tamoxifen if estrogen receptor positive.
  - ▹ Postmenopausal women with positive lymph nodes and a positive estrogen receptor assay are commonly treated with tamoxifen and less likely to benefit from chemotherapy.
  - ▹ Controversial whether women with negative lymph nodes would benefit from chemotherapy (but modest success demonstrated in postmenopausal women with positive estrogen receptors)

Special Considerations

- ▶ Toremifene (Fareston); fulvestram (faslodex), raloxifene (Femara), and aromatase (arimidex) inhibitors may be given to women at high risk for prevention of breast cancer recurrence.

When to Consult, Refer, Hospitalize

- ▶ Refer all suspicious breast lumps and abnormal mammograms to surgeon for excision biopsy.
- ▶ Additional referrals may be made to medical radiation oncologist.

Follow-up

- ▶ After diagnosis and therapy for breast cancer, a physical examination is indicated every 3–4 months for the first 5 years, and thereafter, every year.
- ▶ Regular follow-up visits include chest X-rays and liver function tests.
- ▶ Yearly mammogram and possible MRI for women who have had breast cancer

Expected Course

- ▶ Highly variable; prognosis is best reflected by stage; Stage I treated with the standard of care has up to 95% survival over 10 years

Complications

- ▶ Metastatic disease

NONINFECTIOUS BREAST DISORDERS

BENIGN BREAST MASSES

Description

▶ Benign mammary dysplasia also referred to as fibrocystic changes; majority not at risk for breast cancer

▶ Fibroadenomas (solid, benign masses) are the most common benign palpable breast lesions seen in adolescents and young adults to age 25.

Etiology

▶ Fibrocystic changes are the most common benign breast condition; caused by ductal dilation, usually 2 mm or less; 20%–40% enlarge to palpable cysts (usually fluid-filled), may increase and decrease with menstrual cycle

▶ Fibroadenomas are made of glandular fibrous tissue, often located in upper quadrant, caused by an inflammatory reaction from ductal irritation, with onset late teens to early 20s.

Incidence and Demographics

▶ Fibrocystic breast: Most common ages 30–50

▶ Cysts and fibroadenomas: Most common benign breast changes, followed by duct ectasia

▶ Up to 50% of women affected

▶ Fibroadenomas often occur in younger women within 10 years of menarche

Risk Factors

▶ Fibrocystic disease: Caffeine, chocolate, tea, coffee, smoking, family history

Prevention and Screening

▶ Avoid methylxanthines; side effects are similar to excessive caffeine intake

Assessment

History

▶ Achy, tender, or painless lumpy breasts

▶ More tender with menses

▶ Any nipple discharge; may be seen in galactocele or ductal ectasia, papilloma, or cancer

Physical Exam

▶ Benign multiple breast masses, size fluctuating with menses (cystic, adenosis, fibrosis, ductal hyperplasia), occasionally with unilateral or bilateral nipple discharge; may feel 1 or 2 dominant cysts, usually 1–2 cm

- ▶ Fibroadenomas: Unilateral mass, often solitary; well-defined, round, rubbery, mobile masses
- ▶ Fibrocystic disease: Multiple masses, tender with menses, fluctuating size, rare nipple discharge
- ▶ Axillary, supraclavicular, infraclavicular lymph nodes for enlarged nodes

Diagnostic Studies

- ▶ Ultrasonography can identify cystic structures vs. solid mass.
- ▶ Suspicious masses should be evaluated by ultrasonography or mammogram.
- ▶ Refer for fine-needle aspiration, biopsy of suspicious areas, bloody fluid, persistent mass, or excision.
- ▶ Cytologic evaluation of nipple discharge

Differential Diagnosis

- ▶ Breast cancer
- ▶ Fibroadenoma
- ▶ Breast abscess
- ▶ Galactocele
- ▶ Fat necrosis
- ▶ Benign cyst
- ▶ Prolactinoma

Management

Nonpharmacologic Treatment

- ▶ Fibroadenoma: Watch, excise, or aspirate.
- ▶ Fibrocystic disease: Reduce caffeine and chocolate in diet, wear a supportive brassiere, take oral contraceptive pills.

Pharmacologic Treatment

- ▶ Vitamin E supplements 400 IU daily (for 2 weeks then discontinue), vitamin B_6 25–50 mg daily, magnesium supplements 200–400 mg/day
- ▶ Oral contraceptives may or may not relieve symptoms of fibrocystic disease.
- ▶ OTC analgesics; NSAIDs: Take with food.

Special Considerations

- ▶ Breast pain in postmenopausal women not on HRT should be worked up for cancer.
- ▶ Despite limitations (for example, reduced mammographic sensitivity), women with implants should continue to be radiographically screened as appropriate for their age and risk factors.

When to Consult, Refer, Hospitalize

- ▶ Refer to a surgeon for fine-needle aspiration to confirm that cyst is fluid-filled, excisional biopsy, or suspicious findings as outlined above.

Follow-up

▶ For fibrocystic disease (with multiple or single small < 1 cm cysts), reevaluate in 1–2 months soon after menses to determine efficacy of therapy, whether further work-up required.

Complications

▶ Usually none if benign process

GALACTORRHEA OR NIPPLE DISCHARGE

Description

▶ Milky nipple discharge not associated with lactation

Etiology

▶ Duct ectasia is a collection of dilated terminal collecting ducts in the breast and is commonly associated with nipple discharge. It is not clear if the discharge causes ectasia or the other way around. The problem commonly presents when the woman is in her 40s.

▶ Nipple discharge is most commonly associated with endocrine alterations, medications (e.g., methyldopa, illicit drugs, neuroleptics, phenothiazines, oral contraceptives, tricyclic antidepressants, opiates), or both affecting hypothalamic inhibition of dopamine.

▶ Galactorrhea may be due to a prolactin-secreting pituitary adenoma (prolactinoma).

▶ The likelihood of malignancy increases when the discharge is unilateral, arises from a single duct, is accompanied by a palpable mass, is associated with a positive mammographic finding or positive cytologic galactotrophic findings, or when the patient is older than 50 years.

▶ Physiologic etiologies for galactorrhea include stress, breast stimulation, exercise, eating, and sleep; bilateral nipple discharge can be expressed in up to 80% of asymptomatic women.

Incidence and Demographics

▶ Occurs in the United States in frequencies as high as 3%–8%

▶ Benign discharge spontaneously resolves in as many as 73% of patients within 5 years.

▶ About 10%–12% of breast cancers are associated with nipple discharge.

Risk Factors

▶ Nipple discharge often results in fibrocystic changes or ductal ectasia.

Prevention and Screening

▶ During clinical breast exam, gently attempt to express any fluid from the nipple.

Assessment

History

▶ Changes may be unilateral or bilateral, causing discharge from one or several nipple ducts.

▶ Color of nipple discharge: Clear, white, milky, gray, brown, green, or bloody

▶ Any association with a lump; tenderness

▶ Medications

▶ Provoked by nipple stimulation or spontaneous discharge

▶ Pregnant or lactating

▶ Relationship with menstrual cycles; menstrual history

▶ Vision problems, headaches

Physical Exam

▶ Nipple discharge varies in color from white to brown.

▶ To be clinically significant, nipple discharge must be true, spontaneous, persistent, nonlactational.

▶ Surgically significant discharge is clear (i.e., watery), serous (i.e., clear yellow), serosanguineous, or sanguineous (i.e., bloody).

▶ Nipple discharge typically green to yellow to black in color if physiologic, coming from multiple ducts versus spontaneous, unilateral

▶ Nipple discharge often associated with duct ectasia, often thick and cheesy

▶ Blood discharge more likely to be associated with cancer

▶ Check vital signs, neurologic exam with visual fields, complete breast exam sitting and lying with hands on hips and above head.

Diagnostic Studies

▶ Mammogram, ultrasound, and possible MRI of breast

▶ Subsequent to negative mammographic findings, galactography or ductography is the procedure of choice. Galactography involves the retrograde injection of water-soluble radiopaque contrast material into a discharging duct with subsequent mammographic imaging.

▶ Hemoccult tests can be used to assess the nipple discharge fluid to confirm or exclude the presence of occult blood.

▶ Cytologic tests of the fluid can be performed; however, false-positive rates and significant false-negative rates have been reported (2.6% and 17.8%, respectively, in Leis' series).

▶ Prolactin, TSH

▶ MRI or CT of brain to rule out pituitary adenoma if prolactin level is elevated

Differential Diagnosis

- ▶ Breast cancer
- ▶ Fibroadenoma
- ▶ Breast abscess
- ▶ Fat necrosis
- ▶ Thyroid disease
- ▶ Benign cyst

Management

Nonpharmacologic Treatment

- ▶ Avoid nipple stimulation.
- ▶ Monthly breast self-exams encouraged

Pharmacologic Treatment

- ▶ None unless specific for treatment of prolactinoma

When to Consult, Refer, Hospitalize

- ▶ As needed for suspicious findings, such as positive occult blood or galactorrhea in a nulliparous woman

Follow-up

- ▶ As indicated by breast specialist or primary care provider

MASTITIS ABSCESS

Description

- ▶ Mastitis is inflammation of the breast tissue with possible infection. An abscess (a collection of pus) may develop but is more likely when treatment has been delayed or inadequate.

Etiology

- ▶ Occurs as a result of milk stasis
- ▶ If infection present, it is usually due to *Staphylococcus aureus,* which is generally penicillin-resistant.
- ▶ Nonpuerperal infection can occur, although less common and is usually due to *S. aureus, Bacteroides*, or *Peptostreptococcus.*
- ▶ A break in the integrity of the nipple or areolar area is a risk factor, but is neither adequate nor necessary for the development of infection.

Incidence and Demographics

- ▶ Puerperal mastitis: 1%–33%
- ▶ Abscess from puerperal mastitis: 5%–11%

Risk Factors

▶ Lactation

▶ During lactation, any event that causes milk stasis, such as inadequate drainage of the breast; rapid weaning; oversupply of milk; pressure on the breast (e.g., from a poor-fitting bra); a blocked duct; or missed, scheduled, infrequent, or timed feeds

▶ Nipple trauma with skin breakdown

▶ Possibly also infant illness or maternal fatigue or stress, anemia, poor nutrition, or illness

▶ Eczema; these mothers prone to colonization with *S. aureus*

Prevention and Screening

▶ Maintain adequate breast drainage to avoid engorgement. Teach the mother to properly latch, position her infant to maximize milk removal, and minimize nipple trauma.

▶ Encourage feeding demonstration.

▶ If weaning is desired, recommend dropping one feeding every 2–3 days, taking 2–3 weeks to complete.

▶ Recommend avoiding abrupt weaning and binding of the breasts.

Assessment

History

▶ Painful, tender, warm, red breast area (classic presentation is a red wedge-shaped area)

▶ Fever (may or may not be present)

▶ Nipple soreness with or with out skin breakdown may be present.

▶ Assess breastfeeding frequency, milk supply.

Physical Exam

▶ Local edema, erythema, induration

▶ Axillary lymphadenopathy

▶ Localized, extremely tender, fluctuant mass may develop.

▶ May be bilateral or unilateral (suspect *Streptococcus* Group B if bilateral in the early postpartum)

▶ Check nipples for increased redness, soreness, skin breakdown.

▶ Examine skin for eczema.

Diagnostic Studies

▶ Clinical diagnosis; culture drainage if treatment failure, recurrent, or abscessed

▶ Should have mammogram, ultrasound, or both if recurrent or nonpuerperal

▶ Ultrasound to evaluate for abscess p.r.n. or if lump does not disappear in a week with massaging

Differential Diagnosis

▶ Breast trauma, breast engorgement, or plugged duct

Management

Nonpharmacologic Treatment

▶ Warm compresses, massage, to promote drainage; cool compresses to reduce local pain and swelling

▶ Continue to breastfeed or express milk and increase the frequency to shorten symptom duration (bacteria in breast milk demonstrated not to be pathogenic to the infant).

▶ If possible, start on affected side, or start on unaffected side and switch after let-down occurs. If direct breastfeeding is not possible, regular pumping instead of breastfeeding should be done with a hospital-grade double electric pump 8–12 times per day for 15–20 minutes. When necessary, pumping or expression can be done after feedings if the infant fails to adequately drain the breast.

▶ While breastfeeding, pointing the infant's chin toward the affected area may improve the drainage.

▶ Encourage mother to rest, eat nutritiously, drink plenty of fluids.

　　» Suspect abscess if mastitis does not respond to antibiotics.

　　» Abscesses: Warm compresses. It is a relative contraindication to discontinue breastfeeding with an abscess because engorgement may lead to worsening of the infection (because the fluid or milk backs up into the interstitial tissue) and abrupt weaning may cause the mother to develop fever, malaise, and achiness. Maintain adequate breast milk drainage either by direct breastfeeding or with a double electric hospital-grade pump.

　　» Monthly breast self-exams encouraged

Pharmacologic Treatment

▶ In terms of antibiotic treatment for infectious mastitis during lactation, generally mothers with acute pain or toxicity, bacterial colony counts, white blood cell counts and culture results consistent with infection, and nipple fissures or severe or classic symptoms (fever; myalgias; chills along with a localized, red, hot, swollen, painful breast) should be treated with antibiotics. Mothers without these criteria should be instructed to feed frequently and maintain regular drainage of the breast as previously described. If symptoms haven't resolved within 12–24 hours, antibiotic treatment should be promptly commenced.

▶ For puerperal *S. aureus* infections: Dicloxacillin (Dycill)) 500 mg p.o. q.i.d. or clindamycin (Cleocin) 300 mg p.o. q.i.d.; may need to consider IV therapy if mother toxic or extensive cellulitis

▶ For nonpuerperal infection, amoxicillin /clavulanate (Augmentin) 875/125 mg b.i.d. or IV therapy

▶ Analgesics: Acetaminophen, NSAIDs (NSAIDs taken with food may be more effective; ibuprofen and acetaminophen are compatible with breastfeeding.)

How Long to Treat

▶ Although there is no standard recommendation for treatment length, most authorities advise a 10–14-day length of treatment.

Special Considerations

▶ When treatment for nonlactational mastitis is unsuccessful (abscess ruled out), consider squamous metaplasia.

▶ Monitor for candidiasis in mother or infant; treat them concurrently if it is present or develops.

▶ If mother is hospitalized, the infant should be in the room with her to facilitate continued breastfeeding.

When to Consult, Refer, Hospitalize

▶ Refer to physician for abscess, toxic mother with persistent fever despite oral antibiotics, extensive cellulites, or if patient needs hospitalization for IV medications.

▶ If abscessed, refer for incision and drainage or ultrasound-guided needle aspiration.

▶ Consult with a lactation specialist for breastfeeding management, including oversupply, latching problems, lowered milk supply, persistent nipple pain, damaged nipples, nipple vasospasm (Raynaud's phenomenon), fussy infant, etc.

Follow-up

▶ Examination to assess for resolution or identify other differentials

▶ Evaluate for an underlying mass if more than 2–3 episodes in same area

Expected Course

▶ Frequent breastfeeding or milk expression successfully resolves puerperal mastitis 96% of the time.

▶ Any lowering of the milk supply will respond to more frequent breastfeeding within a few days.

Complications

▶ Development of sinus tracts

▶ Development of nipple soreness or burning breast pain, which may be a sign of mammary candidiasis, necessitating concurrent treatment of mother and child

▶ Infant thrush

▶ Functional mastectomy due to extensive incision and drainage; 10% of women affected by a breast abscess experience compromised lactation that includes a functional mastectomy

▶ Recurrent infectious mastitis may cause chronic inflammation.

▶ Temporarily lowered milk supply

CONDITIONS OF THE VULVA, VAGINA, AND CERVIX

ABNORMAL CERVICAL CYTOLOGY

Description

▶ Abnormal cervical cytology (most likely via Pap smear) may indicate cervical cancer.

▶ About 85% of cervical cancer is squamous cell carcinoma.

▶ The Pap smear has moved cervical cancer from a top killer (U.S. in the 1940s) to a preventable disease.

Etiology

▶ Preinvasive cancer of the intraepithelial layers (carcinoma in situ or cervical intraepithelial neoplasia [CIN]) is a common diagnosis in women of childbearing age.

▶ There is often a progression of cellular abnormalities in the single-layered cervical epithelium; an area of metaplasia occurs.

  » A variety of factors leads to additional cellular abnormalities.

  » Squamous cell dysplasia or cancer may occur.

  » Self-contained dysplasia may invade the basement membrane and surrounding tissues.

  » Degree of dysplasia can vary; no strong predictor as to which types will extend; some remain stable, others regress, some extend

  » All dysplasias must be observed serially or treated.

Incidence and Demographics

▶ Current lifetime risk for death by cervical cancer in the U.S. is 0.83%.

▶ Average age at diagnosis of precancerous lesions is the mid-30s.

▶ Average age at diagnosis of invasive cancer is the mid-40s.

▶ 25% of invasive cervical cancers, 41% of cervical cancer deaths occur in women over age 65.

▶ Underscreening is the number-one reason 15,700 women get cervical cancer in the U.S. and why 4,900 die from it annually.

▶ Half of women diagnosed with invasive cervical cancer have never been screened, and another 10% have not had a Pap test in 5 years.

▶ Least likely to be screened: Older, poor, Black, Hispanic, and uninsured women

Risk Factors

▶ Early onset coitus, especially within first year of menarche

▶ Three or more lifetime sexual partners (4× risk in prostitutes); virgins almost never get cervical cancer

▶ Male sexual partner who has had other partners (especially one with cervical cancer)

▶ More than three STIs

▶ Long-term oral contraceptive use increases risk of dysplasias and cancer.

▶ Smoking: Nicotine and other substances bind to cells (cancer cofactor)

▶ Clinical history of human papillomavirus (HPV): Documented warts or positive DNA sampling

▶ Low socioeconomic status (less likely to be screened regularly)

▶ DES exposure

▶ HIV: Prevalence of dysplasia without HIV is 3%; with HIV 36%; with AIDS 64%; 1992 CDC surveillance criteria for AIDS include cervical cancer as an AIDS-defining illness (immunosuppression increases the risk of dysplasia). Any woman in her mid-20s or younger with advanced carcinoma in situ (CIS) or cervical cancer needs assessment for HIV.

▶ HPV prevalence accounts for > 90% of abnormal cytology

▶ Herpes simplex virus (HSV), partner circumcision, parity, oral contraceptive use have not been shown to affect risk.

Current Recommendations

U.S. Preventive Services Task Force (USPSTF), American College of Obstetricians and Gynecologists (ACOG), and American Cancer Society (ACS) Cervical Cancer Screening Recommendations 2012 apply to women who have a cervix, regardless of sexual history. These recommendations do not apply to women who have received a diagnosis of a high-grade precancerous cervical lesion or cervical cancer, women with in utero exposure to diethylstilbestrol (DES), or women who are immunocompromised (such as those who are HIV positive). Women of any age with this history need to be screened annually.

▶ Recommend cervical screening for women beginning at age 21 to 65 years with cytology every 3 years or, for women ages 30 to 65 years who want to lengthen the screening interval, screening with a combination of cytology and HPV testing every 5 years.

▶ Recommend against screening for cervical cancer in women younger than age 21 years regardless of sexual history; harm outweighs benefit.

▶ Recommend women between the ages of 21 and 29 should have a Pap test every 3 years. They should not be tested for HPV unless it is needed after an abnormal Pap test result.

▶ Recommend against screening for cervical cancer in women older than age 65 years who have had adequate prior screening and are not otherwise at high risk for cervical cancer. However, women who have been diagnosed with cervical pre-cancer should continue to be screened.

▶ Recommend against screening for cervical cancer in women who have had a hysterectomy with removal of the cervix and who do not have a history of CIN 2, CIN 3, or cervical cancer.

▶ Recommend against screening for cervical cancer using HPV testing, alone or in combination with cytology, in women younger than age 30 years.

▶ Recommend women who have had the HPV vaccine should still follow the screening recommendations for their age group.

▶ Recommend women who are at high risk for cervical cancer may need to be screened more often. Women at high risk include those with HIV infection, organ transplant, or exposure to the drug DES.

Prevention and Screening

▶ Abstinence or safer sex to prevent STIs, which increase risk

▶ HPV vaccine: Gardasil, a vaccine indicated for males and females ages 9 to 26 for the prevention of cervical cancer, precancerous or dysplastic lesions, and genital warts caused by human papillomavirus (HPV) Types 6, 11, 16, and 18; may be administered as early as age 9

   » Also recommended for administration to men up to age 26 who have sex with men

   » HPV vaccine will prevent up to 70% of cervical cancer cases.

   » Contraindicated in individuals who are hypersensitive to the active substances or any of the excipients of the vaccine

   » Does not substitute for routine cervical cancer screening; women who receive Gardasil should continue to undergo screening per standard of care.

   » Not recommended for use in pregnant women

   » May be administered while breastfeeding

   » Vaccination with Gardasil may not result in protection in all vaccine recipients.

   » Not intended to be used for treatment of active genital warts, cervical cancer, cervical intraepithelial neoplasia, vulvar intraepithelial neoplasia, or vaginal intraepithelial neoplasia

   » Has not been shown to protect against diseases, due to nonvaccine HPV types.

   » The vaccine-related adverse experiences observed among recipients of Gardasil at a frequency of at least 1.0% and greater than placebo were pain, swelling, erythema, fever, nausea, pruritus, and dizziness. In addition, common postmarketing reports include vomiting and syncope.

   » Gardasil should be administered in 3 separate intramuscular injections in the deltoid region of the upper arm or the higher anterolateral area of the thigh over a 6-month period, with the first dose at an elected date, the second dose 2 months after the first dose, and the third dose 6 months after the first dose.

▶ Avoid initiation of tobacco use or stop smoking.

▶ Pap smear to collect cells for analysis. Highest risk area on the uterine cervix for cancer is the "transformation zone" (TZ), where stratified squamous epithelial tissue intersects with columnar epithelial tissue.

▶ TZ appears well outside the external os in very young women and migrates into the canal as the woman ages, or as there is disruption in the cervix (childbirth, invasive procedures, cancer treatment). With hormonal stimulation, the TZ may be more visible (hormonal contraception, pregnancy). In DES-exposed women, the TZ may extend into the vagina.

▶ All women who are or have been sexually active should have regular cervical cytologic screening from the time sexual activity begins or they reach 21 years old. If 3 or more normal Paps, examine annually, screen every 3 years. Because of the prevalence of HPV and the false-negative rate of Pap smears, some clinicians will opt to screen women yearly despite this recommendation.

▶ If not screened for 10 years before age 66, screen every 3 years to age 75.

Assessment

History

▶ There are no signs or symptoms of cervical intraepithelial neoplasia. This diagnosis is reached as a result of screening cervical cytology.

▶ Assess the history of cervical cancer screening, management of any abnormalities

▶ Note any colposcopy, biopsy, past ablative or surgical therapy.

▶ Cervical cancer is asymptomatic until well advanced.

▶ Exposure to DES

Physical Exam

▶ Most abnormal changes are picked up on cytologic screening.

▶ Vaginal discharge; vaginal cervical lesions; vaginal bleeding (metrorrhagia, postcoital spotting, cervical lesion or ulceration, abnormal uterine bleeding); and malodorous, bloody, nonpruritic vaginal discharge usually are caused by STIs and other conditions, which bring attention to cervical screening.

  ▹ If evidence of an infectious process, treat condition and defer Pap smear for 3–6 months.

  ▹ If inflammation noted on follow-up, obtain cervical cytology; note this on request slip.

Diagnostic Studies

SCREENING METHODS FOR CERVICAL CANCER

▶ Colposcopy

▶ Recall that false negatives occur from sampling error (poor specimen collection) and from detection error.

▶ Thin prep

  ▹ Specimen obtained from nonmenstruating patient

  ▹ Specimen should include squamocolumnar junction and endocervix

  ▹ Cervical specimen is placed directly into preservative vial.

  ▹ Increases number of cells sampled by removing confounding mucus, blood, and debris

  ▹ Reduces inadequate specimens or sampling error by 50%

▶ Conventional Papanicolaou (Pap) screening

  ▹ Has a sensitivity of 51% and a specificity of 98%

  ▹ Most accurate and very specific for carcinoma or invasive cancer and high-grade lesions

  ▹ Low-grade lesions often overdiagnosed: False-negative rate can be 10%–20% (vs. false-positive rate of < 1%)

▶ Auto Pap

  ▹ Computer-based algorithm classification of standard Pap specimen that reviews the number of abnormal cells per slide

  ▹ Increased sensitivity (picks up more abnormals) and specificity (decreases the number of false positives)

▶ Bethesda Pap Smear Grading System: Last revised in 2001; very comprehensive

   ▸ Specimen adequacy

      ▷ Satisfactory for evaluation

      ▷ Presence or absence of endocervical or transformation zone components or other quality indicators such as partially obscuring blood or inflammation

      ▷ Unsatisfactory for evaluation (specify reason)

      ▷ Specimen rejected or not processed (specify reason)

      ▷ Specimen processed and examined, but unsatisfactory for evaluation of epithelial abnormalities (specify reason)

   ▸ General categorization: Optional

      ▷ Negative for intraepithelial lesion or malignancy

      ▷ Epithelial cell abnormality

      ▷ Other

   ▸ Interpretation or result

      ▷ Negative for intraepithelial lesion or malignancy

      ▷ Organisms

         ▷ *Trichomonas vaginalis*

         ▷ Fungal organisms morphologically consistent with *Candida* species

         ▷ Shift in flora suggestive of bacterial vaginosis

         ▷ Bacteria morphologically consistent with *Actinomyces* species

         ▷ Cellular changes consistent with herpes simplex virus

      ▷ Other nonneoplastic findings (optional to report)

      ▷ Reactive cellular changes associated with:

         ▷ Inflammation (includes typical repair)

         ▷ Radiation

         ▷ Intrauterine contraceptive device

      ▷ Glandular cells status post hysterectomy

      ▷ Atrophy

      ▷ Epithelial cell abnormalities

      ▷ Squamous cell

      ▷ Atypical squamous cells (ASC)

      ▷ ASC of undetermined significance (ASC-US)

      ▷ ASC; cannot exclude high-grade squamous intra-epithelial lesion (ASC-H)

      ▷ Low-grade squamous intra-epithelial lesion (LSIL) encompassing HPV, mild dysplasia, CIN 1

      ▷ High-grade squamous intra-epithelial lesion (HSIL) encompassing moderate and severe dysplasia, CIS/CIN 2, and CIN 3 with features suspicious for invasion

      ▷ Squamous cell carcinoma

▷ Atypical glandular cell:

▷ Endocervical, endometrial, or glandular cells (not otherwise specified [NOS] or specified in comments)

▷ Atypical glandular cell (NOS or specified in comments) favor neoplastic

▷ Endocervical adenocarcinoma in situ (AIS)

▷ Adenocarcinoma

▷ Endocervical

▷ Endometrial cells in a woman 40 years or older

▷ Extrauterine

▷ NOS

▷ Other malignant neoplasms (list not comprehensive)

▷ Automated review and ancillary testing (include if appropriate)

▷ Educational notes and suggestions (optional)

Management

Nonpharmacologic Treatment

▶ Benign with inflammation: Follow up in 3 months.

▶ Cryotherapy (freezing) or cauterization: Appropriate for noninvasive small lesions without endocervical extension

▶ Laser excision: Appropriate for large, visible lesions

▶ Loop Electrosurgical Excision Procedure (LEEP): Appropriate when CIN is clearly visible

▶ Cone biopsy (conization) for higher grade or invasive lesions

▶ Hysterectomy, radiation, or chemotherapy is not indicated unless invasion is suspected.

Special Considerations

▶ Pap screening has a very poor positive predictive value for abnormal vaginal cytology. Vaginal cancers are only 1%–4% of gynecologic malignancies.

▶ Women who have had a hysterectomy (due to other than malignant causes) in which the cervix was removed do not require cytologic screening (< 10% yield on vaginal cuff smears), but should continue to have vaginal inspection annually.

▶ Annual cytology advised if hysterectomy done to treat cervical dysplasia, cervical cancer, uterine cancer

▶ A hysterectomy may *not* remove the cervix. It is important to visualize the vagina and assess for the presence of a cervix.

▶ If a woman happens to have 2 cervices, be sure to collect a Pap on each one and to label the Paps appropriately (e.g., right cervix or right Pap).

▶ Pregnancy changes mimic dysplasia and are sometimes indistinguishable from true neoplasia; 75% of "abnormals" may regress within 6 months after the pregnancy ends. Confer with or refer to obstetrician or pregnancy specialist for abnormal cytology management in pregnancy. Be sure to obtain follow-up Pap smears during the postpartum period.

▶ In women at high risk for endometrial hyperplasia (postmenopausal, chronic anovulation), if endometrial cells are noted on the Pap (even without atypia), refer for endometrial sampling.

▶ Clinical tip: Postmenopausal women with one or more unsatisfactory Pap smears due to atrophy should use topical estrogen cream for 4–6 weeks, then repeat the Pap after more than 1 week without treatment.

When to Consult, Refer, Hospitalize

▶ Refer to gynecologist when signs or symptoms of cervical cancer.

» Abnormal bleeding (either metrorrhagia or postcoital spotting)

» Visible ulcer or mass on cervix, regardless of the Pap result

» Late signs: Anemia, anorexia, urinary frequency, hematuria, weight loss, pelvic or epigastric pain

» Late complications: Vaginal fistulas, urinary and fecal incontinence, back pain, leg edema, ureteral obstruction, eventually renal failure

▶ ⅔ of deaths from cervical cancer are from the uremia; another 10%–20% die from hemorrhage.

▶ Refer to gynecologist for abnormal Pap smear results.

Follow-up

▶ After ablative treatment, screening cytology should be repeated at accelerated intervals; commonly every 3–4 months for the first year, then every 6 months for the next year, then annually once a pattern of normal readings has been established.

▶ Any recurrent abnormals need colposcopic follow-up, repeat endocervical curettage, and biopsy.

Expected Course

▶ With appropriate management, future cancer risk is less than 5%. Many clinicians use automated cytology procedures if the patient has had therapy.

▶ Most treatment failures show up within 1–2 years postprocedure.

▶ If undetected or untreated, 15%–20% of untreated cervical lesions progress while the rest either stay stable or regress; up to 10 years from precancerous changes to invasive disease

Complications

▶ After invasion, death usually occurs in 3–5 years without treatment, or in unresponsive cancers.

▶ Invasion moves from the cervix to the uterus, the pelvis, internal lymphs, ureters, bladder, and rectum.

ATROPHIC VAGINITIS

Description
▶ Thinning fragility of vaginal and vulvar epithelium

Etiology
▶ Estrogen deficiency (estradiol levels less than 20 pg/mL); most common in menopausal and postmenopausal women

▶ Estrogen, along with glycogen, maintains a healthy pH of the vaginal environment between 3.8 and 4.2; estrogen deficiency causes an increased pH, disrupting the normal ecosystem.

▶ Estrogen deficiency also causes thinning and dryness of vaginal epithelium with loss of natural folds (rugae) in vaginal wall, predisposing the vagina to overgrowth of colonizing organisms or invasion of pathogens; vagina becomes friable, prone to inflammation.

Incidence and Demographics
▶ 40% of postmenopausal women not on HRT

▶ Premenopausal women with low estrogen levels

Risk Factors
▶ Menopause, either natural or surgical, leading to a decline in endogenous estrogen

▶ Antibiotic use and anti-estrogenic medications

▶ Stress and conditions suppressing immune function (e.g., diabetes mellitus and HIV)

▶ Lactation: Prolactin, antiestrogenic effects; women who are breastfeeding may be unaware of the possibility of atrophic vaginitis.

Prevention and Screening
▶ All perimenopausal and postmenopausal women should be asked about signs and symptoms during their annual exams.

Assessment

History
▶ Complaints include vaginal itching, thin watery discharge or discomfort with coitus, reduced libido, urinary urgency, dysuria; may be asymptomatic

▶ Obtain history of menopause, use of HRT, vaginal therapies, coital lubricants, UTI history, diabetes

Physical Exam
▶ Exam: Vagina is lighter pink to pallor, fewer rugae, smaller labia, dry to little discharge, overall decreased vaginal moisture, loss of elasticity or turgor of skin and vaginal epithelium.

► Elevated vaginal pH level > 5 ranging pH 5.5–7 (a rise over premenopausal levels of approximately 4.0)

Diagnostic Studies

► Pap, wet prep, maturational index: More parabasal cells and fewer intermediate and superficial cells (changes consistent with reduced estrogen)

► Abnormal amount of WBCs (greater than 10 per high power field [HPF]) on wet prep

► Any vaginal specimen with blood should prompt a work-up for cervical or uterine bleeding sources; there should be minimal trauma during the examination to create vaginal bleeding (except the use of a cytobrush, which often causes slight spotting).

► Urinalysis negative

Differential Diagnosis

► Infectious vaginitis (trichomoniasis, candidiasis)

► Bacterial vaginosis

► Vulvar or vaginal cancer

► Diabetes mellitus

► Trauma or foreign body

► Contact irritation

Management

Nonpharmacologic Treatment

► Use of vaginal water-based lubricants and moisturizers for coitus and general comfort

Pharmacologic Treatment

► Estrogen replacement therapy unless otherwise contraindicated: Intravaginal cream, oral estradiol (Vagifem) 25 mcg estradiol twice a week; transdermal, pessaries; estradiol-impregnated vaginal ring (Estring) delivers 6–9 mcg estradiol daily for 3 months)

► See Menopause entry for oral and transdermal regimens (in lactating women, use topical first because oral and transdermal routes may decrease milk supply).

► Topical regimen is conjugated estrogen cream (Premarin) 2–4 g intravaginally q.d. in cycles of 3 weeks on, 1 week off; maintenance dose is once a week.

How Long to Treat

► Indefinitely as needed

Special Considerations

► Postmenopausal women not on HRT should also be evaluated for other complications from estrogen deficiency.

When to Consult, Refer, Hospitalize

▶ If signs and symptoms do not resolve with treatment, refer for biopsy.

Follow-up

▶ Reevaluate in 1–2 months after treatment to assess for side effects and treatment response.

▶ Reevaluate breastfeeding women after weaning.

Expected Course

▶ Resolves with ongoing or periodic treatment; typically takes 4–6 weeks for symptoms to resolve

Complications

▶ Superimposed infection

BARTHOLIN GLAND CYSTS AND ABSCESSES

Description

▶ Obstruction of a Bartholin gland (greater vestibular gland) causing simple cyst, or possible inflammation and infection; causing pain, swelling, and abscess formation

Etiology

▶ Obstruction of duct with retained mucus, causing simple cyst; contributing factors include trauma, infection, epithelial hyperplasia, congenital atresia

▶ Infection usually polymicrobial

▶ Most cysts remain minimally symptomatic < 4 cm

▶ Infected cysts contain mixed vaginal flora, *N. gonorrhoeae, C. trachomatis, E. coli*; become enlarged, acutely painful

▶ Can result in chronic ductal stenosis and residual distension; frequently recurrent

Incidence and Demographics

▶ Most common vulvar mass

▶ Usually presents ages 20–29

▶ Rare after age 40; presence at that age suspicious for malignancy and requires biopsy, complete excision, or both

Risk Factors

▶ History of gonorrhea or chlamydia, at risk for STIs

▶ Scratching and shaving perineal area

Prevention and Screening

▶ Prevention of STIs

Assessment

History

▶ Previous episodes; prior surgical treatment (incision and drainage, marsupialization, Word catheter placement), STIs; localized edema; erythema and pain of the labia; history of vulvar abrasion, injury, or trauma

▶ Symptoms are pain on sides of introitus, dyspareunia, painful sitting or walking

Physical Exam

▶ Physical exam may show swelling on sides of the introitus, fluctuant mass at 4 o'clock or 8 o'clock or both, but usually unilateral; if active infection, there may be redness, tenderness, edema—size can vary up to 4 cm.

Diagnostic Studies

▶ If drainage present or if incision and drainage performed, wound cultures, perform tests for gonorrhea, chlamydia

▶ Consider cervical testing for gonorrhea and chlamydia.

Differential Diagnosis

▶ Inclusion cysts

▶ Lipoma

▶ Fibroma

▶ Hematoma

▶ Bartholin gland cancer (rare)

Management

Nonpharmacologic Treatment

▶ Warm soaks and sitz baths can alleviate pain, promote spontaneous ductal opening.

▶ Cyst needs no treatment if not symptomatic.

▶ Treatment of large, painful cyst is to perform incision and drainage.

▶ Word catheter can be inserted at time of incision and drainage; it can be sutured or taped into place and is allowed to drain for 2–4 weeks.

Pharmacologic Treatment

▶ Antibiotic treatment for both aerobic and anaerobic bacteria coverage (e.g., ceftriaxone [Rocephin] 125 mg IM one dose plus clindamycin [Cleocin] 300 mg p.o. q.i.d. for 7 days to cover skin bacterial flora, anaerobic bacteria, and possibly gonorrhea); may also need to add metronidazole (Flagyl) 500 mg b.i.d. for 7 days for treatment of trichomonas infection

Special Considerations

▶ For women over 40 or postmenopausal, complex excision under general anesthesia is warranted to rule out carcinoma.

When to Consult, Refer, Hospitalize

▶ Refer as needed for symptomatic or infected cyst that requires incision and drainage or other procedure.

▶ For recurrent cyst, refer for excision of cyst and marsupialization to establish new ductal opening; laser incision can also be used.

▶ Incision and drainage and placement of Word catheters is not a beginner skill. Patients should be referred to either the collaborating physician or a gynecologist.

Follow-up

▶ If incision and drainage are done, follow up in 10 days; if Word catheter inserted, follow up in 4 weeks.

Expected Course

▶ Abscesses often recur after incision and drainage.

Complications

▶ Recurrent abscess

▶ Labial abscesses that start initially as a papule and rapidly expand into a large abscess over 24 hours are highly suggestive of MRSA (methicillin resistant staphylococcus aureus) and require immediate antibiotic coverage and incision and drainage.

BACTERIAL VAGINOSIS

Description

▶ A clinical syndrome caused by replacement of vaginal hydrogen peroxide-producing *Lactobacillus* species by a variety of anaerobic bacteria such as *Gardnerella vaginalis* and *Mycoplasma hominis*; not considered an STI

Etiology

▶ Cause not clearly known, but symptoms caused by an overgrowth of one or more anaerobic bacteria (e.g., *Prevotella* sp., *Mobiluncus* sp., *Gardnerella vaginalis*, *Mycoplasma hominis*, replacing normal flora *Lactobacillus* spp.)

▶ Primarily occurs in sexually active adolescents and adult women; not considered an STI, but is a sexually associated infection

▶ Women who have never been sexually active rarely affected

Incidence and Demographics

▶ *Gardnerella vaginalis* is predominant organism.

▶ The most prevalent vaginitis (symptomatic) in sexually active adolescents, adults

Risk Factors

▶ Sexual activity, increasing with multiple partners and new sex partner

▶ Co-infection with STI

▶ Douching

▶ More common among Black women

▶ IUD use

Prevention and Screening

▶ Wear all-cotton underwear and loose clothes.

▶ Avoid douching or use of tampons to decrease bacteria overgrowth.

▶ Advise use of condoms.

Assessment

History

▶ Malodorous (fishy odor) vaginal discharge, primarily following coitus or before menstruation

▶ Itching and burning usually not present unless co-infection with another pathogen

▶ May report vaginal irritation secondary to presence of discharge

Physical Exam

▶ Introitus, presence of homogenous discharge

▶ Speculum exam, presence of homogenous discharges coating vaginal walls and foul (fishy) odor

▶ Cervix bimanual exam is normal: Cervix without inflammation, discharge, or CMT

Diagnostic Studies

▶ Amsel's clinical criteria positive for diagnosis (must have 3 criteria):

   » Thin, white-gray, homogeneous vaginal discharge adherent to vaginal wall

   » Vaginal pH > 4.5

   » Positive potassium hydroxide (KOH) "whiff" test: Fishy odor when 10% KOH applied to discharge

   » Characteristic clue cells on microscopic exam

Differential Diagnosis

▶ *Trichomonas* vaginitis

▶ Cervicitis caused by chlamydia or gonorrhea

▶ Vulvovaginal candidiasis

Management

▶ Only women with symptomatic disease need treatment.

▶ Intravaginal route may be preferred due to decrease in systemic side effects.

▶ Treatment of men not needed because it has not been shown that treatment alters course or relapse or re-infection rate.

Nonpharmacologic Treatment

▶ Abstain from sexual intercourse during pharmacologic treatment.

▶ Avoid alcohol or any alcohol-containing products while taking metronidazole; interaction produces a disulfiram-like reaction that is very profound.

Pharmacologic Treatment

▶ Metronidazole (Flagyl) 500 mg orally b.i.d. × 7 days, *or*

▶ Metronidazole gel 0.75%, one applicator (5 g) intravaginally h.s. × 5 days, *or*

▶ Clindamycin cream (Cleocin) 2%, on applicator (5 g) intravaginally h.s. × 7 days

▶ Clindamycin 300 mg p.o. b.i.d. × 7 days

Special Considerations

▶ Intravaginal treatment preferred for lactating women

▶ Treatment of high-risk pregnant women (previous premature delivery) who are asymptomatic might reduce premature delivery; screening and treatment suggested early in second trimester

▶ Low-risk pregnant women who have symptomatic bacterial vaginosis should be treated; use lower doses to minimize exposure to fetus.

▶ Clindamycin vaginal gel not recommended during pregnancy; use associated with increase in premature deliveries

▶ Patients allergic to metronidazole should not be given vaginal gel.

▶ Recent meta-analysis of metronidazole does not indicate teratogenicity in humans.

▶ Pregnant women: For high- or low-risk, metronidazole 500 mg p.o. b.i.d. for 7 days, or 250 mg p.o. t.i.d. × 7 days, or clindamycin 300 mg p.o. b.i.d. for 7 days; clindamycin topical should not be used in the 2nd half of pregnancy

When to Consult, Refer, Hospitalize

▶ Consult for recurrent or refractory infection

Follow-up

▶ None needed except for pregnant women, 1 month following treatment

Expected Course

▶ Most respond promptly

Complications

▶ Abnormal vaginal discharge, mucopurulent cervicitis, urinary tract infections, postoperative infections, cervical dysplasia, nonpuerperal endometritis, bacterial vaginosis–related PID

▶ Obstetric: Chorioamnionitis, premature labor, premature rupture of membranes, postpartum endometritis

VAGINAL CANDIDIASIS

Description

▶ Vaginitis caused by the *Candida* species not considered to be a sexually transmitted infection

▶ Also known as moniliasis or vaginal yeast

Etiology

▶ A dimorphic fungi existing as either oval, budding yeast cells, or chains of cells (hyphae)

▶ Normal flora in the vagina and skin

▶ Symptomatic infection typically occuring when the vaginal environment is disturbed, resulting in fungal overgrowth

Incidence and Demographics

▶ About 75% of all women will have at least one episode.

▶ Second most common cause of vaginitis (after bacterial vaginosis); 25% of all vaginal infections

▶ Majority caused by *Candida albicans* (75%–85%) with *C. glabrata C. tropicalis* responsible for remaining

▶ *C. glabrata* and *tropicalis* increasing in prevalence; more often causing recurrent infections

Risk Factors

▶ Antibiotic, corticosteroid, or anti-estrogen medications

▶ Sexual intercourse, oral-vaginal sex, anal-vaginal sex, contraceptives, pregnancy

▶ Douching, tight-fitting undergarments, obesity

▶ Stress, immunosuppressive disorders (e.g., HIV), diabetes mellitus

Prevention and Screening

- ▶ Advise all women of possibility of candidiasis with antibiotic, corticosteroid, and anti-estrogen use.
- ▶ Advise against douching.

Assessment

History

- ▶ Thick, white, nonodorous, cheesy vaginal discharge with or without pruritus
- ▶ Pruritus may be only symptom without discharge
- ▶ Soreness with coitus (dyspareunia); may also be the only symptom
- ▶ Obtain medication history, including recent use of over-the-counter antifungals, vaginal hygiene habits

Physical Exam

- ▶ Varying amounts of thick, white discharge without odor
- ▶ Discharge adherent to vaginal walls
- ▶ Discharge may be scant but vulvar erythema and edema present with excoriations, sometimes severe enough to preclude adequate speculum exam

Diagnostic Studies

- ▶ Litmus paper for pH: Normal pH 4.0–4.5
- ▶ Wet prep: Pseudohyphae may be present on normal saline slide; KOH slide demonstrates fungal hyphae, maybe spores.
- ▶ STI screen as appropriate
- ▶ Fungal cultures only necessary for recurrent episodes
- ▶ HbA1C to evaluate for diabetes mellitus

Differential Diagnosis

- ▶ Bacterial vaginosis
- ▶ Trichomonas
- ▶ Atrophic vaginitis
- ▶ Chlamydia or gonorrhea

Management

- ▶ Pharmacologic treatment required only if symptomatic
- ▶ May presumptively treat (wet mount not very sensitive) if sole complaint is pruritus

Nonpharmacologic Treatment

- ▶ Proper perineal hygiene
- ▶ Wear looser-fitting undergarments (preferably cotton), especially in the summer.
- ▶ Avoid alcohol and large amounts of concentrated sugars.

► Oatmeal baths may reduce itching.

► Sexual hygiene

Pharmacologic Treatment

► Fluconazole (Diflucan) 150 mg p.o., 1 tablet, singe dose

► Clotrimazole 1%, 5 g intravaginally h.s. × 7–14 days

► Miconazole 2% cream, 5 g intravaginally h.s. × 7 days

► Terconazole 0.4% cream, 5 g intravaginally h.s. × 7 days

► Butoconazole 2% cream, 5 g intravaginally h.s. × 3 days

► Many of the above creams can be also given as a 1-, 3-, 10-, or 14-day treatment; also available in suppository form.

► Clotrimazole, miconazole, and butoconazole available over the counter, duration of treatment as per package instructions

Special Considerations

► 7-day treatment recommended for pregnant women with history of recent candidiasis

► Pregnant women should not use fluconazole.

► For acutely symptomatic women, creams and suppositories yield quicker relief than oral fluconazole.

► Test for diabetes mellitus for persistent or recurrent infection.

When to Consult, Refer, Hospitalize

► Refer to gynecologist for persistent or recurrent infection.

Follow-up

► Only indicated if signs and symptoms fail to resolve within 2 weeks or recur

Expected Course

► Usually resolves without problem

Complications

► Refractory candidiasis

ABNORMAL GROWTHS OF UTERUS AND OVARIES

LEIOMYOMAS

Description

- ▶ Uterine fibroids, myomas, fibroid "tumors"
- ▶ Benign uterine smooth muscle connective tissue growth, responsive to estrogens
- ▶ Discrete, firm, roundish, often multiple in various anatomic locations — intramural, submucous, subserous, intraligamentous, pedunculated, and cervical
- ▶ Mostly asymptomatic and found incidentally on examination

Etiology

- ▶ Benign tumors represent localized proliferation of smooth muscle cells surrounded by a pseudocapsule of compressed muscle fibers; etiology unknown.

Incidence and Demographics

- ▶ Occurs in 4%–11% of women; increases with age (20% of women over 35 and 40% of women over 50)

Risk Factors

- ▶ Nulliparity
- ▶ Obesity
- ▶ Black

Assessment

History

- ▶ Occasionally causes menorrhagia (with degeneration calcification), dysmenorrhea, pelvic pain, bladder pressure, back pain (enlargement encroaches on adjacent structures, possible torsion), increasing pain in pregnancy, pregnancy losses (cavity distortion)

Physical Exam

- ▶ Enlarged, firm, irregular uterus; mobile; mostly nontender; and negative other exam findings; clinically useful to document size of uterus comparable to gestational size ("10–12 weeks' size"; "umbilicus minus 1 cm") for comparative evaluation over time

Diagnostic Studies

- ▶ Labs: hCG, CBC (iron deficiency anemia), screening Paps, and other health maintenance as indicated
- ▶ Transvaginal ultrasonography can identify characteristic fibroid changes (hypoechoic, no cysts, uniform structure), map number, location, measure size, assess normalcy of adjacent structures (endometrial thickness); helpful to rule out other concerns (ovarian cysts).

▶ Sonohysterogram to locate intramural lesions

▶ MRI to visualize individual myomas

▶ Hysterosalpingography to define extent of submucuous myomas before surgery or to evaluate uterine cavity and patency of fallopian tubes

Differential Diagnosis

▶ Pregnancy

▶ Endometriosis

▶ Endometrial carcinoma

▶ Ovarian cysts

▶ Uterine cancer

▶ Abnormal vaginal bleeding

▶ Adenomyosis

▶ Cervical cancer

▶ Ovarian cancer

▶ Leiomyosarcoma (0.5% of fibroids; very rare under age 40)

Management

Nonpharmacologic Treatment

▶ Heat, rest, regular complete voiding if causing pressure on bladder

Pharmacologic Treatment

▶ No treatment needed if asymptomatic

▶ Iron replacement therapy if needed; hormonal contraception may reduce bleeding but unclear if reduces fibroid size — may increase size in some

▶ NSAIDs work well for chronic pain.

▶ Analgesics with narcotics only if unremitting pain; needs gynecologic consultation

▶ Reduce size medically using GnRH-agonists such as leuprolide (Lupron) 3.75 mg IM monthly or 11.25 mg IM every 3 months, or Depo-Provera; then surgical treatment may be indicated.

Special Considerations

▶ Patients may become pregnant in the presence of a leiomyoma.

▶ Pregnancy in conjunction with leiomyoma is usually unremarkable with a normal antepartum course, labor, and delivery. These patients need careful surveillance.

▶ The risk of spontaneous abortion or preterm labor following myomectomy is high. Use of prophylactic β-adrenergic tocolytics is sometimes indicated.

▶ Vaginal birth after myomectomy is controversial.

When to Consult, Refer, Hospitalize

▶ Fertility concerns should be referred to a gynecologist for management.

▶ Consult with gynecology about options to reduce bleeding (lepride, surgical excision, myomectomy embolization therapy, hysterectomy) or if endometrial sampling is indicated.

Follow-up

▶ When symptomatic and at yearly exam

▶ Should monitor growth with transvaginal or pelvic ultrasound every 6 months until stable

Expected Course

▶ Reduces in size, symptoms after pregnancy and menopause

Complications

▶ Urinary incontinence, pregnancy loss, anemia

BENIGN OVARIAN GROWTHS

Description

▶ Functional cysts (corpus luteum cysts, theca lutein cysts) and follicular cysts produce hormones.

▶ Very common in adolescents, may have PMS-type prodrome, delayed menses until resolved

▶ Dermoid cysts (benign teratoma) are growths from germ cells; surgical excision prevents rare cancerous changes.

Etiology

▶ Can occur when ovarian follicle enlarges and does not rupture or when the corpus luteum does not regress in the absence of pregnancy

▶ Theca lutein cysts may develop with high levels of hCG or with ovulation induction.

▶ May grow as large as 10–15 cm but rarely larger than 6–8 cm

Incidence and Demographics

▶ 70% of ovarian masses are functional.

Risk Factors

▶ 3-fold increase in risk for smokers

▶ Recent obesity and obesity at age 20

▶ Oral contraceptives and term pregnancies tend to be protective (but benign growths still occasionally occur).

Prevention and Screening

▶ Screening only necessary if undergoing ovulation induction

Assessment

History

▶ Discomfort with or without menstrual cycle alterations; may be incidental to visit

  ▹ Functional or follicular cysts often have hormonal effects.

  ▹ May be bloating, dyspareunia, chronic lower abdominal pain and pressure, menstrual irregularities

  ▹ Always ask about LMP.

Physical Exam

▶ Exam is often unremarkable if growth small; may note unilateral or bilateral adnexal mass; tenderness may be elicited.

Diagnostic Studies

▶ hCG: Rule out ectopic pregnancy; other tests as indicated by history and physical exam.

▶ Transvaginal or pelvic ultrasound: Fluid component, hypoechogenic, single cyst or simple septated area, no free fluid in cul-de-sac

Differential Diagnosis

▶ Ovarian cancer

▶ Pregnancy

▶ Endometrioma

▶ Leiomyoma

▶ Urinary tract disorder

▶ Bowel disorder

▶ PID

▶ STI

▶ Ectopic gestation

▶ PCOS

Management

Nonpharmacologic Treatment

▶ Between menarche and menopause, an asymptomatic, mobile, lateral simple cystic mass less than 5–6 cm confirmed by sonography can be observed; spontaneous resolution is expected. Most functional cysts or follicular cysts will regress or resorb without intervention.

▶ Surgical evaluation should occur for masses that persist > 6 weeks, enlarge, or are > 10 cm for dermoid cysts.

Pharmacologic Treatment

▶ Oral contraceptives may be used to assist regression of functional and follicular cysts.

▶ Manage pain with NSAIDs or other analgesia.

Special Considerations

▶ Some may rupture, causing acute pain.

When to Consult, Refer, Hospitalize

▶ Refer to gynecologist if markedly tender, > 6 cm, increases in size, or persists beyond 6 weeks.

Follow-up

▶ Reevaluate size with ultrasound in 4–6 weeks.

Complications

▶ Usually none

POLYCYSTIC OVARY SYNDROME (PCOS), POLYCYSTIC OVARIAN DISEASE (PCOD), STEIN-LEVENTHAL SYNDROME

Description

▶ Classical presentation of hyperandrogenism (obesity, hirsutism, acne), menstrual irregularities (oligomenorrhea since menarche, amenorrhea, erratic menorrhagia, or metrorrhagia), erratic fertility patterns or infertile, insulin resistance, and hyperinsulinemia

▶ Polycystic ovaries are the end point of the process, not the diagnostic focal point.

Etiology

▶ PCOS is a result of a complex disruption of the hypothalamic-pituitary-ovarian axis and ovarian function, characterized by higher tonic levels of LH and low or low-normal FSH levels.

▶ Familial pattern (autosomal dominant)

Incidence and Demographics

▶ Commonly begins in adolescence (postmenarche)

Risk Factors

▶ Familial: Genetic component

▶ Weight gain with android pattern obesity

Prevention and Screening

▶ No prevention identified; no routine screening

Assessment

History

▶ History of oligomenorrhea, amenorrhea, erratic vaginal bleeding, infertility

▶ Cosmetically disturbing hirsutism; male pattern hair growth, hair thinning or loss, acne, and voice changes

▶ History of gestational diabetes mellitus or hypertension, overweight and weight gain, family history of diabetes mellitus

Physical Exam

▶ Central obesity common, although some are normal weight

▶ May be adnexal mass

▶ *Acanthosis nigricans*, acne, hirsutism, balding, skin tags, increased BMI, clitoromegaly, thyroid enlargement

Diagnostic Studies

▶ Urine hCG or serum β-hCG to rule out pregnancy

▶ TSH, free T4, 17-hydroxyprogesterone, serum total testosterone (elevated), DHEAS (elevated), prolactin (to rule out pituitary tumor), fasting lipids, glucose, and 2-hour GTT after 75-g load

▶ Overnight dexamethasone suppression test

▶ Transvaginal ultrasound shows antral follicles on a single ovary or ovarian volume > 10 cm^3.

▶ MRI is *not* diagnostic; CT and ultrasound may assist in diagnostic process, but are not truly diagnostic alone.

▶ Consider endometrial biopsy when prolonged erratic bleeding to rule out endometrial cancer.

Differential Diagnosis

▶ Adrenal: Tumor, Cushing's, adult-onset adrenal hyperplasia

▶ Hairan syndrome (hyperandrogenism, insulin resistance, acanthosis nigrans)

▶ Ovarian: Tumor, ovarian insensitivity syndrome

▶ Hepatic disease (alters estrogen clearance metabolism)

▶ Thyroid disease (may affect feedback loops)

▶ Prolactinoma

Management

Nonpharmacologic Treatment

▶ Exercise and weight loss: Goal of body mass index < 27

▶ Exercise and weight loss will improve lipid profile, reduce hyperinsulinemia (insulin resistance uncommon with low BMI), improve fertility, improve menstrual cycles, reduce hirsutism

▶ Occasionally, ovarian wedge resection needed

Pharmacologic Treatment

▶ Treatment with oral contraceptives or progestin can minimize menstrual irregularities and decrease risks of endometrial cancer; cycling will occur (reduce endometrial danger), may protect lipids, will not increase glucose

▶ Control of lipids, blood glucose, and hypertension

▶ Bromocriptine (Parlodel) if high prolactin

▶ Metformin (glucophage) improves insulin sensitivity, lowers LH, lowers androgen, improves fertility

Special Considerations

▶ Androgen-excess–related insulin resistance (reduced glucose response to insulin amount or "syndrome X/metabolic syndrome"), which spurs hyperinsulinemia (ratio of fasting glucose to fasting insulin levels less than 3.0), increased risk of diabetes mellitus

▶ Also associated with hypertension, coronary artery disease, increased triglycerides, and decreased HDL levels

When to Consult, Refer, Hospitalize

▶ Consult with gynecologist for fertility issues and treatment with clomiphene (Clomid) to induce ovulation; anti-androgen or other hormonal therapy.

▶ Consult with endocrinologist for obesity, insulin resistance, lipid issues.

Follow-up

▶ Close for screening of excessive endometrial buildup, breast cancer

▶ Lipids, oral glucose tolerance testing at regular intervals

Complications

▶ Osteoporosis risk

▶ Endometrial hyperplasia or carcinoma

▶ Has been associated with failure of lactogenesis II and low milk supply

OTHER CONDITIONS

PELVIC INFLAMMATORY DISEASE (PID)

Description

▶ Ascending infection and inflammation within the upper genital tract in women

Etiology

▶ PID has a polymicrobial etiology with the most common pathogens being *Neisseria gonorrhoeae, Chlamydia trachomatis* in acute PID; mixed with anaerobes, *Bacteroides* spp., staphylococci, streptococci, *Enterobacter* spp., *Haemophilus influenzae*, and others.

▶ Part of an ascending continuum of cervicitis, endometritis, salpingitis, and finally pelvic peritonitis

Incidence and Demographics

▶ Most prevalent at ages 16–25, matching incidence in STI trends

▶ > 100,000 women become infertile each year due to PID.

▶ 1 million women experience an episode of acute PID.

▶ PID is uncommon in pregnancy.

Risk Factors

▶ Sexually active with multiple partners, change in partner within past year

▶ Infected partner, history of or concurrent STI, prior history of PID

▶ IUD, genital surgical instrumentation (D&C, induced abortion)

▶ Lack of condom use

Prevention and Screening

▶ May do STI screen for women with a new sexual partner, especially if < 25 years of age

Assessment

History

▶ Sexual partner practice, history; history of STIs; prior PID; contraception; gynecologic procedures; and vaginal douching

▶ Presentation may be mild or subclinical in nature, which should increase suspicion.

▶ Speed of symptomatology is dependent on the infectious organisms involved.

▶ Mild to moderate: Mid-abdominal pain may be first, with dyspareunia and unusual vaginal discharge; may have some mid-cycle spotting; usually no anorexia. Pain worsens with menses.

▶ Severe: Increasing bilateral pain, fever, and nausea with occasional vomiting as the infection worsens and progresses beyond the salpinges and into the abdominal cavity

▶ Fitz-Hugh-Curtis syndrome: Perihepatitis including fever, chills, and pleuritic right upper quadrant pain; accounts for about 5% of PID

Physical Exam

▶ Classic triad of lower abdominal pain, adnexal tenderness (unilateral or bilateral), cervical motion tenderness; only ⅓ have fever > 101° F

▶ Direct abdominal tenderness (with or without rebound)

▶ Cervix: Cervicitis (edema friability); note blood, ulcerations, nodules

▶ Vaginal discharge may or may not be present, may be mucopurulent.

▶ Mild to moderate uterine tenderness

▶ Adnexal masses may or may not be palpable; consider tubo-ovarian abscess (TOA).

▶ Adnexal tenderness

▶ Pain response to cervical motion may be acute, startling ("chandelier sign").

▶ Enlarged, tender inguinal lymph nodes are often a sign of an STI or a pelvic infection. Diffuse, systemic adenopathy with flu-like symptoms: Consider possibility of primary HIV infection.

Diagnostic Studies

▶ Diagnosis chiefly based on history and physical and less on labs, except for etiologic agent identification

▶ Urine hCG, gonorrhea and chlamydia testing

▶ If lesions noted, assess for herpes, syphilis.

▶ Counsel and recommend HIV screening.

▶ Consider cervical cytology screening after the acute infection phase is passed to minimize confounding changes affecting cytologic accuracy.

▶ ESR nonspecific and not reliable; WBCs not reliable

▶ Vaginal wet preps should have > 10 WBC/HPF; look for trichomonads, which can confound the work-up; confirm sexual transmission, or bacterial vaginosis, which can be an associated condition.

▶ Transvaginal or pelvic ultrasound can rule out pregnancy (ectopic) and identify tubal masses or ovarian abscess.

Differential Diagnosis

▶ Appendicitis

▶ Ectopic gestation

▶ Endometriosis

▶ Ovarian cyst (ruptured)

▶ Leiomyoma

▶ Acute enteritis

▶ Severe UTI or pyelonephritis

▶ Colitis

▶ Renal calculi

Management

Nonpharmacologic Treatment

▶ Counsel on safer sex measures.

Pharmacologic Treatment

▶ 2010 CDC criteria for empiric treatment can be based on finding classic triad; urgent treatment is preferred even without specific lab results rather than risk a lifetime of chronic pelvic pain, scarring, infertility.

▶ Outpatient treatment is best with a multiple drug regimen that covers several pathogens, including *N. gonorrhoeae*, chlamydia:

- Ceftriaxone (Rocephin) 250 mg IM once and doxycycline 100 mg p.o. b.i.d. × 14 days. Consider adding metronidazole (Flagyl) 500 mg p.o. b.i.d. × 14 days or clindamycin 300 mg p.o. b.i.d. × 14 days to cover anaerobes.

- » Concurrent treatment of all sexual partners (and the partners' sexual partners) is highly advisable.
- » Patients who do not respond to oral therapy within 72 hours should be reevaluated to confirm the diagnosis and should be administered parenteral therapy on either an outpatient or inpatient basis.
- » See 2010 CDC guidelines for STI treatment for additional alternative treatment regimens.

How Long to Treat

- ▶ 14 days is standard regimen.

Special Considerations

- ▶ Quinolones should not be used in people with a history of recent foreign travel or partners' travel, infections acquired in California or Hawaii, or infections acquired in other areas with increased quinolone-resistant *Neisseria gonorrhoeaa* prevalence.
- ▶ Minimal signs or symptoms do not correlate with minimal tubal scarring or other adverse sequelae.
- ▶ Avoid alcohol or any alcohol-containing products while taking metronidazole; interaction produces a disulfiram-like reaction that is very profound.
- ▶ 20% of patients with PID do not have positive cervical cultures for gonorrhea or chlamydia.

When to Consult, Refer, Hospitalize

- ▶ Inpatient treatment is best for a very young or unreliable patient, pregnant patient, fever > 101° F, WBC > 11,000/mm³, evidence of peritonitis, suspected pelvic abscess, decreased bowel sounds, and anorexia; for a patient with escalating symptoms despite treatment; for nonresolving symptoms after 72 hours of treatment; or for severely immunocompromised patients.

Follow-up

- ▶ Close within 72 hours to assess treatment efficacy and compliance, again after treatment complete; if no improvement is noted, consider hospitalization
- ▶ Treat all sex partners empirically for both chlamydia and gonorrhea.

Expected Course

- ▶ Signs and symptoms of acute infection should resolve by completion of antibiotic treatment.

Complications

- ▶ If untreated, 15% develop tubo-ovarian abscesses (TOA) and many have chronic infection.
- ▶ After one episode, about 15% of women are infertile; rate doubles with each episode.
- ▶ 6- to 10-fold increase in risk for ectopic gestation following one episode
- ▶ May produce chronic pelvic pain, dyspareunia, adhesion formation, chronic pyosalpinx, or hydrosalpinx

CARE OF THE MATERNITY PATIENT

Preconception Counseling

▶ Offers the opportunity to discuss with the patient planning a future pregnancy her individualized risk factors, perform preconception genetic testing for conditions such as cystic fibrosis and Tay Sachs in specific populations, and teach the patient how to optimize her health and decrease risks in preparation for a healthy pregnancy

▶ To decrease the risks for neural tube defects, provide preconception supplementation with folate 400 mcg daily for all women who plan to become or are at risk for becoming pregnant. The U. S. Public Health Service and CDC recommend that *all women of childbearing age consume 0.4 mg (400 mcg) of folic acid daily* to prevent two common and serious birth defects: spina bifida and anencephaly.

▶ Encourage smoking cessation, limiting alcohol use, avoiding recreational drug use, minimizing use of OTC medications, and, in conjunction with the primary care provider, if possible, lowering prescribed medication dosages while still being therapeutic for the patient's needs.

Prenatal Care

The goal of prenatal care is to ensure the health of both mother and fetus.

▶ Assessment and care of the pregnant woman from conception throughout pregnancy until birth

▶ Prenatal care after conception should begin as soon as possible.

▶ Pregnancy outcome can be improved by early health intervention screening.

▶ U.S. Public Health Service advises intensive intervention in early pregnancy if there are identified risk factors that can be modified (e.g., smoking, poor nutrition, psychosocial disorders, diabetes, drug or alcohol abuse).

▶ Use a biopsychosocial approach with a family focus.

▶ Care during the prenatal period includes primary and secondary prevention.

▶ Health promotion should be emphasized.

▶ Childbirth and parenting education

▶ Adequate nutrition, smoking cessation, drug and alcohol avoidance, exercise

▶ Review of current medications, including over-the-counter drugs

▶ Review benefits of breastfeeding and the recommendation to breastfeed exclusively for the first 6 months and continue breastfeeding with the addition of solids for a minimum of 1 year

▶ Pregnant women should avoid cat-litter boxes and feces, eating uncooked meat (to avoid risk of toxoplasmosis), sushi (hepatitis A), and unpasteurized cheeses. Limit tuna, salmon, and other high-fat fishes to once a week (due to mercury contamination).

Prenatal Screening

▶ To identify the patient at risk for maternal-fetal conditions and complications that require monitoring or may be treatable; identify health status of mother and baby

▶ Estimating the gestational age as accurately as possible

▶ Evaluating the health status of mother and fetus

▶ Empowering and encouraging the patient to care for self and baby

▶ Universal testing for all patients includes Pap smear, urinalysis, urine culture, CBC, blood type, Rh antibody testing, STI screening, hepatitis B surface antigen (HBsAg), rubella immunity, and blood glucose.

▶ These tests are done as part of prenatal blood panel at initial visit, except for blood glucose, which is done at 24–28 weeks' gestation in low-risk patients.

▶ Group B β-hemolytic strep genital culture is done at 34–36 weeks' gestation.

▶ Hemoglobin should be checked again during the last trimester to rule out anemia.

▶ Patient is monitored for weight gain or loss, blood pressure, edema, uterine fundal growth, fetal growth, fetal heart tones, and fetal position.

▶ Consider TSH, antithyroperoxidase (TPO) antibodies for undiagnosed hypothyroidism.

FIRST PRENATAL VISIT

Assessment

History

▶ A complete medical, gynecologic, and psychosocial history, including domestic violence screening, should be obtained at the initial visit and updated throughout the pregnancy.

▶ Obstetrical and gynecologic history: Menstrual—age at menarche, cycle, LMP, contraception, pregnancies, deliveries, abortions, past pregnancy or delivery complication, newborn health and complications, STI history, sexual history, medical history, social history, breastfeeding intentions and history

Physical Exam

▶ Height, weight, blood pressure; screen urine for protein and glucose

▶ Complete physical exam: Check skin, hair, teeth, thyroid, lungs, heart, breasts, spine, abdomen, extremities (note varicosities, edema); check neuro (presence of clonus, tremors).

▶ Pelvic: Cervix (note color, position, status of os, lesions, discharge), vagina, uterus (note size, position, tenderness, shape), ovaries (palpable, size, tenderness)

▶ Assess fundal height in centimeters; size equals dates.

▶ Fetal heart rate if present

▶ Breasts should be evaluated for growth, nipple retraction or inversion, glandular tissue, elasticity of the areola, shape and symmetry in the first and last trimester. Poor growth, nipple retraction, insufficient glandular tissue, inelasticity of the areola, and marked asymmetry are lactation risk factors.

▶ Pelvic and cervical exam

Diagnostic Studies

▶ Frequently ordered as prenatal panel

- » CBC; hemoglobin electrophoresis to rule out sickle cell anemia in women of African descent
- » Blood type, Rh antibody screen
- » Serology: VDRL or RPR titers
- » Rubella titer
- » Hepatitis B screen
- » Urinalysis, urine culture
- » Pap smear
- » STI screening: Chlamydia, gonorrhea, herpes if indication, HIV
- » Cystic fibrosis screening (CDC, 2004)
- » Uterine and fetal ultrasound as indicated: To confirm presence of viable intrauterine pregnancy, evaluate a suspected ectopic or molar pregnancy, provide most accurate estimate of gestational age, assist with chorionic villus sampling, and evaluate for pelvic masses

Management

Nonpharmacologic Treatment

▶ Patient education as appropriate to stage of pregnancy, nutrition, exercise, psychosocial evaluation, smoking cessation

Pharmacologic Treatment

▶ Prenatal vitamin with folic acid 400 mcg daily until 3–4 months postpartum during breastfeeding

▶ Iron supplements (200–300 mg/day) for patients with iron deficiency anemia (Hgb < 11.0 g/dL)

When to Consult, Refer, Hospitalize

▶ Consult with physician for all high-risk patients for all abnormal findings during visits.

▶ Consult with lactation specialist for history of lactation failure or abnormal breast exam.

Follow-up

▶ Usual schedule of prenatal visits: Every 4 weeks until 28th week of gestation, then every 2 weeks until 36th week, then weekly until delivery

▶ Patients with identified risk factors can be seen as frequently as needed for careful monitoring.

▶ Weight checks, blood pressure, urine screen for protein and glucose, fundal height measurement and Leopold maneuvers, fetal heart tones, edema

RETURN PRENATAL VISITS

First Trimester: < 13 Weeks

- ▶ Review of family and social conditions
- ▶ Genetic testing, chorionic villous sampling, α-fetoprotein serum levels, amniocentesis
- ▶ Weeks 11–20: Multiple markers screen should be offered; some prenatal sites offer screening for Down syndrome risk during first trimester, measuring serum free hCG and pregnancy-associated plasma protein A (PAPP-A).

Second Trimester: 13–28 Weeks

- ▶ Fetal heart tones
- ▶ Fundus at umbilicus at 20 weeks
- ▶ Quickening: Fetal movement felt by mother at 18–20 weeks
- ▶ May order ultrasound if dates are in doubt or fetal growth in question
- ▶ Weeks 13–20: If not already done, offer second-trimester screening for Down syndrome, trisomy 18, and neural tube defects (NTDs) after 15 completed weeks of gestation using maternal serum, hCG, uE3 and inhibin A.
- ▶ Refer for childbirth education classes.
- ▶ Discuss infant feeding: Breastfeeding, bottle-feeding.
- ▶ Discuss symptoms to report: Bleeding, cramping, fever, decreased fetal movement, dysuria.
- ▶ Weeks 24–28: Diabetes screening with glucose challenge test (50-gram oral glucose load with blood glucose test 1 hour later); if abnormal, may be followed by a 3-hour glucose tolerance test (100-gram oral glucose load with blood drawn fasting 1, 2, 3 hours after ingestion of glucose); hematocrit and hemoglobin; repeat antibody screen in Rh-negative mothers before giving prophylactic Rh immunoglobulin.
- ▶ Optimal timing for a single ultrasound evaluation in absence of specific indications is at 16–20 weeks, at which time dating can be confirmed and anatomy assessed.

Third Trimester: 28 Weeks to Birth

- ▶ Weeks 35–36: Repeat hemoglobin, blood glucose; high-risk patients should be screened again for gonorrhea, chlamydia, HIV, and syphilis; vaginal and rectal cultures for group B streptococcus (linked to preterm delivery and neonatal sepsis); women testing positive for group B streptococcus will need treatment during labor before delivery.
- ▶ Evaluate blood pressure, weight gain or loss, edema, fundal height, and fetal heart tones.
- ▶ Teach signs of labor.
- ▶ Repeat breast exam.
- ▶ Discuss plans for birth control postpartum.

POSTPARTUM VISIT

Usually at 6 weeks postpartum; sooner if delivery, postpartum, or breastfeeding problems

Assessment

History

▶ Review labor and delivery record.

▶ Assess breastfeeding: Milk supply adequacy, nipple or breast pain; encourage exclusive breastfeeding for 6 months; ask about infant's weight and growth, and number of wet diapers per day, to assess adequacy of mother's milk production.

▶ Bowels: Constipation, change in elimination pattern, hemorrhoids

▶ Episiotomy repair: Healed, problems, dehiscence, swelling

▶ Sexual relations: Resumed, problems, dryness

▶ Contraception: Evaluate and prescribe p.r.n.

▶ Bladder: Voiding problems, incontinence, Kegel exercises

▶ Lochia (vaginal bleeding): Resolved, clots, still bleeding

▶ Menses: Resumed or lactational amenorrhea

▶ Sleeping pattern

▶ Nutrition

▶ Psychological adaptation to newborn: Mother, family members

▶ Screen for symptoms of postpartum depression

Physical Exam

▶ Vital signs, blood pressure

▶ Weight

▶ Urine: Screen for protein and glucose.

▶ Breast exam: Look for mastitis, redness, tenderness, masses.

▶ Thyroid exam: Postpartum thyroiditis not uncommon

▶ Pelvic exam: Episiotomy, uterus (involution should be nearly completed)

▶ Rectal exam: Tone, rectoceles, hemorrhoids

Diagnostic Studies

▶ Pap smear

▶ Hemoglobin if history of anemia

Management

▶ Estrogen-containing contraceptive methods can safely be initiated 6 weeks to 6 months postpartum for women who are breastfeeding their infants and three weeks postpartum for women who are not breastfeeding.

▶ Because of a concern about hypercoagulability during the postpartum phase, many clinicians withhold hormonal contraceptives from women after childbirth, whether or not the women are breastfeeding. The World Health Organization (WHO) reviewed available evidence on this issue and suggests that the risks of estrogen-containing contraceptives may outweigh the benefits during the first 3 weeks postpartum. After 3 weeks, however, when thrombosis risk returns to normal, postpartum women who are not breastfeeding can use estrogen-containing oral contraceptives without additional restrictions.

▶ Since low-dose progestins are not associated with thrombosis, the WHO recommends initiating progestin-only contraceptives at any point postpartum.

▶ Breastfeeding mothers may use progestin-only contraception beginning 6 weeks postpartum.

▶ Continue prenatal vitamins for 3–4 months or while breastfeeding.

Follow-up

▶ Routine well-woman care: Pap smear in 6–12 months

▶ Contraception as indicated

CASE STUDIES

CASE 1. A 39-year-old sexually active woman presents with a 3-week history of white vaginal discharge, no itching, but notices a fishy odor.

HPI: Denies abdominal pain, nausea and vomiting, fever, genital lesions, lymphadenopathy, dysuria. Patient is in a monogamous relationship with same partner for 6 years.

► What additional history would you obtain?

Exam: Thin, white-gray vaginal discharge coating vaginal walls, cervix without inflammation or discharge, no cervical motion tenderness on bimanual examination.

► What might you find on examination of vaginal fluid if this woman has bacterial vaginosis?

► Should her partner be evaluated and treated?

► What is the standard treatment for nonpregnant women?

► What does the patient need to know regarding use of this medication?

CASE 2. Jane S. comes to your office for her first prenatal visit. She has had a positive home pregnancy test. This is her third pregnancy. She reports that she has made frequent attempts to stop smoking without success.

► What further history do you need from Jane?

► What would you include in her physical assessment?

► What screening tests would you order?

► What prenatal education would she need?

CASE 3. A 52-year-old woman presents with complaints of hot flashes and no menstrual period for 4–5 months. She asks if there is a blood test to determine if she has gone through menopause and would like your advice on hormone replacement therapy.

HPI: LMP 4–5 months, two periods before that were late and scantier than usual. Hot flashes occur daily with profuse sweating, but denies mood change or vaginal dryness. Has tried an herbal over-the-counter product without relief.

► What additional history would you like before advising her on treatment?

► What laboratory tests would you do to confirm menopause?

► What information would you review about hormonal treatment in menopause?

► What other recommendations should you provide?

REFERENCES

American Cancer Society. (2013). *Cervical cancer screening recommendations.* Retrieved from www .cancer.org/Cancer/news/News/new-screening-guidelines-for-cervical-cancer

American College of Obstetricians and Gynecologists. (2010). ACOG practice bulletin: Clinical management guidelines for obstetrician-gynecologists: Number 112, April 20, 2010: Emergency Contraception. *Obstetrics and Gynecology, 115,* 1100–1109.

American Society for Colposcopy and Cervical Pathology. (2012). *2012 updated consensus guidelines for the management of abnormal cervical cancer screening tests and cancer precursors.* Retrieved from www .asccp.org/Portals/9/docs/ASCCP%20Updated%20Guidelines%20%20-%203.21.13.pdf

Bland, K. I., & Copeland, E. M. (2009) *The breast: Comprehensive management of benign and malignant disorders, volumes I & II* (4th ed.). Philadelphia: W. B. Saunders.

Berek, J. (2011). *Berek & Novak's gynecology* (15th ed.). Philadelphia: Lippincott Williams & Wilkins.

Centers for Disease Control and Prevention. (2004). Newborn screening for cystic fibrosis. *MMWR: Morbidity and Mortality Weekly Reports, 53*(No. RR13), 1–36. Retrieved from www.cdc.gov/mmwr/ preview/mmwrhtml/rr5313a1.htm

Centers for Disease Control and Prevention. (2010). Sexually transmitted diseases treatment guidelines, 2010. *MMWR: Morbidity and Mortality Weekly Reports, 59*(No. RR-12). Retrieved from www.cdc.gov/ STD/treatment/2010/STD-Treatment-2010-RR5912.pdf

Centers for Disease Control and Prevention. (2012). Youth risk behavior surveillance — United States, 2011. *MMWR: Morbidity and Mortality Weekly Reports, 61*(No. SS-4). Retrieved from www.cdc.gov/mmwr/ pdf/ss/ss6104.pdf

Committee on Adolescence. (2012). Emergency contraception. *Pediatrics.* Retrieved from http:// pediatrics.aappublications.org/content/early/2012/11/21/peds.2012–2962

Domino, F. J. (2013). *The 5-minute clinical consult.* St. Louis, MO: Lippincott Williams & Wilkins.

Fisher, M., Alderman, E., Kreipe, R., & Rosenfeld, W. (2011). *Textbook of adolescent health care.* Washington, DC: American Academy of Pediatrics.

Gabbe, J., Steve, G., & Simpson, L. (2007). *Obstetrics: Normal and problem pregnancies* (5th ed.). Philadelphia: Churchill Livingstone.

Gilbert, D. N., Moellering, R. C., Eliopoulos, G. M., Chambers, H. F., & Saag, M. S. (2013). *The Sanford guide to antimicrobial therapy* (43rd ed.). Vienna, VA: Antimicrobial Therapy.

Goroll, A., & Mulley, A. (2009). *Primary care medicine: Office evaluation and management of the adult patient* (6th ed.). Philadelphia: Lippincott Williams & Wilkins.

Hatcher, R., Trussell, J., Nelson, A., Cates, W., Kowal, D., & Policar, M. S. (2011). *Contraceptive technology* (20th ed. rev.). New York: Ardent Media Trade, Inc.

King, T., Brucker, M., Kriebs, J., Fahey, J., Gegor, C., & Varney, H. (2013). *Varney's midwifery* (5th ed.). Sudbury, MA: Jones & Bartlett.

Kliegman, R. M., Stanton, B. F., St. Geme, J. W., Schor, N. F., & Behrman, R. (2011). *Nelson's textbook of pediatrics* (19th ed.). Philadelphia: W. B. Saunders.

LeFevre, M. L., Calonge, N., Dietrich, A. J., & Melnikow, J. (2010). Mammography screening for breast cancer: Recommendation of the U.S. preventive services task force. *American Family Physician, 82*(6), 602–609.

Pickering, L. K., Baker, C. J., Kimberlin, D. W., & Long, S. S. (2012). *Red Book: 2012 Report of the committee on infectious diseases* (29th ed.). Elk Grove, IL: American Academy of Pediatrics.

Riley, L. E., & Stark, A. R. (2012). *Guidelines for perinatal care (AAP/ACOG)* (7th ed.). Washington, DC: American Academy of Pediatrics.

Riordan, J. (2009). *Breastfeeding and human lactation* (4th ed.). Sudbury, MA: Jones & Bartlett.

Rowan, S. P., Someshwar, J., & Murray, P. (2012). Contraception for primary care providers. *Adolescent Medicine, 23,* 95–110.

Saslow, D., Solomon, D., Lawson, H.W., Killackey, M., Kulasingam, S. L., Cain, J., ... Myers, E. R. (2012). American Cancer Society, American Society for Colposcopy and Cervical Pathology, and American Society for Clinical Pathology screening guidelines for the prevention and early detection of cervical cancer. *CA: A Cancer Journal for Clinicians, 62*(3), 147–172.

Trussell, J. (2011). Contraceptive failure in the United States. *Contraception, 83*(5), 397–404.

Trussell, J., & Raymond, E. G. (2010). Emergency contraception: A last chance to prevent unintended pregnancy. *A Review of Available Evidence.* Retrieved from http://ec.princeton.edu/questions/ec-review.pdf

U.S. Preventive Services Task Force. (2010). *Screening for breast cancer.* Retrieved from www.uspreventiveservicestaskforce.org/uspstf/uspsbrca.htm

U.S. Preventive Services Task Force. (2012). *Screening for cervical cancer: Clinical summary of the U.S. Preventive Services Task Force Recommendation.* Retrieved from www.uspreventiveservicestaskforce.org/uspstf11/cervcancer/cervcancersum.htm

U. S. Department of Health and Human Services. (2012). *The guide to clinical preventive services 2012: Recommendations of the U.S. Preventive Services Task Force.* Washington, DC: Agency for Healthcare Research and Quality.

MALE REPRODUCTIVE SYSTEM DISORDERS

Barbara Seibert, DNP, CRNP, FNP-BC, CNE

GENERAL APPROACH

Description

Many complaints of the male genitourinary system are of a sensitive nature, and men are less inclined to initiate discussion or seek help for them. The nurse practitioner should take an active role in screening for such problems with an approach that is open and nonjudgmental.

General areas for screening: Sexuality, safer sex practices, high-risk behaviors

General history questions: Past infections (sexually transmitted infections [STIs], urinary tract infections [UTIs], prostatitis), normal voiding patterns; current symptoms in more detail

Exam: Assessment of the male genitalia should be part of the screening or annual physical exam, even if there are no complaints, since many male genitourinary problems are asymptomatic.

RED FLAGS

Testicular torsion: Rule out with any complaint of scrotal pain: acute onset of severe scrotal pain, in males of any age (peak ages 12–18); requires treatment within 4–12 hours surgically to preserve fertility and prevent loss of the testicle

Paraphimosis: Inability of the foreskin to be retracted over the glans can be a surgical emergency.

Testicular mass: Any mass in the testicles or attached to the testicles is cancer until proven otherwise.

Right-sided varicoceles: Rare; associated with obstruction of the right spermatic vein and retroperitoneal neoplasms

Recurrent UTIs in men: Evaluate for prostatitis.

Prostatic massage: Avoid performing until acute prostatitis ruled out or treatment initiated to prevent hematogenous spread of infection.

OTC medications: Anticholinergics, parasympatholytics, and sympathomimetics precipitate or worsen urinary conditions such as benign prostatic hyperplasia; antidepressants can affect full sexual function.

CONTRACEPTION

Condoms

- ▶ A method of pregnancy prevention used by the male to prevent the spillage of semen into the vaginal vault. A latex or polyurethane sheath applied before sexual intercourse or penetration that fits snugly over the entire length of the penis, with a mildly constricting ring at the base to prevent slipping off. After detumescence, the condom holds ejaculated semen that is discarded with the condom.
- ▶ Condoms reduce risk of exposure to STIs in male-to-female or male-to-male contact.
- ▶ Approximately 21% of males use condoms as a contraceptive; more commonly used for prevention of STI transmission or exposure
- ▶ Effectiveness averages 88% typically, up to 97% if used properly.

Factors Contributing to Unsuccessful Use and Resultant Pregnancy

- ▶ Allergy to latex or rubber
- ▶ Failure to use during genital foreplay when pre-ejaculate can be introduced into or near the vagina
- ▶ Breakage or slippage of the condom during intercourse
- ▶ Limited education about reproduction or contraception; limited access to medical care
- ▶ Dissatisfaction with method and subsequent failure to use

Instruction on Use

- ▶ Apply to penis when in the erect state, before contact with partner's genitals since pre-ejaculate discharge near or in the vagina can contain semen adequate for fertilization.
- ▶ Roll the condom to the base of the penis, leaving a small space at the tip to allow for collection of ejaculate and decrease pressure on the condom (decreased risk of breakage).
- ▶ Use only water-based lubricants if needed. Spermicidal cream or jelly on the penis before application of the condom and penetration or used intravaginally enhances effectiveness and reduces pregnancy risk. Do not use the same condom more than once.

Sterilization

▶ A surgical method of eliminating the transport of semen in ejaculate as a means to prevent pregnancy, which, although possibly reversible, should be considered permanent

▶ An outpatient surgical procedure performed via a scrotal incision that severs and seals the vas deferens; does not require general anesthesia

▶ The most popular method of sterilization in the U.S.

▶ Approximately 12% of men are surgically sterilized via vasectomy.

▶ Failure rate is 0.1% in the first year postoperatively.

▶ Sperm counts are obtained at postprocedure follow-up to confirm success of the procedure before resuming sexual intercourse.

▶ Complications include potential infection and failure of sterilization.

DISORDERS OF THE PROSTATE GLAND

BENIGN PROSTATIC HYPERPLASIA (BPH)

Description

Nonmalignant generalized enlargement of the periurethral prostate gland related to a variety of triggers for cell growth; believed to be under endocrine control; enlargement mechanically obstructs urination by compressing the urethra

Etiology

▶ Cause unknown; universally seen in aging

▶ Hyperplasia of gland due to an abnormal increase in the number of cells in prostate tissue

▶ Hormonal changes: Accumulation of dihydrotestosterone (DHT) and increased estrogen in aging male seem to interact in a way that causes cell proliferation.

Incidence and Demographics

▶ Affects approximately 8% of men age 31–40; 50% of men age 50–60; and nearly 90% of men > 80 years old.

▶ Initially asymptomatic for men in 40s; many develop urinary symptoms by age 60

Risk Factors

▶ Increased age

▶ First-degree relative with BPH

▶ More common in Black population

▶ History of sexually transmitted infections

Prevention and Screening

▶ No prevention other than reducing risk factors (safer sex, change in diet)

▶ Early screening starting in the 40s (patient history, digital rectal exam) may allow for earlier treatment, slowing the progression of hyperplasia, and possible reduction of symptoms.

Assessment

History

▶ General: Fever, malaise, back pain, hematuria, pain with voiding indicate infection.

▶ Obstructive symptoms: Difficulty starting or stopping stream, hesitancy, dribbling, weakening force or size of stream, sensation of full bladder after voiding, retention

▶ Irritative symptoms: Urgency, frequency, nocturia, urge incontinence, dysuria

▶ American Urological Association (AUA) Symptom Index for Benign Prostate Hypertrophy:

　» 35-point scale to assess symptom severity: Incomplete emptying, frequency, intermittency, urgency, weak stream, straining, nocturia

　» Seven categories rated from 0 to 35 points: 0–7 = mild; 8–19 = moderate; 20–35 = severe

　» The higher the points, the more severe the symptoms

　» Should be completed for all patients before therapy begins

▶ Medications, especially cold and sinus medications: Anticholinergics impair bladder contractility, sympathomimetics increase outflow resistance and worsen symptoms.

▶ Date of last digital rectal exam (DRE), prostate-specific antigen (PSA), and results

▶ PMH: Explore for other conditions that may be associated with these symptoms: Surgery, urethral instrumentation or trauma, history of type 2 diabetes, neuromuscular disease (multiple sclerosis), sexual dysfunction, psychogenic disorder, cardiovascular disease, and hypercalcemia.

Physical Exam

▶ Digital rectal exam (DRE): Intact anal sphincter tone; prostate should be nontender, firm, smooth, and rubbery and measure 4×3×2 cm; blunting or obliteration of midline median sulcus indicates BPH; finding of enlarged prostate does not always correlate with symptoms.

▶ Enlargement may be symmetric, nodular, or asymmetric. Any nodules should be considered possibly malignant and fully evaluated; indurated prostate requires cancer evaluation.

▶ Abdomen: With urinary retention, possible distended bladder on percussion or palpation; costovertebral tenderness (CVAT) if renal sequelae

▶ Neurologic: Screening exam to note nonprostate etiology for symptoms of neurogenic or myogenic etiology, detrusor muscle impairment, compression of nerves

Diagnostic Studies

▶ Urinalysis should be negative for hematuria, glycosuria, or infection; their presence indicates secondary UTI or other problem.

▶ Catheterization for a postvoid residual (PVR) illustrates volume remaining in bladder after patient's usual void.

▶ Serum BUN and creatinine are helpful in assessing renal function; may be abnormal if urinary retention or obstruction has affected upper urinary tract, as well as with underlying renal disease.

▶ Prostate-specific antigen (PSA) to distinguish cause (BPH or prostate cancer) of large gland; use of this test is *controversial* if patient is asymptomatic and results are 4–10 ng/mL. Results > 10 ng/mL may be associated with cancer, but not necessarily correlated. PSA increases as gland enlarges, but do not assume increases are due only to gland enlargement. Acute urinary retention, prostatitis, urinary tract instrumentation, or prostatic infarction may elevate the PSA. *Increased levels may also be noted 1–24 hours post-DRE, so avoid lab work during this time period.*

▶ Advanced workup includes urinary flowmetry studies (flow rate), postvoid residual urine, urodynamic studies, transrectal ultrasound, intervenous pylogram (IVP), and abdominal ultrasound.

Differential Diagnosis

Medical

▶ Diseases associated with increased urination (chronic heart failure [CHF]

▶ Type 2 diabetes mellitus

Obstructive

▶ Prostate cancer

▶ Urethral strictures or valves

▶ Bladder neck contracture (usually secondary to prostate surgery)

▶ Inability of bladder neck or external sphincter to relax appropriately during voiding

Infectious or inflammatory

▶ Prostatitis

▶ Cystitis

▶ Urethritis

Neurologic

▶ Spinal cord injury

▶ Stroke

▶ Parkinsonism

▶ Multiple sclerosis

Pharmacologic

▶ Diuretics

▶ Sympathomimetics (cold medication, decongestants, antihistamines)

▶ Anticholinergics

Management

Nonpharmacologic Treatment

▶ The American Urological Association (AUA) recommends "watchful waiting": monitoring of symptoms associated with mild BPH or without bothersome lower urinary tract symptoms or development of serious complications (AUA scores < 7)

▶ Avoid bladder irritants such as coffee, alcohol, decongestants, antihistamines, anticholinergics, and tricyclic antidepressants.

▶ Encourage frequent voiding to keep bladder volume low.

▶ Monitor voiding; watch for signs of retention.

► Limit intake of fluids in the evening; avoid large quantities over a short time.

► Eliminate prescription and OTC meds that may worsen symptoms.

► In men with moderate to severe symptom presentation (> 7 points on AUA scale)

» First-line medical management with alpha-adrenergic antagonists is more effective than other methods alone.

» Use 5-alpha-reductase inhibitors to reduce prostatic volume if prostatic enlargement is present.

» Combination therapy using alpha-adrenergic antagonists and 5-alpha-reductase inhibitors is superior to monotherapy when used for very large prostates.

► Adverse effects

» Alpha-adrenergic antagonists can cause orthostatic hypotension.

► Phytotherapy

» Saw palmetto berry, bark of *Pygeum africanum*, roots of *Echinacea purpurea*, *Hypoxis rooperi*, pollen extract, and leaves of trembling poplar—all still being researched. Saw palmetto may provide mild improvement of peak flow rates and appears to work by blocking 5-alpha-reductase.

► Surgical options

» For those with severe symptoms, large postvoid residual, upper tract infections, or failure of medical therapy

» Transurethral resection of the prostate (TURP) is gold standard

» Transurethral incision of the prostate (TUIP)

» Open prostatectomy

► Minimally invasive therapy

» Nonsurgical procedures to reduce the size of the prostate include the use of heat via transurethral needle ablation (TUNA) and transurethral microwave therapy (TUMT), transurethral laser ablation using holmium laser ablation of the tissue (TULA), transurethral laser resection or enucleation, the use of transurethral electrovaporization of the prostate (TEVP), fiber optics or laser technology, high-intensity focused ultrasound, transurethral balloon dilation of the prostate, and UroLume intraprostatic stent placement.

Pharmacologic Treatment

► For mild to moderate symptoms, see Table 12–1 for primary drugs.

► Less commonly used drugs: GnRH agonists, progestational antiandrogens, flutamide (Eulexin), and testolactone (Teslac)

► Saw palmetto (160 mg b.i.d.) is an alternative herbal therapy; decreases testosterone uptake to decrease size of gland

► Tolterodine (Detrol) to decrease bladder contractions

How Long to Treat

► Dependent upon type and severity of symptoms and impact on daily functioning

► Medications may be prescribed until symptoms no longer manageable and surgery considered

TABLE 12–1

PHARMACOLOGIC MANAGEMENT OF BPH

DRUGS	DOSAGE	COMMENT
α-Adrenergic Blockers		
Terazosin (Hytrin)	Progressive dosing over 1 month: 1 mg × 3 days 2 mg × 11 days 5 mg × 7 days 10 mg daily	Relaxes smooth muscle around urethra Drug of choice for smaller prostate and acute irritative symptoms Decreased smooth muscle tone in bladder neck and prostate Improvement dose-dependent; takes 4–6 weeks for maximal therapeutic effect In nonhypertensive patient, may cause postural hypotension, dizziness, palpitations, or syncope May be beneficial for those with concomitant BPH and hypertension (HTN); can reduce number of medications needed
Doxazosin (Cardura)	1 mg q.d.; h.s., may double every 1–2 weeks to max of 8 mg/day	Similar to terazosin
Tamsulosin HCL (Flomax)	0.4 mg q.d. 30 min. before meal at same time each day. May increase to 0.8 mg after 2–4 weeks	Selective; may produce fewer side effects; no cardiovascular side effects, postural hypotension not common May cause dizziness, abnormal ejaculation, rhinitis Generally more expensive
Alfuzosin (Uroxatral)	10 mg/day p.o.	Selective; may produce fewer side effects; generally more expensive
5α-Reductase Inhibitors		
Finasteride (Proscar)	5 mg q.d. No titration needed	Blocks conversion of testosterone to DHT; gland shrinks Drug of choice for large prostate and men with contraindications or failed treatment with alpha-adrenergic medication Decreased hormonal (androgen) effect on prostate shrinks prostate size and symptoms, resulting in increased peak urinary flow rate Improvement not noted for up to 6–12 months, must be used indefinitely to sustain effect Decreased libido and ejaculate volume; erectile dysfunction Decreased PSA by up to 50%, blocking effectiveness of PSA as screening tool for cancer; screen for cancer with DRE and PSA before initiating treatment
Dutasteride (Avodart)	0.5 mg/day p.o.	Similar to finasteride

Special Considerations

In presence of concomitant diseases (diabetes mellitus; cardiovascular or neurologic disease), particularly with aging of the patient, care should be coordinated with regard to medications, ability for self-care, and recommendations for procedural or surgical treatment.

When to Consult, Refer, Hospitalize

Referral to a urologist is indicated for AUA index score of 8 or more, symptoms not responsive to medications, recurrent infections (epididymitis, repeat UTIs), elevated PSA, obstruction or acute urinary retention, bladder calculi, recurrent hematuria, renal disease, or suspicion of malignancy.

Follow-up

▶ Annual evaluation, including DRE and PSA as indicated for asymptomatic or minor symptoms

▶ Patients who opt for the "watchful waiting" strategy should be followed every 3–12 months.

▶ Patients on medications should be seen every 2–4 weeks until symptoms stabilize, then every 6 months.

▶ Patients receiving surgical or procedural treatments are followed by the treating urologist or surgeon.

Expected Course

May have prolonged course of mild or stable symptoms before advancing to stage of needing nonpharmacologic treatment

Complications

Potentially serious sequelae: UTI, obstructive uropathy, urine retention, renal disease

PROSTATITIS

Description

▶ An inflammation or infection of the prostate gland traditionally categorized as acute bacterial, chronic bacterial, nonbacterial, or prostatodynia

▶ New National Institutes of Health (NIH) prostatitis classification:

　» NIH class I: Acute bacterial prostatitis

　　▷ Febrile illness with perineal pain, dysuria, and obstructive symptoms

　» NIH class II: Chronic bacterial prostatitis

　　▷ Recurrent infection with pain and voiding disturbances

　» NIH class III: Chronic nonbacterial prostatitis or chronic pelvic pain syndrome

　　▷ NIH class IIIa: Inflammatory: significant inflammatory cells in prostatic secretions, postprostatic massage urine, or semen

　　▷ NIH class IIIb: Noninflammatory: insignificant number of inflammatory cells

    » NIH class IV: Asymptomatic inflammatory prostatitis

        ▷ Incidental finding during prostate biopsy for infertility, cancer workup

Etiology

▶ Various causes: Allergic, inflammatory, infectious, related to instrumentation, UTIs, STIs, prostatic abscess or calculi

▶ Acute infectious causes: Generally Gram-negative bacilli; primarily *E. coli;* may also be *Enterobacter, Klebsiella, Proteus mirabilis, Pseudomonas aeruginosa, Staphylococcus aureus, Streptococcus faecalis, Serratia, Neisseria gonorrhoeae, Ureaplasma, Trichomonas vaginalis, Chlamydia trachomatis, Gardnerella vaginalis*

▶ Nonbacterial prostatitis causes: Unknown; leading theory suggests nonrelaxation (spasm) of the internal urinary sphincter and pelvic floor striated muscles leading to increased prostatic urethral pressure and intraprostatic urinary reflux

▶ Infectious causes usually occur by direct invasion from the urethra, typically a UTI.

▶ Younger men (≤ 35 years) have an increased likelihood that the infectious organism is an STI (*C. trachomatis* or *N. gonorrhoeae).*

Incidence and Demographics

▶ 2 million cases annually in the United States

▶ Chronic bacterial primarily in older men ages > 50

▶ All others primarily in sexually active men ages 30–50

▶ Nonbacterial: Most common type, 8× greater than bacterial type, with an increased prevalence in younger males

▶ Acute bacterial: Least common type, occurs in younger or older male

▶ Bacterial prostatitis occurs more frequently in patients with HIV.

▶ Prostatodynia most commonly affects ages 22–56.

Risk Factors

▶ History of or exposure to STIs (multiple sexual partners or recent new partner)

▶ Age over 50: More common cause from recurrent UTI or prostatic calculi

▶ Prostate biopsy, TURP, urethral dilatation, cystoscopy, urethral stricture, chronic indwelling catheter

▶ Instrumentation of urinary tract

▶ Sexual abstinence

▶ Trauma (e.g., bicycle, horseback riding, falls affecting the sacrum)

▶ Abscess elsewhere in the body

▶ Recurrent UTIs

▶ May be associated with autoimmune or neuromuscular problems, stress, allergic conditions

Prevention and Screening

▶ Avoidance of unsafe sex decreases exposure to STIs

▶ Frequent voiding

▶ Screen with good history and DRE

Assessment

▶ See Table 12–2.

TABLE 12–2
CLINICAL PRESENTATION OF PROSTATITIS

	SYMPTOMS	PHYSICAL FINDINGS
Acute bacterial	Chills, fever, malaise Dysuria, urgency, burning, frequency Hematuria Pain: Pelvis, perineum, lower back, scrotum, with defecation, with intercourse	Fever Prostate very tender, boggy, warm, swollen, firm, or irregular ± Urethral discharge
Chronic bacterial	± Low-grade fever Dysuria, hesitancy Hematuria, hematospermia Pain mild: Perineum, scrotal, abdominal, with ejaculation	No systemic findings Prostate may be normal, indurated, mildly tender, boggy, or irregular ± Prostatic stones Scrotum ± edema, erythema, and tenderness
Nonbacterial	No fever Gradual onset: Dysuria, frequency, urgency Pain mild: Perineum, with ejaculation Decreased libido or impotence	Urethral discharge common Prostate enlarged, boggy, and tender
Prostatodynia	No fever Dysuria, hesitancy, decreased flow, post-void dribbling Pain: Perineum, back, testicle(s)	None

History

▶ All presentations have common symptoms of dysuria related to compression of the urethra by the inflamed prostate. All are associated with some degree of pain that is variable and may be associated with intercourse, ejaculation, and defecation.

▶ Acute bacterial prostatitis

  » Low back pain, fever, chills malaise, prostatodynia, perineal pain, obstructive voiding symptoms, frequency, urgency, dysuria, or nocturia

▶ Acute bacterial prostatitis

» Characterized by its acute onset with systemic symptoms and pattern of pain and dysuria

▶ Chronic bacterial prostatitis

» Characterized by remissions and exacerbations with recurrent UTIs, prostatodynia, perineal pain, dysuria, irritative voiding, lower abdominal pain, low back, scrotal or penile pain, pain on ejaculation, hematospermia

▶ Current medications (e.g., anticholinergics), other medical illness, and sexual history to assess risk of infection

Physical Exam

▶ Evaluate for fever; abdominal exam to check for tenderness or distended bladder; examine genitalia and scrotum, and for urethral discharge, CVA tenderness to assess kidneys, and rectal exam.

▶ *Warning regarding prostate examinations:* Due to exquisite tenderness of the prostate gland and the risk of spreading bacterial infection into the bloodstream, examination of the prostate should be done very gently or avoided when acute prostatitis is suspected until after treatment has been initiated. Massage of the prostate is contraindicated when acute bacterial infection is suspected, because this action can spread infection systemically.

▶ In the nonacute patient, prostatic massage is indicated to carry out the sequential urinalysis and culture for evaluation of prostatic secretions and as part of therapeutic treatment.

Diagnostic Studies

▶ Suspected acute prostatitis: Urinalysis, urine and blood cultures, urine Gram stain, CBX with differential

▶ Suspected chronic bacterial prostatitis or nonbacterial prostatitis: Traditional sequential urinalysis and culture test for voided bladder (VB) specimens and expressed prostatic secretions (EPS; see Table 12–3)

TABLE 12-3
SEQUENTIAL LABORATORY TESTS IN PROSTATITIS (FRACTIONAL URINE EXAM)

	SPECIMEN (Culture each sample also)	LOCATION
VB_1	1st 10 mL urine	Urine from urethra
VB_2	Next 200 mL discarded; then midstream urine	Urine from bladder
EPS	Urethral secretions *after* prostatic massage	Prostatic fluid
VB_3	1st 10 mL urine after prostatic massage	Prostatic fluid and urine from bladder

▶ 2-sample method:

1. Clean catch, midstream urine specimen

2. Urine specimen after prostatic massage

▶ Culture any penile discharge for STIs; wet mount of EPS

▶ Blood cultures may be ordered for acute prostatitis.

▶ Chronic prostatitis is additionally evaluated with CBC, serum BUN, and creatinine, and possible IV pyelogram, transrectal ultrasound, or both.

▶ In older men, bladder cancer screening via urine cytology is indicated.

▶ PSA will be elevated with acute prostatitis; do not order PSA until at least 1 month after prostatitis is treated.

▶ Urodynamic testing may be helpful in evaluating suspected prostatodynia.

Differential Diagnosis

▶ Any of the 4 types of prostatitis

▶ Cystitis (bacterial, interstitial), epididymitis, urethritis

▶ Pyelonephritis

▶ Malignancy

▶ Obstructive calculus

▶ Foreign body

▶ Acute urinary retention

▶ Urethral stricture

▶ BPH

▶ Renal colic

Management

Nonpharmacologic Treatment

▶ Avoidance of known irritants: Caffeine, alcohol, OTC antihistamines or decongestants

▶ Avoidance of sex during first 2 or more weeks of acute illness

▶ Increased frequency of ejaculation in nonacute states

▶ Hydration maintenance (force fluids)

▶ Rest and sitz baths 20 minutes 2–3 times a day for pain p.r.n.

Pharmacologic Treatment

▶ The prostate gland is difficult to penetrate with antibiotics; therefore, first-line treatment with antibiotic therapy for acute prostatitis is required for a minimum of 30 days (Table 12–4).

▶ Those < 35 years of age are more likely to be infected with *C. trachomatis* or *N. gonorrheae*, requiring antibiotics according to the current recommended choices of the health department or CDC (updated annually).

▶ NSAIDs are recommended for anti-inflammatory effects as well as pain relief.

▶ Stool softeners p.r.n.

TABLE 12-4
DIAGNOSIS AND MANAGEMENT OF PROSTATITIS

MICRO-SCOPIC	URINE CULTURES	DIAGNOSIS	TREATMENT	DURATION (variable recommendations)
+WBC, bacteria in VB_1, few in other specimens	# bacteria VB_1 > than VB_2 or VB_3	Urethritis	Ceftriaxone 125 mg IM × 1 or Cefixime 400 mg p.o. × 1 or Ciprofloxacin 500 mg p.o. × 1 **PLUS** Azithromycin 1 g p.o. × 1 or Doxycycline 100 mg b.i.d. × 1	Single-dose therapy
+WBC/RBC, bacteria in VB_2, possibly VB_1	# bacteria VB_2 > VB_1 or VB_3	Cystitis	Quinolone q.d. or b.i.d., or Trimethoprim-Sulfamethoxazole (TMP/SMX) 1 DS tab b.i.d. p.o.	3-7 days if uncomplicated
+WBC, bacteria in all specimens	# bacteria EPS, VB_3 > VB_1 or VB_2	Acute prostatitis	Fluroquinolone (Ciprofloxacin 500 mg p.o. q12h or levofloxacin 500 mg p.o. once q.d., or	4-6 weeks
			Trimethoprim-Sulfamethoxazole (TMP/SMX) 1 DS tab b.i.d. p.o.	4-6 weeks
+ WBC, bacteria in EPS and VB3 only	Little/no growth in VB_1 or VB_2	Chronic bacterial prostatitis	Fluroquinolone (e.g., Levofloxacin 500 mg p.o. once daily, or	4 weeks
			Ciprofloxacin 500 mg b.i.d. p.o., or	4-12 weeks
			Organism-specific	
			Chlamydia: Doxycycline 100 mg b.i.d. p.o.	7-14 days
			Ureaplasma: Tetracycline 500 mg b.i.d. PO	7-14 days
			Trichomonas: Flagyl 2.0 g ×1 or 500 mg b.i.d. p.o.	7 days
+ WBC in EPS, VB_3 Nonbacterial organisms in EPS or VB_3	No bacterial growth	Chronic nonbacterial prostatitis	No universally effective treatment Antibiotic therapy not proven to be effective	
No WBC, bacteria or other organisms in any specimen	No bacterial growth	Prostatodynia	NSAIDs & supportive treatments	

Special Considerations

▶ Patients may have concomitant urinary symptoms and infection; recurrent UTI diagnoses warrant chronic prostatitis in the differential.

▶ Older men: Increased incidence of concomitant disease in the genitourinary (GU) system indicates greater need for advanced testing and screening for BPH, prostate or bladder cancer, and UTI.

When to Consult, Refer, Hospitalize

▶ Hospitalization is indicated for all patients who have systemic involvement for IV antibiotics and treatment of possible septicemia.

▶ Refer to a urologist if no improvement within 48 hours of treatment.

▶ Refer older patients (> 50 years) who are symptomatic, have recurrent prostatitis, or acute bacterial prostatitis to a urologist; BPH may be a compounding problem.

Follow-up

▶ *Acute prostatitis:* Reevaluation is done within 48–72 hours, then 2–4 weeks later (1 month after completion of treatment) for urinalysis, urine and prostatic secretion cultures 30 days after initiating treatment to monitor treatment effectiveness and assess for signs of complications.

▶ *Chronic bacterial prostatitis:* Check urinalysis, culture and sensitivity every 30 days. Sequential urine tests and EPS should be repeated 4–6 weeks after initiation of therapy.

▶ Follow-up may be sooner as indicated based on the patient's responsiveness to treatment and changes in symptoms.

Expected Course

▶ Prostatitis requires long-term antibiotic therapy for optimal outcomes. Nonchronic prostatitis may be resolved within 6 weeks; however, chronic prostatitis requires treatment for up to 6 months. In chronic cases, treatment suppresses but does not eradicate the offending organism, hence the recurrence of symptoms.

Complications

▶ Potential for serious sequelae, including development of prostatic abscess, stones, ascending UTIs, epididymitis, urinary retention, renal infection, bacteremia, progressive STI complications

PROSTATE CANCER

Description

▶ Malignant neoplasm of the prostate gland

Etiology

▶ Unknown cause

▶ 95% develop in acinar glands of prostate (acinar adenocarcinoma)

▶ 2 types:

　» Poorly differentiated and fast-growing

　» Androgen-dependent, well-differentiated, and slow-growing

▶ Metastasizes primarily to bone

Incidence and Demographics

▶ Most common cancer in men; second most common cause of cancer deaths in men

▶ Average age at diagnosis is 71 years.

▶ About 80% of all clinically diagnosed cases of prostate cancer are men > age 65.

▶ In the U.S., 200 cases/100,000 men/year

▶ There is a 40% greater incidence in Black men; they are diagnosed with prostate cancer at later stages and die of the disease at higher rates than White men.

Risk Factors

▶ Age > 50, exposure to chemical carcinogens, history of STIs, baseline PSA above median for age group

▶ Family history of carcinoma of the prostate; 2 times increase in risk with first-degree relative affected at age < 50 years

▶ Blacks at greatest risk

Prevention and Screening

▶ Avoid exposure to chemical carcinogens; practice safer sex to prevent STIs.

▶ U.S. Preventive Services Task Force (USPSTF) current recommendations for prostate cancer screening are:

　» Screening for prostate cancer is currently assigned a grade "D" recommendation.

　» Evidence does not support screening for prostate cancer using the prostate specific antigen (PSA) test and DRE (digital rectal exam); risks of morbidity and mortality outweigh survival benefit.

Assessment

History

▶ Early disease is asymptomatic.

▶ With enlargement, frequency, nocturia, and dribbling develop (see BPH).

▶ Symptoms of urethral obstruction and bone pain occur with advanced metastatic stage.

▶ Constitutional symptoms: Anorexia, weight loss, fatigue, weakness, back pain

TABLE 12-5
USPSTF GRADE DEFINITIONS AFTER JULY 2012

GRADE	DEFINITION	SUGGESTIONS FOR PRACTICE
A	The USPSTF recommends the service. There is high certainty that the net benefit is substantial.	Offer or provide this service.
B	The USPSTF recommends the service. There is high certainty that the net benefit is moderate or there is moderate certainty that the net benefit is moderate to substantial.	Offer or provide this service.
C	The USPSTF recommends selectively offering or providing this service to individual patients, based on professional judgment and patient preferences. There is at least moderate certainty that the net benefit is small.	Offer or provide this service for selected patients, depending on individual circumstances.
D	The USPSTF recommends *against* the service. There is moderate or high certainty that the service has no net benefit or that the harms outweigh the benefits.	Discourage the use of this service.
I Statement	The USPSTF concludes that current evidence is insufficient to assess the balance of benefits and harms of the service. Evidence is lacking, of poor quality, or conflicting, and the balance between benefits and harms cannot be determined.	Read the clinical considerations section of USPSTF Recommendation Statement. If the service is offered, patients should understand the uncertainty about the balance between benefits and harms.

Physical Exam

▶ If symptomatic, perform a DRE to assess for prostatic masses and firmness.

▶ Depending on stage of the cancer, the prostate on DRE may be normal on the palpable lateral and posterior portion of the gland, or may be asymmetrical, generally firmer with hard induration, localized nodules, and obliterated median sulcus.

▶ Lower-extremity edema may develop due to lymph node metastases and pathologic fractures.

Diagnostic Studies

▶ PSA levels > 4 ng/mL indicate possible cancer; do not always correlate with DRE. Increased levels may be noted 1–24 hours post-DRE, so avoid lab work during this time period if possible.

▶ Ejaculation may alter total and free PSA levels. Men should abstain from sex for 24 hours before serum PSA levels being drawn.

▶ Prostatitis and BPH can cause an increase in PSA levels.

▶ PSA is discredited as screening test because PSA is normal in 40% of patients with cancer.

▶ CBC, urinalysis, urine culture, and sensitivity for work-up of urinary symptoms

▶ Serum alkaline phosphatase increased with late stage (metastatic) to bone

▶ Ultrasound with guided prostate biopsy is indicated with abnormal DRE or increase in PSA; bone scan.

Differential Diagnosis

▶ BPH

▶ Prostatitis

▶ Prostatic or bladder stones

▶ Bladder cancer

Management

Treatment choice is based on stage of the disease and age of patient.

Nonpharmacologic Treatment

▶ Asymptomatic patients with life expectancy < 10 years: Watchful waiting is an option.

▶ If localized, treatment options include watchful waiting, radical prostatectomy, and radiation therapy.

▶ Disseminated disease is treated with surgical or chemical castration (hormonal therapy) or chemotherapy.

Pharmacologic Treatment

▶ Hormonal treatment: Androgen deprivation or chemical castration—flutamide (Eulexin) 250 mg p.o. t.i.d. or leuprolide (Lupron) 1 mg SQ q.d. along with flutamide 7.5 mg IM monthly

How Long to Treat

▶ Radiation and chemotherapy treatments vary depending on staging.

Special Considerations

▶ Concurrent with treatment of the cancer is the need for addressing the effects of the diagnosis, sequelae of the disease, and side effects of treatments. These include coping with a chronic terminal illness, loss of self-image or self-esteem, transient or permanent incontinence (2%–5%), loss of libido, and impotence. Impotence occurs in 40% post-operatively and 25%–35% postradiation; hormonal treatment may additionally result in gynecomastia, cardiovascular complications, or hot flashes.

When to Consult, Refer, Hospitalize

▶ All patients with PSA > 10, abnormalities on DRE, or symptomatic are referred to specialist for advanced work-up, TRUS (transurethral ultrasound) with biopsy, chest X-ray, and bone scans.

Follow-up

▶ Urologist or oncologist

▶ For early stages, initially every 3–6 months for 5 years for PSA and DRE; annual bone scan if indicated; Hgb and liver function tests (LFT) for monitoring status and potential progression

Expected Course

▶ May be cured if detected and treated early; terminal if late staging

Complications

▶ Incontinence

▶ Erectile dysfunction

▶ Pain

▶ Pathologic fractures related to bone metastases

▶ Death

DISORDERS OF THE SCROTAL CONTENTS

CRYPTORCHIDISM

Description

▶ Failure of one or both testicles to descend into the scrotum

Etiology

▶ Partial lack of or response to gonadotropic and androgenic hormones during fetal development (testes descend by 7th fetal month)

▶ Mechanical factors, including elevated intra-abdominal pressure and retraction of the epididymis by the cremasteric muscles and gubernaculum

▶ May also have neural involvement

▶ Ectopic sites: Superficial inguinal canal (most common site); perineal, femoral, penile, transverse or paradox descent, pelvis—all rare

Incidence and Demographics

▶ 3%–4% full-term males, decreases to 0.8%–1.0% by 1 year of age

▶ 20%–30% of premature males

▶ 6% of fathers of boys with undescended testicles had cryptorchidism; increased incidence in siblings

▶ 20% are nonpalpable, with 25% of those absent at surgical exploration

▶ Can be unilateral or bilateral

▶ Spontaneous testicular descent occurs by age 1–3 months in 50%–70% of full-term males with cryptorchidism.

Risk Factors

▶ Prematurity; small for gestational age (SGA)

▶ Twins

▶ Family history

Associated Conditions

▶ Inguinal hernia or hydrocele; abnormalities of vas deferens and epididymis; intersex abnormalities; hypogonadotropic hypogonadism; germinal cell aplasia; prune-belly syndrome; meningomyelocele; hypospadias; Wilms' tumor; Prader-Willi syndrome; Kallmann syndrome; cystic fibrosis

Prevention and Screening

▶ Careful examination during newborn exam and well-child visits: Important to document presence and position of testicle

Assessment

History

▶ Has parent noted both testicles in scrotum during bath or while changing diaper?

▶ Prematurity

▶ Family history of cryptorchidism

Physical Exam

▶ Warm hands and the position of the patient (tailor position or sitting cross-legged, standing, or kneeling) may facilitate examination.

▶ Examine scrotum: Testicles palpable and asymmetric size or nonpalpable; differentiate between retractile or gliding testis vs. true undescended testis (0.5%–1%)

▶ Position of testicle if palpable outside scrotum (ectopic)

▶ Check for hernias and hydrocele.

Diagnostic Studies

▶ In boys ≤ 3 months of age with bilateral nonpalpable undescended testicles, hormone levels are helpful to determine whether the testes are present; check leuteinizing hormone (LH), follicle stimulating hormone (FSH), and testosterone.

  ▷ 3 months of age, use a human chorionic gonadotropin (hCG) stimulation test to determine presence or absence of testicular tissue, hCG 2,000 IU/day × 3 days, and check testosterone before and after stimulation.

▶ Lab studies: Urinary 17-ketosteriods, gonadotropins, and serum testosterone may help in tracing the cause.

▶ Various radiographic studies may be used on an individualized basis; however, CT scan findings in children have been found to be inconsistent; ultrasound does not reliably localize nonpalpable testes and does not rule out an intrabdominal testis; MRI has a sensitivity of 86%, a specificity of 79%, and an accuracy of 85%.

▶ Laparoscopy is useful to confirm testicular absence and locate abdominal testis and is a first and final step in surgical correction.

▶ Chromosome analysis if bilateral (may be ambiguous genitalia)

Differential Diagnosis

▶ Retractile testicle

▶ Atrophic testis

▶ Endocrine or chromosomal disorder

▶ Anorchia

Management

Nonpharmacologic Treatment

▶ Surgical correction: Orchiopexy should be performed by age 1. Orchiopexy permits accessible examination to monitor for malignancy. Alterations in germ-cell count in the cryptorchid testis have been identified by age 2. Laparoscopy is performed first if testis is nonpalpable.

Pharmacologic Treatment

▶ Hormone stimulation (hCG or GnRH) is off-label use of hCG and has variable results; may even be harmful to testes.

When to Consult, Refer, Hospitalize

▶ Referral to a pediatric urologist if bilateral nonpalpable undescended testicles or if one or more testis has not descended by 6 months to 1 year of age.

Follow-up

▶ Routine well-child visit schedule: Document presence of testicles, monitor for spontaneous resolution; post-op initial follow-up within 1 month of surgery and periodically thereafter to assess testicular size and growth.

▶ Children need to be taught regular testicular self-exam once they enter puberty, to assess for tumors.

Expected Course

▶ 80% of retractile testicles descend by age 12 months.

Complications

▶ Risks if not corrected: Testicular cancer 35–48 times more common, decreased fertility due to higher intra-abdominal temperature, cryptorchid testicle more prone to torsion, associated inguinal hernia in 25% of patients with maldescent, approximately 20% of males with unilateral undescended testis remain infertile even after age-appropriate orchiopexy

HYDROCELE

Description

▶ A painless enlargement of the scrotum due to accumulation of clear fluid within the tunica vaginalis, surrounding the testicles, may be unilateral or bilateral

Etiology

▶ True etiology is unknown; possible causes include closure of the processus vaginalis, closure of the distal processus, failure of closure of processus vaginalis, infection, tumors, trauma

▶ Two types

- *Communicating* (associated with inguinal hernias): Incomplete closure of tunica vaginalis; fluid descends from the peritoneal cavity

- *Noncommunicating:* Increased fluid production or decreased reabsorption within the scrotum; may be secondary to other scrotal disorders such as hernia, epididymitis, orchitis, tumors, trauma, or radiation

Incidence and Demographics

▶ Occur in 0.5%–1.0% of male population; approximately half coincide with a hernia

▶ Predominantly in childhood (up to 6% of male infants), but may occur at any age

Risk Factors

▶ Previous scrotal or genitourinary disorder (epididymitis, orchitis, trauma, testicular tumor)

▶ 50% associated with inguinal hernia

▶ Peritoneal dialysis, Ehlers-Danlos syndrome, ventriculoperitoneal shunt, exstrophy of the bladder

Associated Conditions

▶ Testicular tumors, trauma, ventriculoperitoneal shunt, nephrotic syndrome, renal failure with peritoneal dialysis

Prevention and Screening

▶ Prevention only by repairing inguinal hernia

▶ Examination of scrotum on well-child visits; periodic genital exam in adults

Assessment

History

▶ Acute or subacute onset of scrotal swelling or swelling in the inguinal canal

▶ Sensation of heaviness and bulkiness of the scrotum

▶ Duration of symptoms, including presence during childhood, recent trauma or infection

▶ Usually not painful

▶ Absence of other symptoms such as fever, dysuria, pain, impotency, or altered urinary patterns helps determine diagnosis

Physical Exam

▶ Nontender, scrotal firmness variable from soft to tense, depending upon amount of fluid in the sac

▶ Swelling in scrotum or inguinal canal; fluid collection in scrotum that transilluminates

▶ Pear-shaped, fluid-filled sac with the smaller pole superiorly, usually located behind the testicles

▶ May be unilateral or bilateral

Diagnostic Studies

▶ Transillumination: Transilluminates as translucent red glow with visible testicular shadow

▶ Doppler ultrasound indicated if any doubt of diagnosis, to rule out testicular torsion, incarcerated hernia, or cancer, particularly in a young male with sudden development and no apparent cause

▶ Aspiration of a hydrocele for diagnosis is not recommended and should be discouraged.

Differential Diagnosis

▶ Varicocele

▶ Spermatocele

▶ Epididymitis

▶ Testicle trauma

▶ Indirect inguinal hernia

▶ Tumor

▶ Cryptorchidism

▶ Orchitis

▶ Testicular torsion

Management

Nonpharmacologic Treatment

▶ Many hydroceles will resolve spontaneously during the first year of life.

▶ Surgical correction is considered in cases of extreme size, discomfort, cosmetically bothersome, or if a hernia is present.

▶ Aspiration of the hydrocele with instillation of a sclerosing agent (talc) has been successfully used in adults.

▶ Aspiration of the hydrocele is frequently followed by re-accumulation (recurrence rate of 34%) or infection, so it is not done routinely.

Special Considerations

▶ Occurs with inguinal hernias

When to Consult, Refer, Hospitalize

▶ Referral to a urologist or surgeon is recommended if large

▶ Refer to urologist if persists past 6–8 months of age

Follow-up

▶ Initially every 3–6 months to assess for changes and determine if surgery is necessary

▶ Patients or parents monitor for symptoms (i.e., pain or changes in hydrocele size, contour, or weight; new symptoms)

Expected Course

▶ Pediatric: Noncommunicating hydrocele present at birth usually resolves during first year of life.

▶ Adult: Usually does not resolve on own, but may not need treatment unless causing discomfort or in the presence of an underlying tumor

Complications

▶ For patients with surgical treatment, there is the potential for recurrence of hydrocele, wound infections, hematoma, or hematocele.

SPERMATOCELE

Description

▶ A painless cyst in the scrotal sac containing milky fluid with sperm

▶ Most are small, measuring < 1 cm, but can be as large as 8–10 cm, which are easily mistaken for hydrocele.

Etiology

▶ Unknown etiology

▶ Diverticulum in epididymis, leading to accumulation of spermatic fluid

Incidence and Demographics

▶ Incidence < 1%

Risk Factors

▶ None

Prevention and Screening

▶ No prevention

▶ Periodic genital exam in adults

Assessment

History

▶ Often asymptomatic; often a random finding by the patient or examiner

▶ May be similar to hydrocele in that the patient notes an increased bulk or weight to the scrotum; rarely, can become twisted (torsion) or infected, with subsequent symptoms of pain, edema, and warmth

Physical Exam

▶ Spermatoceles are attached to the epididymis, located above and behind the testicle.

▶ Palpable as round, mobile, and nontender cysts < 1 cm

▶ One or more may be present.

Diagnostic Studies

▶ Transillumination will reveal the mass.

▶ Ultrasound is indicated to clarify if any suspicion of cancer exists (age 18–35 with lump newly developed or sudden onset) or if thorough scrotal examination is hindered by the lump or edema.

Differential Diagnosis

▶ Varicocele   ▶ Hydrocele   ▶ Tumor

Management, Special Considerations, Consultation, and Follow-up

▶ Same as hydrocele

VARICOCELE

Description

▶ Abnormal venous dilatation in the scrotum (varicose veins in the scrotum)

Etiology

▶ Etiology is unknown, but there are several theorized causes:

» Incompetent valves in the scrotal veins

» Increased hydrostatic pressure in the left renal vein, inferior vena cava, and internal spermatic veins

» Increased mechanical pressure from the superior mesenteric artery

▶ *Note:* Right-sided varicoceles are rare and associated with obstruction of the right spermatic vein and retroperitoneal neoplasms.

Incidence and Demographics

▶ Affects 20% of the general male population

▶ Usually seen in older adolescents but can occur in any age group

▶ Almost always left-sided

▶ Can be associated with pathology in adult and prepubescent males

Risk Factors

▶ None

Prevention and Screening

▶ No prevention

▶ Monthly testicular self-exam (TSE) and periodic clinical genitalia exam in the adult male

Assessment

History

▶ Asymptomatic or a sense of heaviness or dull aching in the scrotum

Physical Exam

▶ The characteristic presentation is a scrotum with a soft, irregular mass that feels like a "bag of worms" located above and behind the testicle and epididymitis.

▶ It is nontender, worsens in the standing position, and often improves in the reclining position.

▶ Coughing or performing the Valsalva maneuver will accentuate the varicocele.

▶ If only palpable during a Valsalva maneuver, it is graded I; if palpable on standing, it is graded II; and, if visible on inspection alone, it is graded III.

▶ 97% occur on the left side of the scrotum.

Diagnostic Studies

▶ No testing may be needed to make the diagnosis in its classic presentation.

▶ Studies used to confirm the diagnosis include ultrasound, thermography, echo Doppler, and others, but these are done when a referral to an urologist is indicated.

Differential Diagnosis

▶ Hernia   ▶ Hydrocele   ▶ Tumor

▶ Epididymitis   ▶ Spermatocele   ▶ Epididymal cyst

Management

Nonpharmacologic Treatment

▶ Athletic supporters may provide increased comfort for patients with varicoceles.

▶ Surgery to correct the blood flow may be an option, depending on the grading of the varicocele. Options include ligation, laparoscopic varicocelectomy, percutaneous varicocele occlusion, and others, and are done upon referral to a urologist or surgeon.

Special Considerations

▶ Right-sided varicocele is uncommon; can indicate retroperitoneal malignancy

▶ Sperm concentration and motility are significantly decreased in 65%–75% of patients. Infertility is often a result and can be reversed in a high percentage of patients by correction of the varicocele as soon as identified.

When to Consult, Refer, Hospitalize

▶ Referral is indicated for patients who have suspected infertility, a varicocele that doesn't disappear in the supine position, and — most importantly — if it occurs on the right side.

Follow-up

▶ No firm guidelines; return if there is an increase in pain, size, change in urinary patterns, pain with bowel movements, fever, warmth to scrotum, interference with sexual intercourse

▶ Early treatment and close monitoring for the younger patient (adolescents) may improve long-term fertility

▶ Annual exam is adequate for asymptomatic patients.

▶ Postprocedure monitoring is indicated for recurrence of symptoms or development of complications.

Expected Course

▶ Variable and unpredictable

▶ Varicoceles have been found in 37% of patients with infertility, suggesting an association.

▶ Not associated with sexual dysfunction or increased risk of testicular cancer

Complications

▶ Infertility

▶ Postprocedure (i.e., wound infection)

EPIDIDYMITIS

Description

▶ An acute bacterial intrascrotal infection associated with painful enlargement of the epididymis

▶ Most cases of acute epididymitis are infectious and can be divided into two categories with different age distributions and causes.

  ▹ Sexually transmitted forms typically occur in men < 40 years, are associated with urethritis, and result from *Chlamydia trachomatis* or *Neisseria gonorrhoeae*.

  ▹ Nonsexually transmitted forms typically occur in older men, are associated with urinary tract infections and prostatitis, and are caused by Gram-negative rods. The route of infection is probably via the urethra to the ejaculatory duct and then down the vas deferens to the epididymis.

Etiology

▶ In the younger (< 35 years) male, STIs are the most common cause; primarily *C. trachomatis*, then *N. gonorrhoeae*.

▶ Assess for serous urethral discharge (chlamydia) or purulent discharge (gonorrhea).

▶ In homosexual males practicing anal intercourse, *E. coli* or *H. influenzae* is the common etiology; in heterosexual males > 35, causative organisms are those associated with UTIs.

▶ Sterile epididymitis is linked to vigorous physical activity (bicycle riding), trauma, and TB (rare causes).

▶ Gram-negative rods, *E. coli*, *Pseudomonas aeruginosa*, or coliform bacteria are common causes in men who have epididymitis that is associated with UTI (reflux of infected urine), are over age 35, have had instrumentation, or have anatomic abnormalities.

Incidence and Demographics

▶ Most common intrascrotal inflammation in males in the U.S.

▶ More than 600,000 healthcare visits per year

Risk Factors

▶ Exposure to STIs up to 30 days before onset of symptoms

▶ Anatomical abnormalities

▶ Instrumentation or surgery

Prevention and Screening

▶ Safe sex practices

▶ Antibiotics prior to instrumentation or urethral manipulation

Assessment

History

▶ Presents equally on left or right

▶ Testicular pain and edema that is commonly gradual in onset; symptoms may follow acute physical strain (heavy lifting), trauma, or sexual activity; associated symptoms of urethritis (pain at tip of penis and urethral discharge) or cystitis (irritative voiding symptoms) may occur; pain develops in scrotum and may radiate along spermatic cord or to flank. On occasion, edema may double the size of the testicle in 3–4 hours.

▶ Half of all cases present with fever, urethral discharge, or voiding complaints. Associated nausea and vomiting are unusual.

▶ Explore the PMH for previous urinary symptoms or diagnoses, procedures, instrumentation of the urinary tract, or trauma to the scrotum.

▶ Explore the social history for information on new sexual partners, sexual practices, and use of scrotal support or protectors during sports.

Physical Exam

▶ Scrotal pain radiates up spermatic cord or into groin region; may begin acutely over several hours; there is scrotal swelling and heaviness.

▶ Epididymis is cord-like and palpable separately from the testicle; initially normal size, consistency, and position on exam, but later the two may appear as one enlarged, tender mass becoming less distinguishable with time

▶ Epididymis is markedly tender to palpation.

▶ Pain may be relieved by elevating the scrotum (Prehn's sign—elevation of the scrotum above the pubic symphysis improves pain from epididymitis), but is not reliable.

▶ Cremasteric reflex present (contraction of scrotum after light stroke to thigh) on affected side (differentiates epididymitis from testicular torsion); if cremasteric reflex is absent, suspect testicular torsion.

▶ The prostate may be tender on rectal examination.

Diagnostic Studies

▶ Gram stain of urethral exudate or intraurethral swab to diagnose gonococcal infection if present; culture of same specimen for *N. gonorrhoeae* and *C. trachomatis*, white cells without visible organisms on urethral smear represent nongonococcal urethritis, and *C. trachomatis* is the most likely pathogen

▶ Urinalysis, possible urine culture to diagnose concurrent UTI particularly in nonsexually transmitted types

▶ Syphilis serology; CBC shows leukocytosis

▶ HIV testing with counseling

▶ Ultrasound of the scrotum or radionuclide scanning may also be needed to rule out other possibilities.

Differential Diagnosis

▶ Tumor

▶ Abscess

▶ Cyst

▶ Testicular torsion

▶ Testicular infarction

▶ Testicular cancer

▶ Mumps orchitis

▶ Hydrocele

▶ Varicocele

Management

Nonpharmacologic Treatment

▶ Bed rest and restriction of activity

▶ Scrotal elevation (place a folded towel under genitals and across thighs)

▶ Ice pack or warm compress

▶ Athletic scrotal supporter

▶ Avoidance of sexual activity and physical strain until resolved

Pharmacologic Treatment

▶ Initiate treatment empirically, before culture results are available (see Table 12–6).

▶ Treat sexual partners if condition is likely due to an STI and contact was within last 60 days preceding symptoms.

TABLE 12-6
PHARMACOLOGIC TREATMENT OF EPIDIDYMITIS

INDICATION	MEDICATION
Age < 35 with high likelihood of *N. Gonorrhoeae* or *C. Trachomatis*	Ceftriaxone (Rocephin) 250 mg IM single dose *and* Doxycycline 100 mg p.o. b.i.d. × 10 days If penicillin-allergic or participates in insertive anal intercourse: Ciprofloxacin (Cipro) 500 mg p.o. b.i.d. or ofloxacin (Floxin) 200 mg p.o. b.i.d. × 10 days Treat sexual partner(s)
Age > 35 with high likelihood of enteric organisms *or* Allergies to cephalosporins or tetracycline	Levofloxacin (Levaquin) 500 mg p.o. every day for 7–10 days or Ofloxacin (Floxin) 300 mg p.o. b.i.d. × 10 days or Ciprofloxacin (Cipro) 500 mg PL b.i.d. × 10–14 days
Fever and inflammation	Analgesics (e.g., NSAID, acetaminophen)

How Long to Treat

▶ Until fever and local inflammation have subsided, bed rest and elevation of scrotum should be maintained. Antibiotic therapy should be continued for 10 days.

Special Considerations

▶ Differentiate from other cause of acute scrotal pain, testicular torsion

▶ Prostatic massage is contraindicated in epididymitis due to potential risk for spread of local infection systemically.

When to Consult, Refer, Hospitalize

▶ Referral to urologist is indicated for the patient who is not improving within 3 days or has worsening symptoms.

Follow-up

▶ In 72 hours to ensure infection is resolving

Expected Course

▶ Failure to improve within 3 days requires reevaluation of both the diagnosis and therapy.

▶ Swelling and tenderness that persist after completion of antimicrobial therapy should be re-evaluated, noting that swelling may take weeks to months to resolved.

Complications

▶ Prompt treatment usually results in a favorable outcome; delayed or inadequate treatment may result in:

   ▸ Epididymo-orchitis

   ▸ Chronic pain (chronic epididymitis)

- » Abscess formation
- » Infertility (possibly up to 50% if bilateral)
- » Testicular atrophy

TESTICULAR TORSION

Description
▶ Spermatic cord compression by twisting of the spermatic cord within the scrotum, resulting in compromised blood flow to the testicles. Constitutes a surgical emergency to prevent necrotic testicle.

Etiology
▶ Congenital, anatomically abnormal, free-floating testicle without fixation in the scrotum, which twists around blood supply to testicle, resulting in ischemia and potential infarction of the testicle
▶ May be precipitated by trauma, sudden movements that pull on the cremasteric muscle (jumping into cold water, riding bicycle), sexual activity, cold, exercise
▶ May occur when contents of scrotum shift in the relaxed state during sleep
▶ Torsion usually spontaneous and idiopathic
▶ ⅓ have had prior episode of testicular pain

Incidence and Demographics
▶ Most commonly occurs in ages 12–18 with peak incidence at age 14, but can occur at any age; 1 in 4,000 males < 25 years old
▶ Occurs from newborn period to seventh decade
▶ 40% occur during sleep

Risk Factors
▶ Age
▶ Paraplegia
▶ Previous contralateral testicular torsion

Prevention and Screening
▶ No prevention except surgical correction of defect if discovered
▶ High index of suspicion in young male with acute scrotal pain

Assessment

History

▶ Typically presents with sudden onset of acute, profound pain that is localized to the testicles or radiating to the groin and lower abdomen; nausea and vomiting in 50% of patients

▶ No dysuria, fever, or urethral discharge; no irritative voiding symptoms

▶ A quick history should explore precipitating events (e.g., exercise, sleep, cold exposure), current medical history and medications, sexual partners, and STI exposure.

▶ Torsion of the testicular appendage (not entire testicle) presents with less severe pain and more gradual onset of symptoms, and is not a surgical emergency.

Physical Exam

▶ Typically lying still, in acute distress; first symptom is pain, usually sudden, but may have a gradual onset

▶ Acute tenderness of testicle with swelling and erythemia

▶ Scrotum is enlarged, red, edematous, and painful.

▶ Testicle is horizontal, elevated in the scrotum, with negative (absent) cremasteric reflex.

▶ Prehn's sign is negative (no relief with elevating testicle above pubic symphysis).

▶ Epididymis very tender, out of normal position due to twisting of spermatic cord

▶ If only the testicular appendage is twisted, there will be a "blue dot" sign at the superior aspect of the testicle—a small, palpable lump on superior pole of the epididymis when skin pulled taut.

▶ Nausea and vomiting common due to pain

▶ Fever may occur, but not typical

Diagnostic Studies

▶ Begin immediate surgical treatment in unequivocal cases. Consider risk of time lost for testing vs. preservation of testicle.

▶ Urinalysis usually not helpful unless to quickly rule out infectious component in differentiating diagnosis

▶ Doppler ultrasound with color is best; radionuclide scrotal imaging also used.

Differential Diagnosis

▶ Epididymitis

▶ Torsion of testicular appendage

▶ Trauma

▶ Orchitis

▶ Hernia (incarcerated or strangulated)

Management

▶ An acute urologic emergency can result in loss of the testicle.

▶ 80% salvage rate of testicle if corrected within 4 hours; only 20% if within 12 hours; necrosis of the testicle usually occurs after 6–8 hours

Nonpharmacologic Treatment

▶ Preoperatively, elevate the scrotum, apply ice pack.

▶ Manual reduction followed by surgical treatment (orchidopexy)

Special Considerations

▶ Advise patients that both testicles will be surgically secured within the scrotum to prevent reoccurrence and that there is a risk of decreased fertility or infertility.

When to Refer, Consult, Hospitalize

▶ Immediate surgical consult

Follow-up

▶ The surgeon follows the patient 1–2 weeks post-op.

▶ Annual visits to evaluate atrophy of testicles, particularly before puberty

Expected Course

▶ Potential outcomes depend on timing of treatment. The testicle may be gangrenous and removed, saved but atrophied, or minimally affected. Atrophy of the twisted testicle or the unaffected testicle may occur, affecting spermatogenesis and fertility, but testosterone production is unchanged.

Complications

▶ Impaired fertility; abnormal spermatogenesis

▶ Atrophy of the salvaged testicle in up to ⅔ of patients within 2–3 years

TESTICULAR CANCER

Description

▶ Carcinoma of the testicles that is categorized as germinal or nongerminal.

Etiology

▶ While the cause of testicular cancer is unknown, both congenital and acquired factors have been associated with tumor development. The strongest association has been with cryptorchid testis. Approximately 7%–10% of testicular tumors develop in patients who have a history of cryptorchidism. Seminoma is the most common form (95%) of tumor rising from this condition. Almost all cases of germ cell tumors (GCTs) show chromosome 12p abnormalities; increased expression of p53 protein is found in many GCTs.

Incidence and Demographics

▶ Testicular cancer is rare in children, but 66% of testicular tumors in children are malignant.

▶ 1%–2% of all male cancers; most common cancer of males age 15–35 years

- ► Germinal tumors account for 95% of all cases and are subcategorized as seminomatous (⅓ to ½) or nonseminomatous.
- ► Leydig cell neoplasms account for 5%.
- ► Most commonly occurs in 20–40 year age group but also in > 60 and childhood

Risk Factors

- ► White, Scandinavian, and Swiss; higher social class, rural resident, and unmarried
- ► History of undescended testicles (cryptorchidism)
- ► Family history
- ► Klinefelter syndrome, XY dysgenesis, Down syndrome, testicular atrophy
- ► Exposure to maternal intrapartum estrogen (diethylstilbestrol [DES]), infertility, preterm birth

Prevention and Screening

- ► Teach adolescent males to do regular testicular self-exams (TSE).
- ► Teach adolescent males to tell parents about any abnormal findings and seek treatment immediately.
- ► Encourage annual clinical screening with testicular exam.
- ► Screen patients with risk factors.

Assessment

History

- ► Frequently incidental finding on routine exam or patient notes are painless swelling, sense of heaviness, or thickening in scrotum or testicle.
- ► Testicles may be tender, especially if associated with bleeding within the tumor, or if epididymitis is present concurrently.
- ► Associated symptoms reflective of metastasis include gynecomastia; supraclavicular lymphadenopathy; abdominal or neck mass; or pain in the groin, flank, or back.
- ► Less than 10% with seminomal tumor have symptoms of distant metastases at time of diagnosis.
- ► Inquire about medications and past medical history, particularly relating to the associated symptoms.

Physical Exam

- ► Scrotal exam reveals hydrocele in up to 20% of patients with testicular cancer.
- ► Tumors are often found on the lower pole, but can be anywhere on the testicles.
- ► Tumors are firm, +/- tender, one or more present, on one or both testicles.
- ► Transillumination will not reveal the normal rosy glow; there is darkness of the tumor.
- ► Inguinal lymphadenopathy may or may not be present.

Diagnostic Studies

▶ Serum alpha-fetoprotein reflects presence of nonseminomatous germ cell tumors, LDH, hCG, and CXR

▶ Serum beta-human chorionic gonadotropin (β-hCG) positive in 70%–100% of seminomatous testicular carcinoma

▶ Scrotal ultrasound is gold standard; distinguishes between most of the differential diagnoses

▶ Staging determined with chest X-ray, CT scan of abdomen and pelvis, pedal lymphangiography; MRI of brain and lung and bone scan for patients with metastasis or elevated alkaline phosphatase

Differential Diagnosis

▶ Inguinal hernias

▶ Epididymitis

▶ Orchitis, hematomas

▶ Hydrocele

▶ Spermatocele

Management

▶ Treatment is dictated by the type of tumor, staging, and associated symptoms.

Nonpharmacologic Treatment

▶ Seminomas: Radiation and radical inguinal orchiectomy

▶ Nonseminomatous: Surgery, radiation, and combination chemotherapy

▶ Metastasized cancer is treated with both radiation and chemotherapy.

Pharmacologic Treatment

▶ Chemotherapy directed by the oncologist

How Long to Treat

▶ Directed by the oncologist

Special Considerations

▶ Testicular cancer in older patients most likely metastatic, usually lymphoma

When to Consult, Refer, Hospitalize

▶ Pediatric: All testicular masses or tumors should be referred to a pediatric urologist and oncologist.

▶ Adult: All undiagnosed testicular masses should be referred to a urologist.

▶ Management and follow-up are directed by the oncologist.

Follow-up

Expected Course

▶ Localized seminomatous cancer has 5-year survival rate > 95%.

▶ Disseminated disease 5-year survival is 20%.

▶ Nonseminomatous germ cell tumors treated aggressively have 5-year survival rate of 60%–90%.

Complications

▶ Metastases to lung and abdomen

▶ Side effects of treatment (radiation, chemotherapy)

▶ Post-op wound infection, urinary tract infections related to instrumentation

PENILE DISORDERS

PHIMOSIS

Description

▶ In the uncircumcised male, a tightness of the distal penile foreskin that prevents it from being retracted back over the glans penis

▶ Paraphimosis occurs when foreskin is retracted and remains proximal to the glans, constricting the glans penis.

Etiology

▶ Occurs when the orifice of the prepuce is too small to allow retraction of the foreskin

▶ Most cases occur in uncircumcised males, although excessive skin left after circumcision can become stenotic and cause phimosis.

▶ Acquired from trauma, prior infection, or poor hygiene (retained smegma and dirt) that results in inflammation and the development of adhesions.

▶ Can be physiologic until age 7–10 years

▶ Foreskin is physiologically adherent to the glans in the newborn. In the uncircumcised male, the foreskin naturally separates as the boy gets older; forcible retraction can cause scarring.

▶ Geriatric patients may develop phimosis with use of condom catheters.

Incidence and Demographics

▶ Age 16 or older have 1% incidence

▶ Adolescence is predominant age of occurrence

Risk Factors

▶ Uncircumcised penis

▶ Poor hygiene

▶ Trauma; diabetes

▶ Infection of the glans (balanitis) or prepuce (posthitis)

▶ Sickle cell disease

Prevention and Screening

▶ Teach parents proper care of uncircumcised penis; no need to retract until foreskin does so naturally

▶ Examine foreskin at routine well-child visits

▶ Hygiene of the genitalia with retraction of the foreskin during washing

Assessment

History

▶ Inability to retract foreskin when it was previously retractable

▶ Ballooning of foreskin with urination

▶ Urinary tract infection

▶ Painful urination

▶ Patients may be asymptomatic, with phimosis discovered on examination.

▶ When related to an infectious or inflammatory process, patient complains of irritation and tenderness of the glans, discomfort with voiding, or pain on erection.

▶ *Note:* If severe enough, outflow of urine may be compromised, presenting as a urologic emergency.

Physical Exam

▶ The glans is nonretractable and the prepuce is pallid, striated, and thickened.

▶ If actively infected, there will be erythema, smegma, exudate, or tenderness.

▶ In paraphimosis, there will be swelling or edema of the glans; possible ulceration; and drainage.

Diagnostic Studies

▶ None

Differential Diagnosis

▶ Balantitis

▶ Penile trauma; penile lymphedema; penile tourniquet syndrome due to foreign object around penis

Management

Nonpharmacologic Treatment

▶ Teach parents appropriate care of uncircumcised penis — gentle retraction only as far as foreskin will easily move.

▶ Treat the underlying cause, such as infection or inflammation, with good hygiene, sitz baths, and warm compresses.

▶ Surgical release or circumcision

Pharmacologic Treatment

▶ If concurrent infection or inflammation, treatment with topical antifungals or steroids may be sufficient to allow for retraction. To reduce swelling: Topical 0.05% betamethasone (Beta-Val) b.i.d. for 1 month to soften phimosis and gradual traction placed on foreskin. Within 4–6 weeks, the phimotic ring should open.

▶ Use of a triple antibiotic ointment (Neosporin or Bacitracin or generic brands) applied to the tip of the foreskin can act as a protective barrier to fecal contamination.

How Long to Treat

▶ Topical treatment for underlying infection or inflammation for 1–2 weeks

Special Considerations

▶ Phimosis is normal in uncircumcised infant; however, once foreskin is retractable, it is not normal for it to spontaneously adhere again.

When to Consult, Refer, Hospitalize

▶ Refer to urologist for surgical release or circumcision if nonresponsive to topical treatment and hygiene, urinary flow is compromised, or asymptomatic phimosis remains.

▶ Paraphimosis is a true *surgical emergency*; should be referred to urologist for immediate evaluation and circumcision. Unreduced paraphimosis can lead to gangrene of the glans.

Follow-up

Expected Course

▶ Resolves completely with treatment

▶ No sexual activity following circumcision until healing is complete

Complications

▶ If there is associated infectious precipitant, complications such as meatal stenosis, UTI, or premalignant changes may occur.

ERECTILE DYSFUNCTION (ED)

Description

▶ Inability to achieve or maintain a satisfactory erection more than 25%–50% of the time (although may be defined by patients as premature ejaculation or the loss of orgasm, emission, libido, or erections)

Etiology

▶ Psychological origin is likely with loss of orgasm when libido and erection are intact, and with premature ejaculation concurrent with anxiety, depression, relationship problems, new partner, or emotional disorders.

▶ Medications such as anabolic steroids, digoxin (Lanoxin), cimetidine (Tagamet), centrally acting antihypertensives (reserpine, clonidine, methyldopa [Aldomet]), beta-blockers and spironolactone (loss of libido), antidepressants (MAO inhibitors, tricyclics, SSRIs)

▶ Lifestyle issues of alcohol, drug, and cigarette use

▶ A gradual loss of erections over time is indicative of organic causes.

» Hormonal and endocrine disorders of the thyroid, hypogonadism, kidney, pituitary gland or testicular function, diabetes, Addison's disease, and Cushing's syndrome

» Vascular disorders such as hypertension, arterial insufficiency, venous disease, atherosclerosis

» Neurologic disorders, structural problems, spinal cord injury, and post-treatment of prostate disorders

» When ED occurs in younger men, it is associated with a significantly increased risk of future cardiac events and should be a warning sign for the primary care provider to investigate further underlying conditions.

Incidence and Demographics

▶ Widely underreported, estimated that 10% of the male population affected; 10–20 million men in the United States

▶ 52% of men age 40–70 years

▶ Age-related increase, ranging from 12.4% in men age 40–49 years to 46.6% in men age 50–69 years

Risk Factors

▶ Advancing age

▶ Cardiovascular disease

▶ Diabetes mellitus

▶ Metabolic syndrome

▶ History of urologic surgery, radiation, trauma or injury to the pelvic area or spinal cord

▶ Medications that induce ED

▶ Use or abuse of alcohol, cigarettes, and drugs

▶ Psychological conditions: Lifestyle with high levels of stress, anxiety, depression, or relationship problems

Assessment

History

▶ Determine the patient's perception or definition of erectile dysfunction (impotence) to clarify the problem and symptoms, timing, circumstances, and frequency of occurrence.

▶ Detailed sexual history: Determine the nature of the patient's relationship, sexual partners, lifestyle, and stress.

▶ Complaints include any of the following: Reduced size and strength of erection, lack of ability to achieve or maintain erections adequate for intercourse, rapid loss of erection with penetration, or lack of libido.

▶ Inquire if there are nocturnal or morning erections; their presence reflects an intact blood supply, nervous system, and sexual apparatus, and reduce the likelihood of organic cause.

▶ Associated symptoms indicative of underlying disease: Decreased body hair; gynecomastia; neuropathies; anxiety; headaches; vision changes; decreased circulation; excessive dryness or skin changes; changes in testicle size, consistency or shape; and changes in penis such as rash, discharge, or phimosis.

▶ Review past medical history for other diseases; testicular infections or insults; medications (Rx, OTC, and herbal); and history of smoking, drug, alcohol use.

Physical Exam

▶ Complete screening physical noting general appearance, generalized anxiety or hyperactivity, vital signs for postural hypotension, dry hair, loss of secondary sex characteristics, spider angiomas, hyperpigmentation, palmar erythema, or goiter.

▶ Chest, abdomen, and extremities for cardiac abnormalities, gynecomastia, aortic or femoral bruits, peripheral vascular deficits

▶ Genital examination for penile circulation, discharge, fibrosis or lesions; testicles for size, masses, varicoceles or atrophy; DRE for prostate abnormalities, sphincter tone, assess for Peyronie disease (penile plaques)

▶ Neurologic screening for cortical, brainstem, spinal, or peripheral neuropathies, noting especially bulbocavernosi reflex, cremasteric reflex, pinprick or light touch to genital and perianal area, focal tenderness of spine, vision abnormalities

Diagnostic Studies

▶ Key studies to screen for underlying etiology: Fasting serum glucose, prolactin, morning total testosterone level, CBC, urinalysis, and lipid profile

▶ If testicular atrophy is suspected, include luteinizing hormone and follicle-stimulating hormone.

▶ If hypothyroidism is suspected, measure TSH.

▶ Other tests are added depending on findings of history and physical and results of preliminary tests.

▶ Nocturnal penile tumescence and rigidity testing

▶ Urologist may include duplex ultrasonography, penile angiography, nerve conduction studies, or a trial injection of prostaglandin E1 phentolamine, and papaverine intracorporeally to assess vascular integrity, noting penile response.

Differential Diagnosis

Endocrine Origin

▶ Altered thyroxine

▶ Testosterone

▶ Prolactin

▶ Insulin

▶ Estrogen levels

Neurologic Origin

▶ Cortical

▶ Brainstem

▶ Spinal cord

▶ Peripheral neuropathies

Psychological

▶ Anxiety

▶ Depression

▶ Schizophrenia

▶ Personality or relationship problems

Vascular Origin

▶ Arterial insufficiency

▶ Venous insufficiency

▶ Cavernosal insufficiency

Structural

▶ Peyronie's disease

▶ Microphallus

▶ Hypospadias

▶ Scarring

▶ Trauma

Other

▶ Medication side effects

▶ Renal failure

▶ Zinc deficiency

Management

Nonpharmacologic Treatment

▶ Modify lifestyle: Stress reduction techniques; stop alcohol, drugs, and smoking

▶ Use of vacuum constriction device for men with venous disorders of the penis or nonresponsiveness to vasoactive injections

▶ Surgical treatment

Pharmacologic Treatment

▶ Sildenafil (Viagra): 25–50 mg 1 hour before desired erection (works within 30 min–4 hours) on an empty stomach, at least 2 hours before meals. Dose variable, dependent upon concurrent disease, age; may increase dosage up to 100 mg/day. Contraindicated for patient taking nitrites; used cautiously with unstable angina and history of stroke, MI. Side effects: Headache, flushing, nasal congestion from vasodilation; abnormalities in vision (color changes, light sensitivity, blurred vision), priapism.

▶ Tadalafil (Cialis): 5–20 mg at least 2 hours before sex; may take without regard to meals; may provide longer action (up to 36 hours)

▶ Vardenafil (Levitra): Usual daily dosage 5–20 mg 1 hour before sexual activity, on an empty stomach, at least 2 hours before meals; claims to provide faster onset, have fewer adverse effects

▶ Other oral agents controversial, include yohimbine, trazodone (Desyrel), ginkgo biloba

▶ Substitute or discontinue medications known to cause erectile dysfunction.

  ▹ Alternative antihypertensives include calcium channel blockers, angiotensin-converting enzyme (ACE) inhibitors, selective beta-blockers (atenolol).

  ▹ Trial of antidepressants other than tricyclics: Nortriptyline (Pamelor), desipramine (Norpramin)

  ▹ Substitute ranitidine (Zantac) or other H2 blocker for cimetidine (Tagamet)

▶ Treat abnormal hormones as follows:

  ▹ Insufficient testosterone treated with a 3-month testosterone trial (if indicated by androgen deficiency and patient does not have prostatic cancer), using testosterone injections 200 mg IM q 3 weeks or topical patches of 2.5–6 mg/day

  ▹ Hyperprolactinemia treated with bromocriptine (Parlodel) initially 2.5 mg b.i.d., up to 40 mg/day

▶ Penile injections such as alprostadil (Caverject), first dose in office setting 1.25–2.5 mcg with repeat dose after 1 hour if no response. Patient to remain in office until detumescence completed. Partial response may have 2nd injection in 24 hours.

▶ Alternatives to alprostadil (Edex) are papaverine (Papacon) or phentolamine (Rogitine).

▶ Urethral suppository of alprostadil (Muse) in various strength pellets

How Long to Treat

▶ Variable depending on treatment methods

Special Considerations

▶ Nitrates should be withheld for 24 hours after sildenafil or vardenafil administration and for 48 hours after use of tadalafil.

▶ Reasons for seeking care and etiology are age-related.

  ▹ Age adolescence to 30: Concerns often psychological or gender-related, as well as with primary organic origin

  ▹ Age 50–60 with relationship problems; most concerned about medical problems

  ▹ Age 70+ rarely seek help, most likely have physical problems

▶ Use of injections or oral agents requires thorough patient teaching on proper use, frequency of use, side effects, and risk of priapism, and when to seek medical help, such as erection lasting > 4 hours.

When to Consult, Refer, Hospitalize

▶ Patient should notify primary care provider for immediate attention if erection lasts > 4 hours.

▶ Psychotherapist for individual or couples therapy, sex therapy

▶ Urologist, endocrinologist, cardiologist, neurologist referrals as indicated by diagnosis and requirements for further evaluation or advanced treatment

Follow-up

▶ Varied, depending on diagnosis, underlying etiology, response to treatment, and need for therapy. Patients should be seen initially at shorter intervals to adjust and monitor responsiveness to treatment, then every 3 months.

Expected Course

▶ Improvement in many patients with oral medications, vacuum devices, suppository, and penile implants; 15% improve spontaneously

▶ 20% failure rate with vacuum device, 10%–30% dissatisfaction with penile implants

▶ Alprostadil injections have 85%–90% response rate; urethral suppository method rates are 40–60%; oral agent sildenafil is effective for 70% of patients at maximal dose..

Complications

▶ Variable, depending on underlying etiology and treatment method side effects: Priapism, penile bruising, hypotension, headache, flushing, nausea, side effects of testosterone (urinary retention, acne, vomiting), penile pain and irritation, and testicular pain

CASE STUDIES

CASE 1. A 17-year-old male is brought to your office by his mother complaining of several days of unilateral testicular pain and swelling thought to be caused by injury while wrestling with a friend. The patient is reluctant to give more information.

▶ How can you elicit more information from this patient?

▶ What additional information would you like?

Exam: Edematous, tender hemi-scrotum with indistinguishable, tender epididymis; positive Prehn's sign; positive cremasteric reflex; no urethral discharge; temp 101° F.

▶ Can testicular torsion be ruled out?

▶ What is the most likely diagnosis?

▶ Is diagnostic testing necessary to initiate treatment?

▶ What additional intervention is needed?

CASE 2. Parents bring in their 1-week-old, full-term male infant, reporting that his penis is red and swollen. He has been crying continuously since his bath several hours ago. Previously, the baby had been healthy; nursing well, gaining weight.

HPI: Previously healthy baby has been crying for several hours.

▶ What additional history would you like?

Exam: Unremarkable except for moderately edematous and reddened glans penis with retracted prepuce

▶ What is the differential diagnosis?

▶ How would you treat this patient?

▶ What follow-up is necessary?

▶ What infant care teaching do parents need?

CASE 3. A 67-year-old retired postal worker presents with a 3-month history of difficulty urinating. He denies urinary burning, hematuria, foul-smelling urine, or abdominal pain. He does complain of hesitancy, dribbling, and a sensation of still needing to urinate at the end of urination. He wakes up 2–3 times each night to urinate.

PMH: No history of UTIs, prostate issues, or renal disease. He worked as mail carrier for 30 years. He has been living a sedentary lifestyle since retirement 5 years ago. HTN was identified 3 years ago and treated until about 1 year ago, when he felt better and stopped his blood pressure medication. He has not return to his healthcare provider for follow-up. He does not smoke and drinks 3–4 beers a week.

▶ What additional history would you like to obtain?

Exam: BP 168/102, pulse 72 regular, afebrile. Abdomen: non-tender with no bladder distension; no CVA tenderness. DRE: Good sphincter tone; prostate smooth, firm, non-tender with obliteration of median sulcus.

▶ What diagnostic tests would you perform?

▶ What does the clinician need to know regarding the indicated diagnostic test necessary for this patient?

▶ Can you make a diagnosis?

▶ What is your treatment plan?

▶ What follow-up and screening recommendations would you give this patient?

REFERENCES

American Urological Association (AUA) Guidelines. (2012). *Guideline for the management of clinically localized prostate cancer.* Retrieved from www.auanet.org

American Urological Association (AUA) Guidelines. (2012). *Guideline on the management of benign prostatic hyperplasia (BPH).* Retrieved from www.auanet.org

American Urological Association (AUA) Guidelines. (2009). *Guideline on the management of erectile dysfunction: Diagnosis and treatment recommendations.* Retrieved from www.auanet.org

Boyle, P., & Brawley, O. W. (2009). Prostate cancer: Current evidence weighs against population screening. *CA: A Cancer Journal for Clinicians, 59,* 220–224.

Centers for Disease Control and Prevention. (2010). Sexually transmitted diseases treatment guidelines, 2010. *MMWR: Morbidity and Mortality Weekly Report, 59,* No. RR-12. Retrieved from www.cdc.gov/mmwr/preview/mmwrhtml/mm6131a3.htm?s_cid=mm6131a

Domino, F. J. (2013). *The 5-minute clinical consult.* St. Louis, MO: Lippincott Williams & Wilkins.

Edmunds, M. W., & Mayhew, M. S. (2009). *Pharmacology for the primary care provider* (3rd ed.). St. Louis, MO: Mosby.

Goroll, A., & Mulley, A. (2009). *Primary care medicine: Office evaluation and management of the adult patient* (6th ed.). Philadelphia: Lippincott Williams & Wilkins.

Hatcher, R., Trussell, J., Nelson, A., Cates, W., Kowal, D., & Policar, M. S. (2011). *Contraceptive technology* (20th ed. rev.). New York: Ardent Media Trade.

Heidelbaugh, J. J. (2010). Management of erectile dysfunction. *American Family Physician, 81,* 305–312.

Hutson, J. M., Balic, A., Nation, T., & Southwell, B. (2010). Cryptorchidism. *Seminars in Pediatric Surgery, 19,* 215–224.

Kapoor, S. (2008) Testicular torsion: A race against time. *International Journal of Clinical Practice, 62,* 821–827.

Lao, O., Fitzgibbons, R., & Cusick, R. (2012). Pediatric inguinal hernias, hydroceles, and undescended testicles. *Surgical Clinics of North America, 92*(3), 487–504.

Lipsky, B. A., Byren, I., & Hoey, C. T. (2010). Treatment of bacterial prostatitis. *Clinical Infectious Diseases, 50,* 1641–1652.

McAninch, J. W., & Lue, T. F. (2013). *Smith & Tanagho's general urology* (18th ed.). New York: McGraw-Hill.

Motzer, R. J., Agarwal, N., & Beard, C. (2009). National Comprehensive Cancer Network (NCCN) Clinical practice guidelines in oncology: Testicular cancer. *Journal of the National Comprehensive Cancer Network, 7,* 672–693.

National Comprehensive Cancer Network. (2009). *Clinical practice guidelines: Prostate cancer.* Retrieved from www.nccn.org

National Comprehensive Cancer Network. (2011). *Clinical practice guidelines: Testicular cancer.* Retrieved from www.nccn.org/professionals/physician_gls/f_guidelines.asp#site

Neal, R. H., & Keister, D. (2009). What's best for your patient with BPH? *Journal of Family Practice, 58,* 241–247.

Tracy, C. R., Steers, W. D., & Costabile, R. (2008). Diagnosis and management of epididymitis. *Urologic Clinics of North America, 35,* 101–108.

Trojian, T. H., Lishnak, T. S., & Heiman, D. (2009). Epididymitis and orchitis: An overview. *American Family Physician, 79,* 583–587.

U.S. Preventive Services Task Force. (2012). *Screening for prostate cancer: U.S. Preventive Services Task Force Recommendation Statement.* Retrieved from www.uspreventiveservicestaskforce.org/prostatecancerscreening/prostatefinalrs.htm

U.S. Preventive Services Task Force. (2008). *U.S. Preventive Services Task Force grade definitions.* Retrieved from www.uspreventiveservicestaskforce.org/uspstf/grades.htm

SEXUALLY TRANSMITTED INFECTIONS

Debra Shearer, EdD, MSN, FNP-BC

GENERAL APPROACH

Description

▶ Sexually transmitted infections (STIs) are also known as sexually transmitted diseases.

▶ 20 million new infections annually in the United States

▶ On January 18, 2013, the Food and Drug Administration (FDA) announced a shortage of doxycycline, which is recommended for chlamydia, nongonococcal urethritis, epididymitis, and pelvic inflammatory disease, as well as an alternative treatment for syphilis when there is penicillin allergy. Tetracycline is not available.

Prevention

▶ Counsel the adolescent or adult patient regarding sexual abstinence, the only certain method of prevention; followed by mutual monogamy,

▶ Consistent use of the male latex condom is highly protective if used consistently and correctly (see Chapter 12).

▶ Use of female condoms and other barrier methods of contraception for women may be somewhat protective against some, but not all, STIs.

▶ Safer sex practices are aimed at reducing risk of HIV transmission for patients at highest risk through partner reduction and avoidance of certain practices (see Chapter 4).

Risk Assessment

▶ Risk assessments and screening tests help reduce the incidence of STI and must be done on every sexually active adult and adolescent patient.

▶ Adolescents are at a higher risk for STIs.

▶ Obtain accurate, detailed history from patients to determine risk for STIs. Most people do not know they are infected with STI and underestimate their own risk level. Ask specific questions regarding type of sexual exposure in "lay terms" in order to obtain accurate information. Maintain confidentiality by asking partners and parents to leave the room. No parental consent is needed for adolescents to seek treatment for STI; the age of consent for adolescents varies by state.

▶ High-risk factors for STI are current STI(s), including HIV and history of STI(s); multiple sexual partners (or a new partner); exchanging sex for money or drugs; drug user or partner of drug user; homosexual or bisexual men and their partners; and lack of consistent use of barrier contraceptives.

Screening

▶ Routine steps for all sexually active (ever) women and men:

  » Explain importance and context of screening, since many STIs are asymptomatic: "We review this information and screen all patients because many people with infections do not have symptoms and therefore have no idea that testing might be needed. Routine review is recommended by the CDC."

  » Give prevention information and encourage wise decisions and prevention behavior.

  » Review personal history for high-risk behaviors.

  » Provide annual *Chlamydia* test for men and women ≤ 25 years (urine or swab).

  » Women age 21–29 should have a Pap test every 3 years.

  » Women age 30–65 should have a Pap test every 3 years and co-test for cervical cytology and high-risk human papillomavirus (HPV) every 5 years.

  » Provide annual gonorrhea test if in an area of high *Gonococci* (GC) prevalence and age ≤ 25 years.

  » If in an area with high syphilis prevalence and age ≤ 25 years, or high-risk behavior, initial syphilis serology.

▶ Routine steps for high-risk women and men should include offering and encouraging HIV testing, reviewing history, and providing hepatitis B vaccination.

▶ Patients with known STI exposure or symptoms should be cultured from areas of exposure or penetration (e.g., anal, vaginal, oral pharyngeal, penile, or urethral), then treated.

▶ Routine screening in < 25 years (high-risk) pregnant women in first trimester should include syphilis serologic test, hepatitis B antigen, GC; offer HIV test, Pap smear. Repeat screening for high-risk women in third trimester or at delivery: Syphilis, hepatitis B antigen, GC and *Chlamydia,* and bacterial vaginosis (BV).

Management

▶ Follow Centers for Disease Control and Prevention on treatment guidelines for gonoccal infections (including 2011 update) for evaluation and management of all STIs.

▶ With patients who are likely not to return for follow-up, consider empiric treatment with CDC-recommended one-dose regimen when appropriate.

▶ Patients treated for STI should be counseled to have their sexual partners evaluated and treated.

▶ Sexually active patients should be counseled regarding dual protection against unintended pregnancy and STIs. The male latex condom is effective in providing dual protection if used correctly.

RED FLAGS

▶ Consult, refer, or hospitalize with unusual presentation of STI; serious complication such as PID, pregnancy, HIV infection, recurrent infection, unable to tolerated oral medication, allergy to medication

▶ Refer to infectious disease specialist for pregnant women with hepatitis B virus (HBV), primary cytomegalovirus (CMV), primary genital herpes, or Group B streptococcal infection, and women with syphilis and allergic to penicillin.

▶ With STIs in pediatric or adolescent populations, suspect child abuse.

▶ If patient reports sexual assault, consult local law authorities regarding procedures for obtaining evidence. Test for *Trichomonas vaginalis,* bacterial vaginosis, yeast, *Chlamydia,* GC, HIV, hepatitis B, and syphilis. Empiric antimicrobial regimen for *Chlamydia,* gonorrhea, *Trichomonas,* and BV is suggested, as well as prophylactic treatment for Hep B, pregnancy testing, and emergency contraception, if indicated.

INFECTIONS THAT CAUSE VAGINITIS AND CERVICITIS IN WOMEN AND URETHRITIS IN MEN

TRICHOMONIASIS

Description

▶ An inflammatory process of the vagina, cervix, and vulva in women and lower genitourinary tract in man caused by a flagellate protozoan

Etiology

▶ The causative organism is *Trichomonas vaginalis.*

▶ Usually sexually transmitted; *rarely* transmitted by fomites

▶ Men can be asymptomatic carriers.

Incidence and Demographics

▶ Estimated 6 million women and partners infected annually

Risk Factors

▶ Risk factors listed under General Approach

Prevention and Screening

▶ Prevention listed in General Approach

▶ No routine screening

▶ Trichomoniasis screening should be conducted yearly for HIV-infected women

Assessment

History

▶ Incubation period is 4–20 days with an average of 1 week

▶ Women

  » May be asymptomatic

  » Severe pruritus; malodorous, profuse, gray-yellow or green vaginal discharge

  » Dysuria, dyspareunia, postcoital spotting, possible menorrhagia and dysmenorrhea

  » Onset of symptoms following menses

▶ Men

  » Usually asymptomatic

  » Dysuria, clear penile discharge, slight penile itching

Physical Exam

▶ Women

  » May have inguinal adenopathy

  » External genitalia may be irritated from scratching.

  » Vulva is erythematous and edematous.

  » Introitus, urethra, vagina, and cervix are coated with profuse malodorous, frothy, gray-yellow or green discharge.

  » Cervix or vagina has petechiae or strawberry patches appearance (characteristic).

▶ Men

  » Slight penile erythema with clear discharge

Diagnostic Studies

▶ Women

  » Saline wet mount of vaginal discharge to identify motile trichomonads

  » Vaginal pH > 4.5; Pap smear sometimes shows trichomonads

  » Potassium hydroxide (KOH) wet mount to rule out *Candida albicans;* positive whiff test (fishy odor) when KOH applied in BV

▶ Men

  » Microscopic exam of urine (first void in morning) positive for trichomonads

Differential Diagnosis

- Bacterial vaginosis
- Vulvovaginal candidiasis
- Gonorrhea
- Pelvic inflammatory disease (PID)
- *Chlamydia trachomatis*

Management

Nonpharmacologic Treatment

- Concurrent treatment of sex partners
- Patients and sex partners should avoid sex until treatment completed and asymptomatic
- Screen for other STIs.
- Avoid alcohol with metronidazole (Flagyl) and for 72 hours after due to disulfiram-like reaction (severe nausea and vomiting).

Pharmacologic Treatment

- First treatment choice: Metronidazole (Flagyl) 2 g p.o. as single dose or tinadazole (Tindamax) 2 g p.o. as a single dose
- Alternative: Metronidazole (Flagyl) 500 mg p.o. b.i.d.

How Long to Treat

- Single dose or 7-day regimen; if regimen fails and patient remains symptomatic, re-treat with metronidazole (Flagyl) 500 mg p.o. b.i.d. for 7 more days or tinidzaole (Tindamax) 2 g in a single dose. If there is frequent treatment failure, treat with metronidazole (Flagyl) 2 g p.o. daily for 3–5 days; consider culture for possible resistant stain of *T. vaginalis.*

Special Considerations

- Pregnancy: Metronidazole (Flagyl) 2 g p.o. in a single dose
- Allergy to metronidazole: There is no effective alternative. Clotrimazole (Lotrimin) may inhibit growth of *T. vaginalis* but does not eradicate it.

When to Consult, Refer, Hospitalize

- Consult on refractory cases not responding to treatment in 2 weeks.

Follow-up

- None indicated if asymptomatic following treatment
- Evaluate the patient's sex partner.

Expected Course

- Response prompt, although symptoms will return with re-infection

Complications

▶ Nausea or vomiting from oral metronidazole, disulfiram-like reaction from ingestion of alcohol and metronidazole, vulvovaginal candidiasis infection following 7-day treatment course

▶ Associated with preterm labor and premature rupture of membranes

▶ Pelvic inflammatory disease, bartholinitis, skenitis, cystitis

GONORRHEA

Description

▶ A sexually transmitted bacterial infection caused by *Neisseria gonorrhoeae*

Etiology

▶ *Neisseria gonorrhoeae* is a Gram-negative diplococci present in exudate and secretions of infected mucous secretions occurring only in humans.

▶ Causes localized inflammatory conditions: Urethritis, epididymitis, proctitis, cervicitis, bartholinitis, pelvic inflammatory disease (salpingitis or endometritis), and pharyngitis in adults; vulvovaginitis in children; and conjunctivitis in newborns and adults; presence in children almost always a result of child sexual abuse

▶ Gonococcal bacteremia results in the disseminated systemic condition; arthritis-dermatitis syndrome sometimes associated with endocarditis or meningitis

Incidence and Demographics

▶ Transmission through intimate contact such as sexual intercourse; also parturition

▶ 60%–90% of women become infected following exposure.

▶ Greatest incidence in sexually active 15–29-year-olds

▶ Approximately 15% of infected women may develop PID with possible sterility if untreated.

▶ Most infections in men have symptoms that cause them to seek treatment before serious outcome. Many infected women do not have symptoms until complications are present.

▶ Common sites in women are the urethra, endocervix, upper genital tract, pharynx, and rectum.

▶ Common sites in men are the urethra, epididymis, prostate, rectum, and pharynx.

Risk Factors

▶ Risk factors listed under General Approach

▶ Homosexual males have 10× greater incidence.

Prevention and Screening

▶ Prevention methods listed under General Approach

▶ Yearly screening for sexually active and women ≤ 25 years if in an area of high GC prevalence

▶ Yearly screening for sexually active gay men, bisexual men, and men who have sex with men. Screen more frequently for men who have sex with multiple men or anonymous partners.

▶ Screen all pregnant women at initial prenatal visit and again early in third trimester.

▶ Prophylactic treatment to contacts of infectious patients

Assessment

History

▶ Incubation is short: Urethritis is 2–5 days, cervicitis is 5–10 days.

▶ Women: Often asymptomatic; dysuria, frequency, purulent urethral discharge, vaginal discharge, pelvic pain, spotting or abnormal menses; adolescent girls often have dissemination or progression within a week of menses

▶ Male: Could be asymptomatic; dysuria, urinary frequency, copious purulent (blood-tinged) penile discharge, testicular pain. Rectal symptoms: Erythematous, discharge, pain with defecation.

▶ Both may have conjunctivitis or pharyngitis as well.

Physical Exam

▶ Women: Purulent discharge from cervix, inflammation of Bartholin's glands; positive cervical motion tenderness (CMT) and signs of PID if untreated

▶ Men: Purulent urethral discharge, signs of prostatitis or epididymitis if untreated

▶ Disseminated gonorrhea: Stage 1, bacteremia with chills, fever, skin lesions (petechial or pustular skin rash); endocarditis or meningitis may occur; Stage 2, septic arthritis; knees, ankles, and wrists show erythema, edema, and pain.

Diagnostic Studies

▶ Cervical or urethral culture for *N. gonorrhoeae* using modified Thayer-Martin media

▶ Nucleic acid amplification test on first-void urine in men can be used in women but is less accurate

▶ DNA probe (can diagnose gonorrhea and chlamydia) for men and women

Differential Diagnosis

▶ PID

▶ Nongonococcal cervicitis

▶ Urethritis

▶ Proctitis

▶ Nongonococcal pharyngitis

▶ *Chlamydia* infections

▶ Arthritis

▶ Vaginitis

Management

Pharmacologic Treatment

▶ Uncomplicated gonococcal infections (genital, rectal and pharyngeal)

- Ceftriaxone (Rocephin) 250 mg IM in a single dose *and* azithromycin 1 g orally in a single dose or doxycycline 100 mg orally twice daily for 7 days

- If ceftrixone is not available:

  ▷ Cefixime 400 mg orally, plus either azithromycin 1 g orally or doxycycline 100 mg orally for 7 days is recommended

  ▷ Azithromycin 2 g dose orally for severe allergy to cephalosporins

  ▷ CDC recommends test of cure if alternative regimen is used.

▶ Mild to moderate PID treated as an outpatient: Ceftriaxone (Rocephin) 250 mg IM in a single dose plus doxycycline 100 mg p.o. b.i.d. for 14 days

▶ Gonococcal conjunctivitis: Lavage of infected eye with saline solution once, plus:

- Ceftriaxone (Rocephin) 1 g IM × 1 dose

- Neonates: 25–50 mg/kg IM or IV × 1 dose not to exceed 125 mg

- Infants with gonococcal conjunctivitis: Ceftriaxone (Rocephin) 25–50 mg/kg IV or IM, not to exceed 125 mg in a single dose

- Gonococcal infection in children who weigh > 45 kg: Treat the same as adults.

- Gonococcal infection in children who weigh < 45 kg: Ceftriaxone 125 mg IM in a single dose

Special Considerations

▶ Pregnant women should be treated with a cephalosporin; erythromycin or amoxicillin can be used for presumptive or diagnosed *Chlamydia* infection.

▶ Pregnant and lactating women should not be treated with quinolones or tetracycline. If a pregnant woman cannot tolerate cephalosporins, treat with spectinomycin (Tobicin) 2 g IM × 1 dose alone (not currently available in the U.S.) with effective *Chlamydia* regimen.

▶ All infants born with neonatal ophthalmia should be observed for gonococcal sepsis and disseminated infection.

When to Consult, Refer, Hospitalize

▶ Hospitalize for disseminated gonorrhea.

▶ Hospitalize for severe PID.

▶ Refer patients unresponsive to treatment.

Follow-up

▶ Retest in 1–2 months following treatment if symptomatic.

Expected Course

▶ Usually there is prompt response to therapy.

Complications

▶ PID, sterility, salpingitis, epididymitis, prostatitis, disseminated gonococcal infection

▶ Perinatal postabortal endometritis and salpingitis, acute salpingitis, increased incidence of premature rupture of membranes, preterm delivery, chorioamnionitis, neonatal sepsis, postpartum sepsis, neonatal conjunctivitis

▶ May help facilitate HIV transmission

CHLAMYDIAL INFECTION

Description

▶ A sexually transmitted infection caused by *Chlamydia trachomatis*

Etiology

▶ *C. trachomatis* is an obligate intracellular parasite; transmission is by sexual or perinatal contact.

▶ Infection in women may ascend from cervicitis and urethritis to salpingitis and spread vertically to cause proctitis; in men, it may ascend the urogenital tract to epididymis and prostate.

Incidence and Demographics

▶ The most common sexually transmitted infection; prevalence is highest in persons age < 25.

▶ 4 million cases per year, prevalence 3–4 times greater than GC

▶ Leading cause of infertility, ectopic pregnancy, and PID; reportable to local health authority, case report required in most U.S. states.

Risk Factors

▶ Risk factors listed under General Approach

▶ Presence of concomitant STI, especially *N. gonorrhoeae*

Prevention and Screening

▶ Prevention methods listed under General Approach

▶ Annually screen sexually active men and women ≤ 25 years.

▶ When treating gonococcal infections, include treatment against possible co-infection with *C. trachomatis.*

▶ Screen pregnant women initially and repeat in the third trimester for high-risk women.

Assessment

History

▶ Incubation 6–14 days

▶ May be asymptomatic

▶ Women: Increase in mucopurulent vaginal discharge, low pelvic discomfort, dysuria, urinary frequency, spotting, and possibly dyspareunia; incubation period usually 1 week

▶ Men: Mucopurulent urethra discharge or dysuria

Physical Exam

▶ Cervix is friable, mucopurulent discharge; may have positive cervical motion tenderness, adnexal or uterine tenderness if untreated

▶ Occasional inguinal lymphadenopathy

Diagnostic Studies

▶ *Chlamydia* culture is definitive test but expensive

▶ DNA probe

▶ Nucleic acid amplification (PCR and LCR) in men on first-void urine; can also be used in women but less accurate

Differential Diagnosis

▶ PID   ▶ Gonorrhea   ▶ Salpingitis   ▶ Urethritis

Management

Nonpharmacologic Treatment

▶ Sexual partners should be evaluated and treated.

▶ Patients should abstain from sexual intercourse until they and their sex partners have completed treatment: 7 days following single-dose treatment or after completion of a 7-day regimen.

Pharmacologic Treatment

▶ First choice: Azithromycin (Zithromax) 1 g p.o. single dose *or* doxycycline (Vibramycin) 100 mg p.o. b.i.d.

▶ Alternative choice: Erythromycin base 500 mg p.o. q.i.d. for 7 days *or* ofloxacin (Floxin) 300 mg p.o. b.i.d. *or* erythromycin ethylsuccinate 800 mg p.o. q.i.d.

How Long to Treat

▶ Single dose of azithromycin or 7-day course of treatment with all others

Special Considerations

▶ Neonatal ophthalmia and pneumonia may occur in infant born to infected mother; consult and treat with erythromycin IV.

▶ Doxycycline, ofloxacin, and erythromycin estolate contraindicated in pregnancy

▶ Ofloxacin contraindicated in patients < 17 years

▶ Pregnancy: Azithromycin 1 g p.o. in a single dose or amoxicillin 500 mg p.o. t.i.d.

▶ Children 6 months to 12 years with uncomplicated genital tract infection: Erythromycin 50 mg/kg/day divided q.i.d. × 7 days

When to Consult, Refer, Hospitalize

▶ Consult with physician for PID in pregnant women, recurrent infection, conjunctivitis, or neonatal infection.

Follow-up

▶ Not necessary if symptoms resolve with treatment with doxycycline, azithromycin, or ofloxacin

▶ If treated with erythromycin, reculture in about 3 weeks after initial treatment may be needed if symptoms persist or re-infection suspected

▶ Pregnant women need repeat cultures 3 weeks after therapy completion due to high noncompliance rate and lower efficacy of erythromycin regimens.

Expected Course

▶ Prompt resolution of symptoms

▶ May become re-infected if sexual partners are not treated

Complications

▶ PID, infertility, increased incidence of ectopic pregnancy; may help facilitate HIV transmission

MUCOPURULENT CERVICITIS

Description

▶ A sexually transmitted syndrome characterized by purulent discharge visualized on the cervix or in the endocervical canal, endocervical swab, or sustained endocervical bleeding easily induced by gentle passage of a cotton swab through the cervical os

Etiology

▶ May be caused by *C. trachomatis* and *N. gonorrhoeae*; ⅓ of cases, agent cannot be established

▶ Ureaplasma (related to *Mycoplasma hominis*) may be the responsible organism.

Incidence and Demographics

▶ Common in sexually active, especially young, women

Risk Factors

▶ Same as for *Chlamydia* and gonorrhea

▶ May be associated with frequent douching or exposure to chemical irritants

Prevention and Screening

▶ Prevention methods listed under General Approach

▶ Screening for *Chlamydia* and gonorrhea (see General Approach)

Assessment

History

▶ Often asymptomatic, abnormal vaginal discharge, vaginal bleeding postcoital

Physical Exam

▶ Cervix has purulent or mucopurulent exudate and is friable.

Diagnostic Studies

▶ DNA probe to test for gonorrhoea and *Chlamydia*

▶ Wet mount exam to test for *Trichomonas*

▶ A finding of leukorrhea (> 10 WBC/high power field) on wet mount has been associated with chlamydial and gonococcal infection of the cervix.

▶ Urine for culture and sensitivity

Differential Diagnosis

▶ *Gonorrhoeae*

▶ UTI

▶ *Trichomonas*

▶ *Chlamydia*

▶ PID

Management

Pharmacologic Treatment

▶ Treat according to suspicion for chlamydia, gonorrhea, or both. Wait for test results if prevalence of both organisms is low and chance for follow-up is good.

▶ See treatment for gonococcal and chlamydial infections.

How Long to Treat

▶ Treatment for chlamydia and gonorrhea single dose to 7 days per CDC guidelines

Special Considerations

▶ Treat pregnant women with cephalosporin, erythromycin, or amoxicillin, not with quinolones or tetracycline.

When to Consult, Refer, Hospitalize

▶ Consult for recurrent infection.

Follow-up

▶ Recommended for gonorrhea or chlamydia as appropriate

▶ If symptoms persist, patient should refrain from sexual activity and return for evaluation.

▶ Sexual partners should be examined and treated for STIs.

Expected Course

▶ Prompt response to treatment is expected.

Complications

▶ Depending on organism, same as for gonococcal or chlamydial infections

NONGONOCOCCAL URETHRITIS (NGU)

Description

▶ Inflammation of the urethra caused by a nongonorrheal infection characterized by mucopurulent or purulent discharge and burning

Etiology

▶ NGU if Gram-negative intracellular organisms are not identified on Gram stain

▶ *C. Trachomatis* is the major cause (23%–55%).

▶ Etiology of non-chlamydial NGU is unknown; however, *Ureaplasma urealyticum* and possible *Mycoplasma genitalium* may be present in as many as one third of cases

▶ Sometimes *Trichomonas vaginalis* and herpes simplex virus (HSV) cause NGU.

Incidence and Demographics

▶ Most common STI syndrome in males living in industrialized countries

▶ NGU more common than gonococcal urethritis in most areas of U.S.

▶ Proportion of NGU cases caused by *Chlamydia* has been declining gradually.

Risk Factors

▶ Risk factors listed under General Approach

Prevention and Screening

▶ Prevention methods listed under General Approach

▶ Screening for gonorrhea and chlamydia (see General Approach)

Assessment

History

▶ Patient reports urethral discharge that is purulent or mucopurulent, dysuria, urethral itching

▶ Recent unprotected sexual activity or new sex partner

Physical Exam

▶ Urethra erythematous and positive for purulent or mucopurulent discharge

Diagnostic Studies

▶ Gram stain of urethral secretions has ≥ 5 WBCs/oil immersion field without intracellular Gram-negative diplococci

▶ Positive leukocyte esterase test on first-void urine, or microscopic exam of first-void urine positive for > 10 WBCs/high power field

▶ DNA probe test for *N. gonorrhoeae* and *C. trachomatis*

▶ Nucleic acid amplification test for *Gonorrhoeae* and *Chlamydia* on urine sample

Differential Diagnosis

▶ Gonorrhea   ▶ UTI   ▶ Trichomoniasis

Management

Nonpharmacologic Treatment

▶ Sexual partners should be evaluated and treated appropriately.

Pharmacologic Treatment

▶ Defer treatment if no confirmation of urethritis, until results of DNA probe are back.

▶ Treat for *Chlamydia* (see Chlamydial Infection) as indicated.

▶ Empiric treatment of symptoms for high-risk patients if unlikely to return for follow-up.

▶ Empiric treatment covers infection with *Gonorrhoeae* and *Chlamydia* (refer to those entries).

How Long to Treat

▶ Treatment should be initiated immediately after diagnosis.

▶ A single dose is preferable due to better compliance; other regimens, treat for 7 days.

Special Considerations

▶ None

When to Consult, Refer, Hospitalize

▶ Refer for persistent or recurrent urethritis following adequate treatment.

Follow-up

▶ None necessary if resolves

▶ All sexual partners within the preceding 60 days should be referred for evaluation.

Expected Course

▶ Symptoms should be alleviated soon after treatment initiated.

Complications

▶ Epididymitis, prostatitis, Reiter syndrome, may help facilitate HIV transmission

PELVIC INFLAMMATORY DISEASE, CANDIDIASIS, BACTERIAL VAGINOSIS

See Chapter 11, Female Reproductive Disorders.

VIRAL INFECTIONS

GENITAL HERPES SIMPLEX VIRUS (HSV) INFECTION

Description

▶ Genital infection with primarily type 2 herpes simplex virus (HSV) and, less often, type 1 herpes simplex virus

▶ May present as a primary, latent, or recurrent disease

▶ No cure

Etiology

▶ HSV infection is transmitted through direct contact with mucous membranes and secretions.

▶ Primary infection causes local viral replication, seeding of regional neural ganglia, and possible viremia.

▶ Herpes viruses establish lifelong latency in neural ganglia and periodically reactivate.

▶ Up to 50% of first-episode cases of genital herpes are caused by HSV-1, but recurrences and subclinical shedding are much less frequent for genital HSV-1 infection than genital HSV-2 infection.

▶ Many HSV-2–infected people have not received a diagnosis of genital herpes and are unaware of transmission.

Incidence and Demographics

▶ 50 million people are infected with herpes in the United States.

▶ HSV is endemic in the U.S., with 776,000 new cases per year.

▶ 16.2% of people age 14–49 years have HSV infection.

▶ The highest frequency is in 15- to 29-year-olds.

▶ The incidence of primary or recurrent herpes is about 10% of pregnant women.

▶ Perinatal transmission occurs in 1:3,200 live births with 60% infant mortality.

Risk Factors

▶ Listed under General Approach

Prevention and Screening

▶ Prevention methods listed under General Approach; however, condoms may not block transmission of some lesions.

▶ Infected people should abstain from all sexual activity when lesions or prodromal symptoms are present.

▶ Sexual transmission of HSV can occur during asymptomatic periods. Asymptomatic viral shedding is more frequent in genital HSV-2 infection than genital HSV-1 infection and is most frequent during the first 12 months after acquiring HSV-2.

▶ Advise use of condoms during all sexual exposures; however, may not eliminate possibility of transmission

▶ Patients should be informed about the risks of neonatal infection.

▶ No routine screening

Assessment

History

▶ Genital lesions (occurring 2–14 days after exposure), which are painful papules followed by vesicles, ulceration, crusting, and healing

▶ First-episode symptoms consist of hyperesthesias, burning, itching, dysuria, pain, and tenderness in genital area; fever, myalgia, malaise, lymphadenopathy. Healing of initial lesions takes up to 21 days (average = 12 days).

▶ Recurrent episodes usually have prodrome (unusual sensation in area before eruption of lesions), recur in same region, and length of shedding is reduced (average 7 days). Healing occurs in approximately 5 days.

Physical Exam

▶ Examination of genital area for characteristic herpetic lesions: Tender vesicles on erythematous bases or ulcers in various stages of progression

▶ Enlarged lymph nodes in inguinal area

Diagnostic Studies

▶ Viral detection or culture from early lesion or vesicle is most sensitive and permits viral typing, which is helpful for prognostic information (HSV-1 has much lower risk for symptomatic recurrent outbreaks).

Differential Diagnosis

▶ Syphilis

▶ Chancroid

▶ *Molluscum contagiosum*

▶ Folliculitis

▶ Trauma, burn

Management

Nonpharmacologic Treatment

▶ Cool perineal compresses, sitz baths, loose-fitting clothes to help alleviate pain

▶ Good handwashing and hygiene to reduce autoinoculation to other body regions

Pharmacologic Treatment

▶ Topical acyclovir is less effective than oral; use is discouraged.

▶ First episode: Acyclovir (Zovirax) 400 mg p.o. b.i.d. *or* famciclovir (Famvir) 250 mg p.o. b.i.d. *or* valacyclovir (Valtrex) 1 g p.o. b.i.d. Treat 7–10 days.

▶ Recurrent infection: Acyclovir 400 mg p.o. t.i.d. × 5 days *or* acyclovir 800 mg p.o. b.i.d. × 5 days *or* acyclovir 800 mg p.o. t.i.d. × 2 days, *or* famciclovir 125 mg p.o. b.i.d. × 5 days *or* famciclovir 1,000 mg p.o. b.i.d. × 1 day

▶ Analgesics such as acetaminophen, NSAIDs, and topical astringents

How Long to Treat

▶ For first episode: 7–10 days or longer if lesions not completely healed

▶ For recurrent episode: 1–5 days

▶ Daily suppressive therapy; after 1 year of therapy, consider discontinuation to assess rate of recurrent episodes.

▶ For episodic recurrent infection, start treatment during prodrome or within 1 day after onset of lesions.

Special Considerations

▶ HIV+ or immunocompromised: Acyclovir 400–800 mg p.o. t.i.d. *or* famciclovir 500 mg p.o. b.i.d. *or* Valacyclovir 500 mg p.o. b.i.d. until clinically resolved; if severe, treat as for severe infection. If resistance suspected, consult with HIV specialist.

▶ All acyclovir-resistant strains are also resistant to valacyclovir; most are resistant to famciclovir.

▶ First clinical episode during pregnancy may be treated with acyclovir. Safety of acyclovir, valacyclovir, and famciclovir in pregnancy not established; benefits must outweigh risks.

▶ Prophylactic administration of acyclovir intrapartum for women with a history of HSV is not recommended.

▶ Cesarean delivery not always necessary with history of herpes, only recommended when active lesions visible at onset of labor

▶ Signs of congenital infection may occur from birth to 4–6 weeks (vesicles around eyes, mouth, skin; respiratory distress; central nervous system [CNS] infection; sepsis)

When to Consult, Refer, Hospitalize

▶ Consult if pregnant, serious infection, or infections resistant to treatment

▶ Hospitalize if suspected encephalitis, pneumonitis, or hepatitis, or congenital infection

Follow-up

Expected Course

▶ Most symptoms reduce promptly.

▶ Usually none indicated unless severe recurrent episodes and treatment inadequate

Complications

▶ Encephalitis, blindness, pneumonitis, hepatitis, perinatal transmission

HUMAN PAPILLOMAVIRUS INFECTION

Description

▶ Infection with certain subtypes of the human papillomavirus (HPV or genital warts) causing flat, papular, or pedunculated growths on the genital mucosa

▶ Visible warts are known as condyloma acuminata.

Etiology

▶ Virus enters body during sexual activity, via an epithelial defect, and infects stratified squamous epithelium of lower genital tract; visible genital warts are usually caused by HPV types 6 or 11

▶ HPV infection usually persists throughout patient's life in dormant state and becomes infectious intermittently; generally benign, may be asymptomatic or cause minor symptoms

▶ Highly contagious; 90%–100% of male partners of infected women become infected, mostly subclinically

▶ HPV infections with types 16, 18, and 31 strongly associated with cervical dysplasia

▶ HPV implicated in epithelial cancers, especially anorectal carcinoma, vulvar or penile cancer

Incidence and Demographics

▶ 79 million men and women are currently infected with HPV.

▶ 14 million men and women are infected annually.

▶ About 360,000 people are infected with genital warts yearly.

▶ More than 40 HPV types can infect the male and female genital area.

▶ Prevalent in females 14–59 years of age

▶ Most common viral STI in the U.S.

Risk Factors

▶ Risk factors listed under General Approach

▶ Early coitus and lack of barrier methods for contraception

▶ Growth of warts may be stimulated by oral contraceptives, pregnancy, or immunosuppression.

Prevention and Screening

▶ Prevention methods listed under General Approach; however, condoms may not eliminate risk of transmission entirely; patient with HPV still infectious even after warts removed

▶ Screening of women through annual Pap smear

▶ Gardasil, a quadrivalent vaccine against HPV types 6, 11, 16, and 18, recommended for males and females age 9–26

▶ Cervarix, a bivalent vaccine against HPV types 16 and 18, recommended for females ages 10–25; not recommended for males

Assessment

History

▶ Usually asymptomatic or can cause palpable lesion, itching, burning, local pain, or bleeding

▶ Significant lesions in some people

▶ May be unknown history of contact; incubation period from weeks to a year or longer

Physical Exam

▶ Small, flesh-colored, wart-like lesions; some can become confluent as one large wart

▶ Some warts flat or difficult to visualize, others are vegetative growths

▶ Women: Warts seen on labia, perianal areas, vagina, cervix, or mouth

▶ Men: Warts seen on shaft of penis, penile meatus, scrotum, perianal areas, and mouth

Diagnostic Studies

▶ Most warts are diagnosed by visualization. Applying 3%–5% acetic acid to the vulva of a woman or penis of a man to reveal white coloring of lesions (called acetowhitening).

▶ Pap smear on women detects koilocytosis, indicative of HPV.

▶ Should test for concomitant STIs: HIV, gonorrhea, syphilis, chlamydia

▶ Biopsy for detection of viral DNA available but not used clinically

Differential Diagnosis

▶ Condyloma latum

▶ Neoplasm

▶ Granuloma inguinale

▶ Moles

▶ Herpes simplex

▶ Syphilis

▶ Folliculitis

▶ Skin tags

▶ Keratosis

▶ Scabetic nodules

Management

Nonpharmacologic Treatment

▶ Smoking is a co-factor for cervical cancer with HPV; encourage cessation for woman infected with HPV.

▶ Examination of sexual partners is not recommended, since partner's role in re-infection is minimal.

▶ Encourage continued use of condoms.

Pharmacologic Treatment

▶ Drugs treat symptoms and may decrease size of wart; no treatment available that completely eradicates virus

▶ External/perianal warts

▷ Patient-applied podofilox (Condylox) 0.5% solution or gel (apply b.i.d. × 3 days, then off 4 days); may repeat cycle total of 4 times *or*

▷ Imiquimod (Aldara) 5% cream: Apply q.h.s. 3× week; wash off after 6–10 hours. May use up to 16 weeks, may clear in 8–10 weeks.

▷ Provider-administered cryotherapy with liquid nitrogen, may repeat every 1–2 weeks

▷ Provider-administered podophyllin (Podofin)10%–25% in compound tincture of benzoin (wash off thoroughly 1–4 hours after application); repeat weekly if necessary *or*

▷ Provider-administered trichloroacetic acid (TCA) 80%–90%; apply only to warts. Powder with talc or baking soda to remove acid. Repeat weekly if necessary.

How Long to Treat

▶ Depending on the size of wart and response to treatment, could take one to several treatments

Special Considerations

▶ Pregnancy: Podophyllin, imiquimod, podofilox are contraindicated.

▶ Some specialists recommend removal of visible warts during pregnancy.

▶ HIV patients may not respond well to treatment.

When to Consult, Refer, Hospitalize

▶ Vaginal and cervical warts: Consult with gynecologist; dysplasia must be excluded before treatment instituted.

▶ Warts on rectal mucosa should be referred to proctologist.

▶ Refer women with large warts (> 2 cm) to gynecologist for treatment with CO_2 laser, electrodesiccation, electrocautery, cryocautery, or LEEP (loop electrosurgical excision procedure [gynecologic surgery]).

Follow-up

▶ During therapy, women should continue to have regular, annual Pap smears.

Expected Course

▶ Treatment of warts may require several visits for provider-administered treatment.

▶ Genital warts can resolve on their own, remain unchanged, or continue to grow untreated.

▶ Reoccurrence of warts is common, especially within the first 3 months following treatment.

Complications

▶ Cervical dysplasia and cervical squamous cell carcinoma; invasive carcinoma of vulva and penis

▶ Anal squamous cell carcinoma of bisexual or homosexual males

▶ Scarring from treatment procedures

OTHER SEXUALLY TRANSMITTED INFECTIONS

SYPHILIS

Description

▶ Sexually transmitted disease affecting many organs throughout body, caused by *Treponema pallidum*

▶ Clinical stages include primary, secondary, early latent (up to 1 year duration), late latent, tertiary

Etiology

▶ *T. pallidum:* Spirochete that invades the human body by penetrating intact skin or mucous membrane during sexual contact

▶ Once inside body, rapidly multiplies and spreads to regional lymph nodes

▶ Congenital: Occurs from transplacental passage of organism occurring any time during gestation; can result in spontaneous abortion (second trimester), stillbirth

Incidence and Demographics

▶ Increase in cases of syphilis in men who have sex with men (MSM)

▶ In 2008, 63% of reported primary and secondary syphilis cases were among MSMs.

▶ Rates of primary and secondary syphilis increased in men and women age 15–24 in 2007.

▶ Approximately 55,400 new cases are reported in the U.S. annually.

▶ The congenital syphilis rate has decreased in recent years.

Risk Factors

▶ Listed under General Approach

Prevention and Screening

▶ Prevention methods listed under General Approach

▶ Early diagnosis and treatment with partner notification and treatment

▶ Routine screening for persons ≤ 25 years in high-prevalence areas; also screen patients with other STIs

▶ Pregnancy: Screening at first prenatal visit, then repeat for high-risk population at 28 weeks and delivery

Assessment

History and Physical Exam

▶ See Table 13–1.

TABLE 13-1
STAGES OF ACQUIRED SYPHILIS

PRIMARY	SECONDARY	LATENT	TERTIARY
Painless ulcer or chancre at site of inoculation 3–4 weeks after exposure	Rash is macular, papular, annular, or follicular (rarely pustular) and often present on palms and soles	Begins with healing of the lesions in secondary stage	Gummatous formation, cardiovascular or neurosyphilis
Extragenital lesions such as lips or breast may be painful	In warm, moist areas, may develop broad flat lesions (condylomata lata)	Early latent < 1 year (infectious)	
Primary chancre is highly infectious, heals spontaneously after 1–5 weeks and patient may not seek treatment	Rash lasts 2–6 weeks, then heals spontaneously	Late latent > 1 year (noninfectious)	
	Mucous patches appear as gray erosions noted in mouth, throat, on cervix	Sometimes difficult to distinguish early latent from late latent stage due to unknown duration of symptoms	
	Generalized lymphadenopathy	Meningitis	
	Arthralgias, myalgias, and "flu-like" symptoms	Cardiovascular disease, arthritis, neurologic lesions	
		Often asymptomatic	

▶ Primary

  » Incubation is approximately 3 weeks and ranges 10–90 days after exposure.

  » Painless, indurated ulcer (chancre) at site of inoculation is highly infectious, heals spontaneously after 1–5 weeks and patient may not seek treatment; may be regional lymphadenopathy

  » Extragenital (lips, breast) lesions may be painful.

▶ Secondary

  » May occur from 6 weeks to 6 months after primary stage; most contagious

  » Rash is macular, papular, annular, or follicular and often present on palms and soles.

  » Rash lasts 2–6 weeks, then heals spontaneously.

  » Moist, raised lesions of the skin (condyloma lata) and mucous patches in mouth and throat, on cervix

  » Generalized lymphadenopathy

  » Arthralgias, myalgias, and "flu-like" symptoms

▶ Latent

  » Asymptomatic, begins with the end of secondary symptoms

  » Early latent < 1 year (infectious)

  » Late latent > 1 year (noninfectious)

  » Difficult to distinguish early latent from late latent stage if unknown duration of symptoms

▶ Tertiary

  » Gummatous formation, cardiovascular or neurosyphilis

▶ Congenital: Asymptomatic until age 2; failure to thrive, skin rash, jaundice, rhinitis, hepatosplenomegaly

Diagnostic Studies

▶ Definitive method: Darkfield microscopy and direct fluorescent antibody tests of lesion exudate or tissue

▶ Serologic tests: RPR, VDRL for initial testing and titers, FTA-ABS, MHA-TP to confirm diagnosis in people with positive RPR or VDRL

▶ For sequential serologic tests, use the same test (VDRL or RPR); titer will decrease with time and treatment.

▶ Four-fold increase in titer indicates new infection.

▶ Failure to achieve four-fold decrease in titer in 1 year indicates failed treatment.

▶ Latent syphilis of > 1 year duration, cardiovascular syphilis, and neurosyphilis: Serologic tests and lumbar puncture with tests on cerebrospinal fluid (CSF)

▶ Test for other STIs: HIV, gonorrhea, chlamydia.

Differential Diagnosis

▶ Genital ulcers

▶ Genital herpes

▶ Chancroid

▶ Neoplasm

▶ Lymphogranuloma venereum

▶ Superficial fungal infections

Management

Nonpharmacologic Treatment

▶ Abstain from sexual activity until treatment is complete.

▶ Early infection (primary, secondary, and early latent) and congenital syphilis reportable in all U.S. states

Pharmacologic Treatment

▶ Patients exposed sexually to a patient who has syphilis in any stage should be evaluated clinically and serologically and treated in the following cases:

  » People exposed within 90 days preceding diagnosis of primary, secondary, or early latent stages in a sex partner, even if seronegative

  » People exposed > 90 days before the diagnosis of primary, secondary, or latent stages in a sex partner and in whom serologic test results are not available immediately and the opportunity for follow-up is uncertain

  » For purposes of partner notification and presumptive treatment of exposed sex partners, patients with unknown duration of illness and high serologic test titers (≥ 1:32) may be considered as having early syphilis.

▶ Patients with symptoms or history of symptoms and positive diagnostic studies, see Table 13–2

TABLE 13–2
RECOMMENDED TREATMENT OF ACQUIRED SYPHILIS

STAGE OF DISEASE	TREATMENT REGIMEN
Primary, secondary, and early latent disease	Benzathine penicillin G 2.4 million units IM in single dose Penicillin-allergic patients: Doxycycline 100 mg b.i.d. × 28 days, or tetracycline 500 mg orally q.i.d. × 28 days
Late latent syphilis or syphilis of unknown duration	Benzathine penicillin G 2.4 million units IM × 3 each at 1-week intervals Penicillin-allergic patients: Doxycycline 100 mg orally b.i.d. for 4 wks, or tetracycline 500 mg orally q.i.d. × 4 wks
Tertiary disease, excluding neurosyphilis	As for late latent disease, with appropriate management of complications
Neurosyphilis	Aqueous cystamine penicillin G, 18–24 million units/day given as 3–4 million units IV every 4 hours for 10–14 days, or procaine penicillin 2–4 million units IM a day *plus* probenecid (Benemid) 500 mg orally q.i.d., both for 10–14 days

Special Considerations

▶ HIV-infected people

▹ Serologic tests and interpretation the same as for HIV-infected patients

▹ When clinical finding suggests syphilis, but serologic tested nonreactive or unclear, use alternative test such as biopsy of lesion, darkfield examination, or direct fluorescent antibody staining of lesion material.

▹ Treatment the same as for HIV-negative people

▹ Neurosyphilis must be considered in differential for HIV+ patients. CSF examination should be performed on HIV-infected people who show mental status changes or have either late latent syphilis or syphilis of unknown duration.

▹ Penicillin must be used to treat; if penicillin-allergic, must be desensitized

▹ Primary and secondary syphilis should have VDRL/RPR serology at 3, 6, 9, 12, and 24 months to evaluate for treatment failure. If titer increased four-fold, fails to decrease four-fold at 3 months, or symptoms persist, retreatment is indicated.

▶ Pregnancy: Treat for appropriate stage of syphilis.

▹ Some experts recommend a second dose of benzathine penicillin 2.4 mil units IM 1 week after initial dose for pregnant women with primary, secondary, or early latent syphilis. If penicillin-allergic, desensitize patient to penicillin.

▹ Women treated in second trimester are at risk for premature labor and fetal distress.

▶ Infants born to mothers with positive nontreponemal and treponemal test

▹ If infant was born to mother who tests positive for syphilis but adequate treatment with penicillin is not documented, the infant should be observed for congenital syphilis (into early childhood).

▹ Routine physical exams for rash, hepatomegaly, lymphadenopathy, persistent rhinitis

▹ Quantitative nontreponemal test on infant's blood (not cord blood)

▹ Cerebrospinal fluid testing, long bone X-rays, and other testing may be indicated.

▶ All patients may experience the Jarisch-Herxheimer reaction.

▹ Upon treatment of primary or secondary syphilis, occurs due to lysis of treponemes

▹ Experience fever, chills, headache, myalgias, rash

▹ Treated with antihistamines and antipyretics

When to Consult, Refer, Hospitalize

▶ Consult with physician or refer to infectious disease specialist for pregnant women, congenital syphilis, neurosyphilis infection, or HIV+ patients.

▶ Hospitalize for parenteral therapy and for penicillin desensitization therapy.

Follow-up

▶ Primary and secondary syphilis: Examine clinically and serologically at 6 or 12 months or more frequently if clinically indicated; if serologic titer (VDRL or RPR) has not declined by four-fold in 6 months after therapy, consider treatment a failure.

» Treatment failure: Reevaluate for HIV infection, provide more frequent follow-up (3 months instead of 6). If additional follow-up cannot be ensured, retreatment recommended (3 weekly IM injections of penicillin G 2.4 million units).

» Consider CSF examination.

▶ Latent syphilis: Serologic testing at 6, 12, and 24 months; evaluate for neurosyphilis and re-treat if titers increase four-fold, initial high titer (> 1:32) fails to decline at least four-fold within 12–24 months, or symptomatic

Expected Course

▶ Primary stage lasts 1–5 weeks, secondary stage lasts 2–6 weeks.

Complications

▶ Tertiary syphilis: Cardiovascular involvement causing aortitis, aortic insufficiency, aneurysm, and neurosyphilis; recurrent secondary symptoms possible within 1 year for 25% cases.

CASE STUDIES

CASE 1. A 23-year-old sexually active male presents with a 4–5 day history of dysuria he feels is caused by a urinary tract infection.

HPI: Denies frequency, fever, flank pain, hematuria, history of urinary tract infections.

▶ What additional information will help you evaluate this patient?

Exam: Mucopurulent urethral discharge, no inguinal adenopathy, no genital lesions.

▶ What is the differential diagnosis?

▶ Should any diagnostic tests be done?

▶ What are your treatment considerations?

CASE 2. A 17-year-old female comes to the family planning clinic for routine pelvic exam and contraception. She has had 4 sexual partners in the past year and only occasionally uses condoms. She requests an HIV test because one of her recent partners is an IV drug user.

PMH: History of 2 pregnancies with 2 abortions, no major illnesses, does not smoke, drinks 2–3 beers on the weekend, lives with mother and grandmother, in 11th grade, failing some classes.

▶ What additional information should you obtain?

Exam: Complete physical exam with no significant findings except flat-topped, fleshy-colored lesions on labia minora and thin yellow vaginal discharge.

▶ What screening tests should be done?

▶ What treatment should be considered today?

▶ What education and prevention topics should be discussed with this patient?

REFERENCES

American Academy of Pediatrics. (2012). *The 2006 red book: Report of the Committee on Infectious Disease*. Elk Grove, IL: Author.

Bartlett, J. G. (2009). *Medical management of HIV infection* (2nd ed.). Cockeysville, MD: PR Graphics.

Centers for Disease Control and Prevention. (2013). *Sexually transmitted diseases.* Retrieved from www.cdc.gov/STI/

Centers for Disease Control and Prevention. (2010). Sexually transmitted diseases treatment guidelines. *MMWR: Morbidity and Mortality Weekly Report, 59* (No. RR-12), 1–116.

Gilbert, D. N., Moellering, R. C., Eliopoulus, G. M., & Sande, M. A. (2013). *The Sanford guide to antimicrobial therapy.* Hyde Park, VT: Antimicrobial Therapy, Inc.

Mandell, G. L., Bennett, J. E., & Dolin, R. (2009). *Mandell, Doublas, and Bennett's principles and practices of infectious diseases.* Philadelphia: Churchill Livingstone.

Sande, M. A., Gilbert, D. N., & Moellering, R. C. (2012). *The Sanford guide to HIV/AIDS therapy.* Hyde Park, VT: Antimicrobial Therapy, Inc.

Siberry, G., & Iannone, R. (2011). *The Harriett Lane handbook.* New York: Mosby.

U.S. Preventive Services Task Force. (2012). *Guide to clinical preventive services.* Retrieved from www.ahrq.gov/clinic/pocketgd1011/pocketgd1011.pdf

MUSCULOSKELETAL DISORDERS

Deborah Gilbert-Palmer, MSN, EdD, FNP-BC

GENERAL APPROACH

Description

▶ In infants and children, obtain history of mother's pregnancy, child's birth and development (musculoskeletal problems comprise ~10% of childhood problems and ~25% of primary care visits).

▶ Obtain history of problem, including mechanism of injury, occupation, any sports or exercise, repetitive use, duration, aggravating and alleviating factors. Age is important in evaluation of any musculoskeletal findings.

▶ Observe gait, posture, guarding, and patient positioning; examine affected side in comparison to unaffected side.

▶ Provocative tests specific to area are important to rule out certain conditions.

RED FLAGS

▶ *Back pain:* Urgent referral if constant, under age 11, lasts several weeks, wakes patient at night, limits motion, fever, neurologic signs, weight loss, or history of malignancy

▶ *Malignant bone tumors* may present as unexplained pain and swelling over a bone, decreased range of motion, night pain, pain with weight-bearing, weight loss, night sweats, pallor, malaise, and fever; or have a high index of suspicion for bone metastasis in patients with previous breast, lung, or prostate cancer.

▶ *Osteomyelitis* may present as pain in bone, fever, difficulty bearing weight, and possible local warmth and swelling following recent trauma. Obtain a CBC, ESR, and C-reactive protein and refer to orthopedist. Be aware that X-ray changes will not occur for 10–24 days after start of infection.

ARTHRITIS

OSTEOARTHRITIS (OA)

Description

▶ Degenerative joint disease with progressive loss of articular cartilage in movable joints, degeneration of cartilage, bone hypertrophy, formation of osteophytes and subchondral cysts, and development of subchondral sclerosis in synovial joints and vertebrae

Etiology

▶ Results from both mechanical and biologic events that lead to degradation of articular cartilage and subchondral bone in joint

Incidence and Demographics

▶ Most common form of arthritis; affects of 25% of adult population; greatest prevalence in Native Americans

▶ Leading chronic condition among adults age ≥ 65 years; incidence increases with advancing age

▶ 80% of adults in U.S. have radiographic evidence by age 75.

▶ Women affected more often than men

Risk Factors

▶ Advancing age; symptom onset typically at 55–65 years

▶ Athletic overuse or repetitive joint use in occupation

▶ Joint trauma from acute injury or metabolic disease

▶ Obesity, heredity, congenital musculoskeletal disorders

▶ Metabolic disorders (e.g., gout) or endocrine disorders (e.g., hyperparathyroidism)

Prevention and Screening

▶ Maintain physical activity.

▶ Maintain ideal body weight, avoid obesity.

▶ Maintain control of metabolic and endocrine disorders.

Assessment

▶ See Table 14–1.

TABLE 14–1
DIFFERENTIATING CHARACTERISTICS OF OSTEOARTHRITIS AND RHEUMATOID ARTHRITIS

CHARACTERISTICS	OSTEOARTHRITIS	RHEUMATOID ARTHRITIS
Radiographic appearance	Joint space narrowing, osteophytes, subchondral bone sclerosis, subchondral cysts	Periarticular osteopenia or osteoporosis, soft tissue swelling, marginal bony erosions
Morning stiffness	Lasts < 30 minutes	Lasts > 1 hour before improving
Joint involvement	Usually weight-bearing (spine, hips, knees), or distal finger joints (DIP)	Multiple joints, symmetric joint involvement (esp. of hands)
Laboratory findings	ESR < 20–40 mm/hr; RF negative	Positive serum RF, may have positive ANA, elevated ESR
Clinical findings	Joint pain, bony tenderness and hypertrophy, crepitus, may have some deformity; no warmth or redness	Joint deformity, muscle atrophy, soft tissue nodules (rheumatoid nodules), soft tissue swelling, warmth, redness of joints

ANA = antinuclear antibody; ESR = erythrocyte sedimentation rate; RF = rheumatoid factor

History

▶ Gradual onset of joint pain, tenderness, and stiffness; worsens with activity and relieved by rest

▶ Morning stiffness common, usually lasts < 30 minutes

▶ Joint instability in later stages, especially with osteoarthritis of knees

▶ Perform review of systems for systemic symptoms to rule out other types of arthritis.

Physical Exam

▶ Usually localized to affected joints

▶ Bony hypertrophy of joint, tenderness at joint line; limited range of motion

▶ Common in hands: Proximal intraphalangeal (PIP) joint swelling = Bouchard's nodes; distal intraphalangeal (DIP) joint swelling = Heberden's nodes

▶ Coarse crepitus in joint with movement; soft tissue swelling may be present

▶ Joint effusion, if present, usually mild

▶ Cardiac and pulmonary exam, as well as other body systems as indicated by history to rule out other types of arthritis

Diagnostic Studies

▶ Plain radiographs: Unequal and narrowed joint space, subchondral bony sclerosis, sharp articular margins, cysts or osteophytes

▶ Bone densitometry (DEXA scans), peripheral ultrasonography, quantitative computed tomography (QCT)

▶ No specific laboratory test; laboratory findings may be normal or show markers of systemic inflammation or autoimmune disease.

Differential Diagnosis

▶ Rheumatoid arthritis

▶ Psoriatic arthritis

▶ Gout, pseudogout

▶ Septic arthritis

▶ Reiter's disease, lupus

▶ Fibromyalgia

▶ Tendonitis, soft tissue injury

▶ Osteoporosis

▶ Multiple myeloma

Management

▶ Goals are to relieve symptoms, maintain or improve function, and avoid adverse effects of medication.

Nonpharmacologic Treatment

▶ Physical activity or therapy with supervised walking

▶ Occupational therapy

▶ Arthritis self-management programs and water aquatics courses

▶ Ambulation aids (canes, braces, walkers)

▶ Weight-loss programs

▶ Consider surgery if all other modalities fail and joint symptoms prevent normal activities.

Pharmacologic Treatment

▶ Simple analgesics, available OTC (acetaminophen, aspirin, ibuprofen, or naproxen) for pain

  ▹ Acetaminophen 2.6–4 g/day considered first-line treatment by American College of Rheumatology due to low toxicity; extended release preparations lengthen duration

▶ NSAIDs taken with food are indicated for failed acetaminophen trial; start with lower doses and use those with shorter half-lives in older adults, increase to full strength if needed, switch to different class if not effective after several weeks. Increased cardiovascular risk, which increases with duration of use. Monitor closely for NSAID-induced renal insufficiency in older patients; renal toxicity can occur in all age groups if recommended dose exceeded.

▶ Selective COX-2 inhibitors: Lower GI toxicity than other NSAIDs, continue to monitor renal function closely with COX-2s

▶ Topical analgesic creams such as capsaicin 0.025% b.i.d. to t.i.d. p.r.n.

▶ Narcotic analgesics rarely indicated; may be used short-term if necessary

▶ Intra-articular corticosteroid injections for joint effusion and inflammation limited to a few joints

▶ Hyaluronic acid injections to rebuild cartilage in a single joint

▶ Nutraceutical (glucosamine, chondroitin, SAM-e) may be beneficial.

How Long to Treat

▶ As long as symptomatic

Special Considerations

▶ Presence of radiographic changes does not correlate with presence or severity of symptoms

When to Consult, Refer, Hospitalize

▶ Consult with physician or orthopedic specialist for intra-articular corticosteroid or hyaluronic acid injections.

▶ Patients with functional impairment (i.e., inability to perform normal activities of daily living) and moderate to severe pain unrelieved by other nonpharmacologic and pharmacologic therapies should be considered for joint replacement; refer to orthopedic surgeon.

Follow-up

▶ Appointments as needed based on pain and disability

▶ If on NSAIDs or acetaminophen, monitor for liver or kidney dysfunction, GI bleeding

Expected Course

▶ Chronic, often progressive

Complications

▶ Joint destruction, chronic pain, limitation of mobility

RHEUMATOID ARTHRITIS (RA)

Description

▶ Chronic, systemic, inflammatory disease that affects mainly synovial joints in a symmetric distribution; small-joint destruction and extra-articular symptoms prominent

Etiology

▶ Probably autoimmune, but no specific inciting factor yet identified

▶ Genetic, environmental factors affect progression and extent of disease

▶ Pathology consists of initial changes in the synovium microvasculature, swelling of endothelial cells, and synovial hyperplasia forming a pannus. Inflammatory cells invade and joint symptoms develop secondary to the inflammatory process.

Incidence and Demographics

▶ Worldwide incidence, involving all ethnic groups; prevalence about 5 times greater in females

▶ In children, bimodal age presentation: 2–4 years, 8–12 years

▶ Juvenile RA diagnosed in children < 16 years old who have chronic synovial inflammation of at least one joint for 6 weeks. JRA has 3 major types:

  » *Pauciarticular* (fewer than 5 joints): Characterized by chronic arthritis of a few joints, usually the large weight-bearing joints, asymmetric distribution

  » *Polyarticular* (5 or more joints): Resembles adult disease with chronic pain, swelling of many joints

  » *Systemic:* Associated with rash, arthritis, fever, or visceral disease

Risk Factors

▶ Possible genetic component, immunologically mediated; strong family history of autoimmune disorders

▶ Occurs in all age groups, more common with increasing age, peak onset in adults in 4th decade of life

▶ 5% of cases begin in childhood.

Assessment

▶ Early diagnosis (within first few months of symptoms) important for improved prognosis

▶ Important to rule out septic arthritis, typical presentation: Sudden onset of pain, swelling, warmth, and redness in one large weight-bearing joint, may have fever

History

▶ Prodromal systemic symptoms: Malaise, fever, weight loss, morning stiffness lasting > 30–60 minutes

▶ Articular inflammation, swelling, pain, erythema, and warmth

▶ Involvement usually symmetrical; 75% of joints involved are knees, followed by ankles and elbows

▶ In children, joint pain, one or more joints affected, swelling or effusion, and 2 of the following: limitation of range of motion, tenderness or pain in motion, warmth; usually involves large joints or hands; if systemic: fever, rash

▶ Perform review of systems to identify any associated symptoms of systemic involvement; physical or emotional stress may trigger

Physical Exam

▶ Edema, erythema, warmth, nodules in any joint; effervescent, pale pink or salmon-colored macular rash

▶ Joints are tender, may feel warm to touch; bright erythema and palpable heat in joint usually indicative of infection

▶ Subcutaneous nodules over bony prominences or extensor surfaces

▶ Soft tissue swelling, vasculitis, palmar erythema

▶ As disease progresses, joint deformities become more pronounced and joint instability develops.

▶ Systemic manifestations may be seen in the pulmonary, cardiac, hepatic, renal, vascular, hematologic systems. and the eyes (dry mucous membranes, ocular problems, splenomegaly, increased lymphocytes)

▶ In children with systemic JRA, may have macular salmon-colored rash, splenomegaly, eye symptoms

Diagnostic Studies

▶ No single test is adequate to make diagnosis.

▶ Positive serum rheumatoid factor (RF) in about 80% of cases; levels hard to correlate with severity of other signs; ANA increased in 20% patients. In children, RF and ANA may be positive.

▶ Erythrocyte sedimentation rate (ESR) correlates with degree of synovial inflammation.

▶ CRP (C-reactive protein) may also be used to monitor inflammation.

▶ Synovial fluid shows inflammatory changes: Sterile leukocytosis, increased PMN, negative culture

▶ CBC may show chronic, mild, normochromic or hypochromic, normocytic anemia

▶ Other: Eosinophilia, hypergammaglobulinemia, thrombocytosis may be present in severe disease.

▶ X-ray shows soft tissue swelling and juxta-articular destruction.

Differential Diagnosis

▶ Systemic lupus erythematosus (SLE)

▶ Seronegative spondyloarthropathy

▶ Psoriatic arthritis

▶ Septic arthritis

▶ Lyme disease

▶ Gout

▶ Osteoarthritis

▶ Lupus

Management

▶ Goals are early diagnosis and early, aggressive treatment to limit, prevent irreversible joint damage, maximize mobility, limit pain, halt disease progression

Nonpharmacologic Treatment

▶ Rest as indicated; may require complete bedrest with acute inflammatory phase

▶ Patient education (Arthritis Foundation self-help courses); physical and occupational therapy to strengthen muscles, improve joint range of motion (ROM) and function, protect≈joint(s)

▶ Regular exercise program; may use alternating heat and cold to increase comfort

▶ Assistive devices (canes, splints)

▶ Surgery to correct joint deformity if necessary

Pharmacologic Treatment

▶ Aspirin is often recommended as a first-line drug.

▶ NSAIDs taken with food have not been shown to alter disease course, but may offer symptom relief.

▶ COX-2s for those with risk of bleeding; COX-1 with misoprostol or proton pump inhibitors

▶ Biologic agents (disease-modifying antirheumatic drugs [DMARDs]): Tumor necrosis factor (TNF) inhibitors may be used if patient fails methotrexate therapy.

▶ Leflunomide (Arava), etanercept (Enbrel), and infliximab (Remicade) may cause hypersensitivity reaction, severe infections or sepsis, and autoimmunity (lupus-type syndrome). Work faster than methotrexate, good response in 60%, more costly.

▶ Hydroxychloroquine (Plaquenil): Monitor eye symptoms, neuropathy, and myopathy.

▶ Methotrexate: Monitor closely for bone marrow, pulmonary, hepatic, and renal toxicity.

▶ Sulfasalazine (Azulfidine): Monitor closely for bone marrow, hepatic, and renal toxicity.

▶ Minocycline: Use in mild disease.

▶ Corticosteroids: Use short-term for severe exacerbations.

▶ Prednisone up to 0.1 mg/kg (2.5–7.5 mg/day) p.o.; may also be used in combination with DMARDs

▶ Methylprednisolone 80–60 mg IM during acute flare

▶ Chronic corticosteroid use decreases bone mineral density.

How Long to Treat

▶ In adults, lifelong therapy usually indicated, may have periods of remission or decreased symptoms

▶ In children, some have periods of long remissions

Special Considerations

▶ Methotrexate, hydroxychloroquine (Plaqenil) known to be detrimental to fetus; should be stopped some time before conception

▶ Pregnancy may result in remission and may allow temporary discontinuation of medications; however, exacerbations common in first 6 months postpartum. Breastfeeding not advised, since antirheumatic medications are secreted in breast milk.

When to Consult, Refer, Hospitalize

▶ Rheumatologic consultation or referral is appropriate. All children should be referred to a pediatric rheumatologist and ophthalmologist at diagnosis.

Follow-up

▶ Clinical course is highly variable; until symptoms are controlled, frequent follow-up visits are indicated, then regular evaluations at 3–6-month intervals.

Complications

▶ May be severe, including carpal tunnel syndrome, pleuritis, pericarditis, vasculitis, iridocyclitis, disability, and adverse reactions from drugs; see joint deformity, hip disease.

GOUT

Description

▶ A group of metabolic diseases producing inflammatory arthritis of peripheral joints caused by deposition of uric acid or monosodium urate crystals in extracellular fluid

Etiology

▶ Inborn error of purine metabolism or uric acid excretion causing hyperuricemia and uric acid crystal deposition in the joint (acute gouty arthritis)

▶ May be primary (hereditary) or secondary (due to other conditions that cause underexcretion or overproduction of uric acid)

▶ Overproduction: High intake of purine-rich foods (organ meats, shellfish, peas, lentils, beans), polycythemia vera, leukemia, multiple myeloma, hemolytic anemia, psoriasis, sarcoidosis

▶ Underexcretion of uric acid: Reduced renal function, lactic acidosis, ketoacidosis, dehydration

▶ Secondary gout also associated with obesity, starvation, lead intoxication, ingestion of drugs (salicylates, diuretics, pyrazinamide, ethambutol, nicotinic acid)

▶ Combined overproduction and underexcretion: Alcohol abuse, glucose-6-phosphatase deficiency (G6PD), hypoxemia

Incidence and Demographics

▶ Affects 2.2 million in U.S.; men affected 9 times as often as women; most common in Asians

▶ Rarely affects men before adolescence or women before menopause

▶ Peak incidence is fifth decade

Risk Factors

▶ Heredity, purine-rich diet, obesity, dehydration, starvation, alcohol ingestion

Prevention and Screening

▶ Correct or control underlying problem.

▶ Avoid foods high in purines, alcohol, and causative medications.

▶ Maintain normal body weight.

Assessment

History

▶ Sudden attack of red, hot, swollen, exquisitely tender joint is common (first metatarsal phalangeal [MTP] joint very susceptible: podagra); feeling of malaise, fever; often no apparent cause

▶ Foot, ankle, knee, shoulder are most common sites; wrist, elbow, fingers also may be affected.

Physical Exam

▶ During acute attack, joint is red, hot, swollen, exquisitely painful; low-grade fever

▶ Skin desquamation and pruritus during resolution of acute attack commonly seen

▶ Tophi (sodium urate crystals deposited in soft tissue) present in chronic tophaceous gout, usually after 2–10 years from onset of acute intermittent gout

▶ Joint swelling, restricted range of movement caused by chronic arthritis

Diagnostic Studies

▶ Joint aspiration: Fluid shows presence of needle-shaped crystals (negatively birefringent) on polarized light microscopy.

▶ Serum uric acid > 7.0 mg/dL supports diagnosis but is not specific; elevated ESR, elevated leukocytes

▶ X-ray: Normal in early disease; shows punched-out lesions in subchondral bone, usually first seen in first MTP joint ("Mickey Mouse" ears); soft tissue tophi may be seen if at least 5 mm in diameter

Differential Diagnosis

▶ Septic joint

▶ Pseudogout

▶ Cellulitis

▶ Fracture

▶ Rheumatoid arthritis

▶ Acute rheumatic fever

▶ Pyogenic arthritis

Management

Nonpharmacologic Treatment

▶ Dietary modification; increased fluid intake ≥ 3 liters/day

▶ Complete bedrest during acute attack

▶ Weight loss in obese patients

Pharmacologic Treatment

▶ Acute attack

» First-line: NSAIDs such as naproxen at full anti-inflammatory dose; naproxen 500 mg t.i.d. p.o. for first 2–3 days (until symptoms subside), then taper to cessation over 3–5 days; or corticosteroids, depending on comorbidities, prednisone 20–40 mg p.o. q.d. for 2–3 days, then taper over 10–14 days; intra-articular methylprednisolone (Depo-Medrol) one 20- to 40-mg dose; IM methylprednisolone, one 80- to 120-mg dose

» Second-line: Colchicine 1.2 mg p.o. as soon as symptoms appear, then 0.06 mg 1 hour later (colchicine used for patients who are not good candidates for NSAIDs: on anticoagulants, congestive heart failure, renal insufficiency); drug has very narrow therapeutic index; maintenance dose is 0.6 mg p.o. q.d. to b.i.d.

► Maintenance

  » Urate-lowering therapy indicated with multiple attacks, development of tophi or urate nephrolithiais, to block renal absorption of uric acid

  » First-line: Start allopurinol 100–150 mg q.d. to b.i.d. p.o., gradually increasing by 100 mg per week until serum uric acid is below 6 mg/dL; maximum dose of 800 mg/day. Contraindicated in patients with renal impairment or febuxostat.

  » Second-line: Probenecid or IV pegloticase

  » Concurrent therapy: Use maintenance colchicine to reduce number of attacks and medications.

How Long to Treat

► Acute symptoms treated until tolerable, then long-term therapy begun

Special Considerations

► Transplant patients (who use cyclosporine) have increased incidence.

► Asymptomatic hyperuricemia with normal renal function: Generally do not treat

► Slightly higher incidence in Black males than White males

► Geriatric patients: NSAIDs less well tolerated, dosages should be reduced

When to Consult, Refer, Hospitalize

► Consult for any complicated presentation, underlying metabolic pathology

► Refer for joint aspiration, unclear diagnosis, new or acute gout in transplant patient

► Hospitalize if intravenous administration of colchicine necessary (rare)

Follow-up

Expected Course

► Decrease in frequency, severity of attacks with appropriate treatment

Complications

► Kidney stones, renal obstruction or infection, joint destruction if undertreated

CONDITIONS OF THE BONES

OSTEOMYELITIS

Description

▶ Local bone infection, usually bacterial; can be acute or chronic

Etiology

▶ Bacteremia with acute or subacute hematogenous spread to bone (most common form in pediatrics)

▶ Direct bacterial inoculation through trauma, contact infected tissue (most common in adults)

▶ Predominant organism *Staphylococcus aureus*

Incidence and Demographics

▶ Occurs in all ages, more common in children < 5 years old

▶ Males 2–4 times more than females; 5–10 cases per 10,000 children

▶ Increases in late summer and early fall

▶ Uncommon in neonatal period

▶ Femur and tibia most often infected, followed by humerus, calcaneus, and pelvis

Risk Factors

▶ General debilitating diseases (cancer, diabetes, hemodialysis); sickle cell disease; *Salmonella*

▶ Intravenous drug abuse

▶ Puncture wound: *Pseudomonas aeruginosa*

Prevention and Screening

▶ Careful treatment of comorbid conditions; appropriate wound care

Assessment

History

▶ 75% report recent trauma, 25% report recent respiratory tract infection

▶ Sudden onset high fever and pain in affected bone or joint; sudden refusal to bear weight or move extremity; localized warmth, swelling

▶ May have drainage from affected area (sinus tract develops)

Physical Exam

▶ Swelling, erythema, possible abscess formation or purulent drainage; decreased ROM; fever; point tenderness over infected bone

Diagnostic Studies

▶ CBC: WBC elevated in 70% of cases

▶ ESR: Elevated by 3rd day of infection

▶ C-reactive protein: Peaks at day 2

▶ Blood cultures: Positive in 50% of cases

▶ Bone cultures: Positive in 65% of cases; wound cultures of no benefit

▶ X-ray shows changes after day 10–14 of infection

▶ If suspicious, MRI defines area of infection, soft tissue pathology; differentiate tumor and infection

▶ Bone scan: Sensitive but not specific

▶ CT: Changes may not be evident (periosteal elevation) until after day 10

Differential Diagnosis

▶ Septic arthritis

▶ Toxic synovitis

▶ Cellulitis

▶ Sickle cell anemia

▶ Myositis

▶ Slipped capital femoral epiphysis

▶ Rheumatic arthritis

▶ Malignancy

Management

Nonpharmacologic Treatment

▶ Surgical debridement, splinting, local wound care, bed rest

Pharmacologic Treatment

▶ Intravenous antibiotics are mainstay of treatment; choice depends on infectious organism

How Long to Treat

▶ Antibiotic therapy for 4–6 weeks, depending on organism; initially use intravenous antibiotics, may change to oral later

Special Considerations

▶ Culture of draining sinus tract or superficial wound does not correlate with actual infectious organism. Bone biopsy should be obtained before starting antibiotics.

▶ Geriatric patients: Constitutional symptoms (fever, elevated WBC) may be less pronounced in older adults; presentation also may be clouded by concomitant chronic illnesses.

▶ Pregnancy or lactation: Choice of antibiotics should be considered carefully.

When to Consult, Refer, Hospitalize

▶ Orthopedics referral necessary immediately

▶ Infectious disease consult if necessary for choice of antibiotic

▶ Hospitalization for central vascular catheter placement, initiation of IV antibiotics

Follow-up

▶ Diagnosis and treatment plan developed by orthopedic specialist

Expected Course

▶ Clinical improvement should be seen within 24–48 hours, then gradual resolution of drainage, pain, WBC, ESR, and fever.

Complications

▶ Chronic osteomyelitis; need for bone, skin grafting, or both; structural weakening of bone

DEVELOPMENTAL HIP DYSPLASIA

Description

▶ Congenital displacement of the femoral head from acetabulum; ranges from subluxation to dislocation

Etiology

▶ Multifactorial (mechanical, physiologic, environmental, genetic)

▶ *Mechanical:* Breech presentation, positioning of fetal hip against mother's sacrum; tight maternal abdomen and uterine musculature causing molding and restriction of fetal movement; first-born

▶ *Physiologic:* Ligamentous laxity due to estrogen exposure; collagen disorders

▶ *Environmental:* Swaddling infant with legs in extension or adduction (Navajo population); cerebral palsy

▶ *Genetic:* 20% have positive family history.

Incidence and Demographics

▶ 0.5%–2% of live births

▶ Females more than males

▶ 60% involves left hip; 20% bilateral

Risk Factors

▶ First-born, female, breech

▶ Positive family history

Prevention and Screening

▶ Avoid swaddling with legs in extension and adduction.

▶ Check hips at birth, 2 week, 2 month, and 4 month well-baby exams.

Assessment

History

▶ Prenatal and birth history

▶ Positive family history

Physical Exam

▶ Limited abduction of hip; hip instability; asymmetry of thigh folds; femoral shortening on affected side

▶ Unequal leg lengths; unequal knee heights when supine (Galeazzi sign); limp or "duck-like" waddle

Diagnostic Studies

▶ Provocation tests: Click (hip relocation) felt with Ortolani's maneuver; clunk felt (hip dislocation) with Barlow's maneuver

▶ Ultrasound useful in neonatal period

▶ If older than 3–6 months, may use radiographs

Differential Diagnosis

▶ Unstable hip in newborn period

Management

▶ Goal is to prevent long-term complications and pathologic changes through early diagnosis and treatment in infancy.

Nonpharmacologic Treatment

▶ Birth – 6 months: Pavlik harness

▶ 6–18 months: Pavlik harness, closed reduction with cast

▶ > 18 months: Open reduction with casting

How Long to Treat

▶ Until corrected

Special Considerations

▶ About 60% of unstable hips in newborns spontaneously become normal in the first 2–4 weeks of life.

▶ In infant > 3 months, muscle tightness may mask click or dislocation.

▶ Standard radiographs difficult to interpret before 3–6 months of age

When to Consult, Refer, Hospitalize

▶ At diagnosis, all children should be referred to a pediatric orthopedist for evaluation.

Follow-up

▶ Orthopedic specialist

Expected Course

▶ Most cases respond to treatment.

Complications

▶ Osteoarthritis, pain, abnormal gait, decreased agility

▶ Even with treatment, avascular necrosis of femoral head may occur.

SCOLIOSIS

Description

▶ Lateral curvature of the spine

Etiology

▶ Functional: Poor posture, leg length discrepancies, muscle spasm

▶ Idiopathic: Unknown cause, but may be due to equilibrium dysfunction, familial causes, or asymmetrical growth

Incidence and Demographics

▶ 65% of all cases idiopathic

▶ Categorized by age

  » Infantile: 0–3 years; rare in U.S.; male-to-female ratio 3:2; spontaneous resolution in 90% of cases

  » Juvenile: 3–10 years; affects males and females equally; may progress during growth spurts

  » Adolescent: 5%–10% of all teens have scoliosis; progression to a significant curve (15°) occurs in < 0.5%; female-to-male ratio 5–7:1; may rapidly progress during growth spurts

Risk Factors

▶ 30% have positive family history

▶ Affects 20% of children with cerebral palsy

▶ Rapid progression during growth spurts: 12-year-old females and 14-year-old males

Prevention and Screening

▶ Screen during routine school age and adolescent physical exams with back fully exposed and no shoes

▶ Observe for asymmetry of shoulders, scapulae, and pelvis.

Assessment

History

▶ Asymmetry of shoulder or hip height; shirts or hemlines may be uneven

▶ Positive family history

▶ Complaints of pain

Physical Exam

▶ Screening done with back fully exposed and without shoes

▶ Observe for asymmetry of shoulders, scapulae, and hip or pelvis.

▶ Check for leg-length discrepancy.

▶ Bend forward at waist to 90° and slowly return to upright (Adams test).

▶ Assess for prominence of scapula or lateralization of spine.

▶ 90% thoracic with right curve; left thoracic curve more likely to progress

Diagnostic Studies

▶ Routine X-rays not required for mild scoliosis

▶ More severe cases require X-ray entire length of spine (Cobb method).

▶ X-ray determines location and direction of curvature, measures degree of asymmetry, and evaluates vertebral bodies; view entire spine from C7 to S1.

▶ Repeat X-rays to monitor progression of curve.

▶ Consider bone age.

▶ Scoliometer may be helpful to detect and follow smaller curves.

Management

▶ Goal is prevent further deformity

▶ Use Cobb method for evaluating degree of curvature; follow every 4–6 months in children < Tanner V.

   » Curves < 14°: Observe, follow every 4–6 months in children < Tanner V.

   » Curves ≥ 15°: Refer to orthopedist to monitor for progression.

   » Curves > 25° – 30° in growing children with 5° – 10° progression may need bracing to stabilize until growth is complete.

   » Curves > 40° in growing children require surgery with rod insertion or spinal fusion (Dormans, 2005).

Special Considerations

▶ Back pain uncommon in adolescents with idiopathic scoliosis so further examination warranted if pain present

▶ Refer to orthopedist immediately for congenital or infantile congenital scoliosis

▶ Scoliosis in older adults seen with deterioration of vertebral disks; often requires surgery to relieve pain, restore stability

Follow-up

▶ Close follow-up essential; can be done in primary care if < 15 (every 4–6 months)

▶ Otherwise followed by the orthopedist with periodic follow-up X-rays

Expected Course

▶ More concern with patients with large curvature at diagnosis and those with curvature before adolescent growth spurt; close follow-up essential

▶ Repeat standing posterior-anterior (PA) X-ray every 6–12 months in young adolescents with mild curvature, every 3–6 months in adolescents with large curves

Complications

▶ Untreated scoliosis results in unacceptable cosmetic appearance and cardiopulmonary impairment.

▶ Spinal osteoarthritis may occur in later life.

OSTEOPOROSIS

Description

▶ Metabolic disease with bone demineralization producing diffusely decreased bone density, diminished strength; predisposes patient to pathologic fractures, severe backache, loss of height

▶ Bone mineral density (BMD) at least 2.5 standard deviations (SD) below peak bone density of young adult (T score); osteopenia T score is −1.5 to −2.5 of standard deviation

Etiology

▶ Bone resorption by osteoclasts occurs faster than new bone matrix formation by osteoblasts and subsequent bone mineralization.

▶ Trabecular bone (spine, ribs, pelvis) turnover is greater than cortical bone.

Incidence and Demographics

▶ Approximately 20–25 million women affected; 5–6 million men in the U.S.

▶ White, Asian women at greater risk

▶ Primarily affects postmenopausal women

Risk Factors

▶ Inadequate calcium intake, vitamin D deficiency; excessive alcohol, protein, or caffeine intake

▶ Genetic predisposition: White or Asian

▶ Petite frame; low weight (< 127 pounds); advancing age

▶ Hyperthyroidism or hyperparathyroidism; rheumatoid arthritis

- ▶ Malignancy (multiple myeloma, leukemia)

- ▶ Early menopause (natural or surgical) with deficiency in estrogen and androgen

- ▶ Steroid use, Cushing's syndrome

- ▶ Renal insufficiency

- ▶ Declining physical activity

- ▶ Smoking

- ▶ Sedentary lifestyle without exposure to sun

Prevention and Screening

- ▶ Balanced diet with adequate intake of calcium and vitamin D; regular weight-bearing exercise; smoking cessation; avoiding high alcohol, protein, or caffeine intake; hormone replacement therapy or raloxifene (Evista) for postmenopausal women

- ▶ Estrogen replacement is drug of choice for first-line prevention (postmenopausal)

Assessment

History

- ▶ Risk factors, fracture after age 40 (spine, hip, wrist), back pain (from vertebral fracture), osteopenia on X-ray

Physical Exam

- ▶ No finding specific to osteoporosis; kyphosis common in elderly; loss of height

Diagnostic Studies

- ▶ Dual X-ray absorptiometry bone densitometry (DEXA) scan shows bone density at least 2.5 standard deviations below peak bone density; biochemical markers

- ▶ Osteopenia on X-ray (indicates loss of approximately 30% of bone mass)

Differential Diagnosis

- ▶ Endocrine disorders
- ▶ Malabsorption syndromes
- ▶ Malnutrition
- ▶ Osteomalacia
- ▶ Metastatic bone disease
- ▶ Connective tissue disorders

Management

Nonpharmacologic Treatment

- ▶ Prevention remains best strategy

- ▶ Regular weight-bearing exercise (20–30 minutes/day, 2–3 days/week); high-impact physical activity

- ▶ Calcium intake or supplementation (1,000–1,500 mg/day), adequate vitamin D intake (400–800 IU/day)

Pharmacologic Treatment

▶ Selective estrogen receptor modulators (SERMs): Raloxifene (Evista) 60 mg/day p.o. or tamoxifen (Nolvadex) 10–20 mg/day p.o.; bisphosphates: alendronate (Fosamax) 10 mg/day p.o., (Binosto) 70 mg q week, risedronate (Actonel) 5 mg/day, ibandronate (Boniva) 150 mg p.o. q month, zoledronic acid (Reclast) 5 mg IV q 12 months, or risedronate (Atelvia) 35 mg p.o. weekly should be taken for no more than 5 years without drug holiday

▶ RANK ligand inhibitors: Denosumab (Prolia) 60 mg SC q 6 mos used when other osteoporosis treatment options have failed

▶ Calcitonin (Miacalcin) nasal spray 200 units/day intranasal or calcitonin-salmon (Fortical) promotes osteoblastic activity.

How Long to Treat

▶ Until bone density is normal

Special Considerations

▶ Men: Treat with calcium supplementation, vitamin D, bisphosphates, or calcitonin nasal spray.

▶ Medications cannot be used in pregnancy.

When to Consult, Refer, Hospitalize

▶ Refer to orthopedist for suspected fracture; hospitalize for any hip fracture.

Follow-up

▶ Regular follow-up for review of diet, exercise, and medications

▶ Repeat DEXA scan every 23 months (covered by Medicare)

Expected Course

▶ Improvement in bone density evident 6–12 months after initiation of therapy

Complications

▶ Fracture (vertebral most common; hip has greatest mortality)

MALIGNANT BONE TUMORS

Description

▶ Neoplastic growth in a bone or bones

Etiology

▶ Malignant tumors of bone may originate in or metastasize to bone

▶ In adults, most often results from seeding of another malignancy

  » Metastasis from breast, lung, prostate, kidney, thyroid cancers

Incidence and Demographics

▶ Chondrosarcoma most common middle to late life

▶ Multiple myeloma most common primary bone tumor in adults, followed by osteosarcoma

▶ Osteosarcoma most common in children and young adults (more common in males)

▶ In the 60–70s age group, metastatic bone cancers more common

Risk Factors

▶ High doses of ionizing radiation

▶ Certain conditions (Paget's disease, von Recklinghausen's disease, enchondromatosis) may undergo malignant transformation.

Prevention and Screening

▶ Early diagnosis, treatment of primary malignancy

Assessment

▶ See Table 14–2.

TABLE 14–2
MALIGNANT BONE TUMORS

MALIGNANT TUMOR	TYPICAL AGE RANGE, INCIDENCE	CLINICAL PRESENTATION	RADIOGRAPHIC FINDINGS
Multiple myeloma Plasma cell malignancy (most common in adults)	Incidence 3/100,000 40 years Male:female 1.6:1	Bone pain Anemia, hypercalcemia, azotemia	Typical "punched-out" lytic lesions Diffuse osteoporosis
Osteosarcoma: 2nd most common malignant tumor in adults, most common malignant bone tumor children	Peak age 10–20 50% leg 2000–3000 per year Male:female 1.5:1	Local pain, tenderness, swelling Night pain, pain with weight-bearing Constitutional symptoms	X-ray findings: "Sunburst" pattern of radiating extensions from bone into soft tissue
Chondrosarcoma (malignant tumor of cartilage)	Middle–late adult life 90% are primary tumors; pelvis, femur, shoulder common sites Slow-growing	Acute or progressive deep pain Muscular weakness or atrophy Soft tissue mass may be palpable	Radiolucent lesions on X-ray Increased uptake on bone scan
Ewing's sarcoma: 2nd most common malignant bone tumor in children	Most common in children, young adults More common in White males	Pain, swelling, tenderness, erythema	Lytic lesion with onion-skin appearance of periosteum 53% occur on extremities

History (see Table 14–2)

► Unexplained pain and swelling over bone, decreased range of motion, night pain, pain with weight-bearing

► Constitutional symptoms: Weight loss, night sweats, pallor, malaise, fever

Physical Exam

► Painful mass, swelling, limited range of motion of joint

► Lymphadenopathy, hepatosplenomegaly

Diagnostic Studies

► X-ray may show aggressive, poorly defined lesion, irregular border, extension into soft tissue

► CT or MRI to determine extent of lesion

► Bone scan to detect metastasis

► Cytologic and pathologic examination

► CBC, liver function tests (LFTs)

Differential Diagnosis

► Benign bone tumor   ► Osteomyelitis   ► Metastatic disease

Management

Nonpharmacologic Treatment

► Surgery

► Radiation

Pharmacologic Treatment

► Chemotherapy

How Long to Treat

► Determined by oncologist

Special Considerations

► Refer for support, hospice, and pain control if necessary.

When to Consult, Refer, Hospitalize

► Refer to orthopedist for any bone lesion seen on X-ray, any constitutional signs of malignancy

Follow-up

Expected Course

▶ Highly variable depending on type of tumor, patient history, tumor stage at diagnosis

Complications

▶ Loss of limb, metastases, death

CONDITIONS THAT CAUSE HIP PAIN

TOXIC SYNOVITIS

Description

▶ Transient synovitis

▶ Self-limited, unilateral inflammation of hip joint

Etiology

▶ Unknown cause resulting in inflammation of the synovium in the hip

▶ Often associated with viral infections, postvaccination, drug-mediated

Incidence and Demographics

▶ Most common disorder causing limp and hip pain in children

▶ 2–10 years of age, average age 6; occurs more frequently in boys than girls

▶ Occurs more frequently in springtime

Risk Factors

▶ Preceding upper respiratory tract infection

▶ Daycare attendance

▶ Recent antibiotic use

▶ Recent immunization (especially MMR)

Assessment

History

▶ Low-grade fever but no other systemic symptoms

▶ Insidious onset of pain, often complaining of vague "leg" pain or knee pain

▶ Antalgic limp or refusal to walk

Physical Exam

▶ Well-appearing child

▶ Hip held in position of flexion, abduction, and external rotation; decreased internal rotation

Diagnostic Studies

▶ CBC, ESR: Usually normal or slightly elevated; ESR may be slightly elevated

▶ Blood culture and sensitivity to rule out infection

▶ Hip aspiration if septic arthritis suspected

▶ X-ray: Unnecessary if hip motion is full; may show capsular swelling

▶ Ultrasound: Can demonstrate if effusion in hip joint

Differential Diagnosis

▶ Septic arthritis

▶ Osteomyelitis

▶ Legg-Calvé-Perthes disease

▶ Slipped capital femoral epiphysis

▶ Juvenile rheumatoid arthritis

Management

Nonpharmacologic Treatment

▶ Bedrest for 1–3 days

Pharmacologic Treatment

▶ OTC analgesics: Acetaminophen or NSAIDs taken with food may be used for 1–2 weeks

Special Considerations

▶ Rule out child abuse.

When to Consult, Refer, Hospitalize

▶ Orthopedic referral needed for hip aspiration if infection is suspected.

▶ Hospitalize for any indication of infection.

Follow-up

Expected Course

▶ Improvement should occur in 24–48 hours.

▶ If symptoms persist beyond 1 week, re-evaluation is important to rule out other diagnoses.

Complications

▶ 2%–5% develop Legg-Calvé-Perthes disease within 1 year.

▶ Rarely, avascular necrosis of femoral head

▶ May experience reoccurrence with subsequent viral infections

LEGG-CALVÉ-PERTHES DISEASE

Description

▶ Idiopathic juvenile avascular necrosis of femoral head

Etiology

▶ Unclear; can be idiopathic or due to slipped capital femoral epiphysis, trauma, steroid use, sickle cell crisis, or congenital dislocation of hip that may cause disruption in blood flow to femoral head

Incidence and Demographics

▶ Children 4–8 years old; male-to-female ratio 4–5:1; low frequency among relatives

▶ 10% bilateral

▶ Increased frequency in urban areas

Risk Factors

▶ Low birth weight, delayed bone age, short stature

▶ 10% breech delivery

▶ 17% with previous trauma

▶ History of steroid use, sickle cell disease, congenital hip dislocation

▶ Older parents, from large families of lower socioeconomic status

Prevention and Screening

▶ If child is obese, weight reduction may reduce risk of developing in other hip

Assessment

History

▶ Either subtle or sudden onset of limp, may be intermittent in early stages

▶ Sudden onset of groin, thigh, or knee pain

▶ Pain worse in morning and after activity

Physical Exam

▶ Presents with painful or painless limp

▶ Resists internal rotation and abduction

▶ Leg kept in position of flexion and external rotation

▶ May have atrophy of quadriceps muscles

Diagnostic Studies

▶ X-ray AP and frog leg views

▶ Early X-ray may be negative or show widening of joint space

▶ Later X-ray with increased density, decreased femoral head size, and flattening of femoral head

▶ Ultrasound may show joint effusion early

Differential Diagnosis

▶ Septic arthritis

▶ Trauma

▶ Slipped capital femoral epiphysis

▶ Neoplasia

▶ Hemophilia

▶ JRA

▶ Acute or chronic infection

Management

Nonpharmacologic Treatment

▶ Bedrest initially, followed by limited activities

▶ Physical therapy to maintain range of motion; may need crutches initially

▶ Containment of the femoral epiphysis with cast, brace, or orthosis

Pharmacologic Treatment

▶ OTC NSAIDs taken with food for pain relief

Special Considerations

▶ Pain often referred to knee

When to Consult, Refer, Hospitalize

▶ All suspected cases require orthopedic consult.

Follow-up

Expected Course

▶ Related to degree of femoral head involvement and age at onset; symptoms slowly resolve over 12–18 months

▶ Children < 6 years old with better prognosis; children > 8 years old have increased risk of degenerative arthritis in adulthood and may need hip replacement

Complications

▶ Hip replacement may be needed.

SLIPPED CAPITAL FEMORAL EPIPHYSIS (SCFE)

Description

▶ Anterior displacement of femoral neck from the capital femoral epiphysis, sudden or gradual dislocation of the head of the femur from its neck and shaft at the proximal epiphyseal plate

Etiology

▶ True etiology unclear; likely a combination of factors

▶ Mechanical factors (motor vehicle accident, fall from height, abuse)

▶ Endocrine (hypothyroidism, pituitary disorders)

▶ Genetic

▶ Inflammatory

Incidence and Demographics

▶ Most common adolescent hip disorder; male-to-female ratio 2:1; 2 cases per 100,000

▶ Peak age 12-year-old girls, 14-year-old boys

▶ 30% present with bilateral involvement

▶ 5% of cases with positive parental history of SCFE

Risk Factors

▶ Obesity

▶ Increased height

▶ Black

▶ Sedentary lifestyle

Assessment

History

▶ Pain in hip, infrequently referred pain to medial aspect of knee

▶ Severe pain in acute displacement

▶ Insidious, dull pain in gradual displacement

Physical Exam

▶ Presents with limp or inability to walk; walks with foot turned outward

▶ Local tenderness over hip

▶ Decreased flexion, abduction, and internal rotation

▶ Muscle atrophy and leg length shortening

Diagnostic Studies

▶ AP, lateral, and frog-leg X-rays diagnostic: Femoral head resembles ice cream falling off cone

▶ Early slippage may be missed on X-ray; if suspicious, order bone scan

Differential Diagnosis

- ▶ Toxic synovitis
- ▶ Legg-Calvé-Perthes disease
- ▶ Osteochondritis dissecans
- ▶ Chondrolysis

- ▶ Tumor
- ▶ Muscle strain
- ▶ Osteomyelitis
- ▶ Juvenile rheumatoid arthritis

Management

- ▶ Goals to prevent increased slippage and maintain hip function

Nonpharmacologic Treatment

- ▶ Early disease: Surgical placement of pin through femoral head and growth plate; rapid recovery with excellent prognosis
- ▶ Late disease: Reconstructive surgery; poor outcome due to degenerative arthritis and need for early hip replacement

Special Considerations

- ▶ Prognosis is good if diagnosed early; avoid delay in diagnosis

When to Consult, Refer, Hospitalize

- ▶ Emergency referral to orthopedist for surgical repair

Follow-up

Expected Course

- ▶ Depends on how quickly it is diagnosed
- ▶ Anatomic position must be maintained postoperatively.
- ▶ In children < 10 years old, monitor for bilateral slip.

Complications

- ▶ Avascular necrosis of femoral head
- ▶ May have slight but persistent leg-length shortening
- ▶ Chondrolysis more common in Black children

CONDITIONS THAT CAUSE KNEE PAIN

OSGOOD-SCHLATTER'S DISEASE

Description

▶ Overuse syndrome causing traction apophysitis of tibial tubercle

Etiology

▶ Repetitive microtrauma causing partial avulsion of patellar tendon insertion site on tibia (tibial apophysis)

Incidence and Demographics

▶ Boys 11–18 years old; girls 10–16 years old; more common in boys
▶ 30% bilateral

Risk Factors

▶ Physically active adolescents

Prevention and Screening

▶ Avoiding overuse
▶ Adequate stretching with exercise

Assessment

History

▶ Pain below knee that begins during or after activity and is relieved by rest

Physical Exam

▶ Local tenderness and swelling over tibial tubercle
▶ Resisted knee extension worsens pain

Diagnostic Studies

▶ Plain X-ray shows characteristic fragmentation of tibial tubercle; also can rule out other conditions if diagnosis uncertain
▶ May show soft-tissue swelling and thickening of patellar tendon

Differential Diagnosis

▶ Osteogenic sarcoma
▶ Patellar tendinitis

Management

Nonpharmacologic Treatment

▶ Avoid activities causing pain

▶ Ice for 20 minutes after exercise

▶ Quadriceps strengthening exercises q.i.d.

▶ If pain interferes with school and sleep, consider knee immobilization.

Special Considerations

▶ Recurrence rate 60%

When to Consult, Refer, Hospitalize

▶ Consult or refer if not improving with conservative treatment after 4 weeks.

Follow-Up

▶ At 2–4 week intervals

Expected Course

▶ Usually self-limited

▶ Resolves when tubercle fuses to diaphysis

Complications

▶ 5%–10% of cases become chronic and may require surgical resection of ossicle.

KNEE INJURY

Description

▶ Damage to the knee or its supporting structures caused by trauma

Etiology

▶ Direct or indirect force to the knee

▶ Common in sports that require rapid changes in direction, acceleration, and deceleration; knee injuries common in outpatient setting

▶ Often tear of ligaments or cartilage in knee

▶ May be fracture of the patella; children's ligaments and tendons are relatively stronger than bones, therefore children are at increased fracture risk

Incidence and Demographics

▶ Common in all ages, especially adults

▶ Meniscus injuries more common in adults than children

Risk Factors

▶ Participation in contact, running sports

▶ Poor conditioning

▶ Osteoarthritis

▶ Poorly fitting footwear, especially if associated with falls

Prevention and Screening

▶ Proper training, protective gear

Assessment

▶ See Tables 14–3 and 14–4.

Diagnostic Studies

▶ Joint aspiration: Diagnostic and therapeutic (presence of fat globules seen with fracture; removal of effusion can improve ROM, increase patient comfort)

▶ X-ray: Diagnose fracture, osteoarthritis

▶ CT: Evaluate extent of fracture depression (if any), position of fracture fragments

▶ MRI: Differentiate ligamentous, cartilaginous injuries

Differential Diagnosis

▶ Worsening osteoarthritis

▶ Septic joint

▶ Gout

▶ Tumor

Management

Nonpharmacologic Treatment

▶ Fracture: Immobilization, no weight-bearing, surgical repair sometimes necessary

▶ Grade I, II collateral ligament sprains: Hinged knee brace; surgery usually not required

▶ Grade III sprains involve complete tearing of ligament: Surgery usually required

▶ Cruciate ligament sprains: Bracing, physical therapy, surgical reconstruction may be necessary

▶ Meniscus tears: Arthroscopic repair (preferred treatment)

▶ Physical therapy for improving ROM, strength

Pharmacologic Treatment

▶ NSAIDs taken with food for 1–2 weeks regularly for inflammation and pain

▶ Analgesics , including narcotic medications for short-term pain management (up to 7–10 days)

Special Considerations

▶ Active younger patients may require functional bracing to return to sports.

TABLE 14-3
SUMMARY OF COMMON KNEE INJURIES

INJURY	DEMOGRAPHICS	HISTORY	PHYSICAL
Fracture	Any age	Trauma Steroid use, osteoporosis Sudden swelling, pain, worse with weight-bearing	Effusion (hemarthrosis) Bony tenderness or pain to palpation Decreased ROM Difficulty bearing weight
Medial collateral ligament (MCL) injury	Adolescents and adults Contact sports	Sudden valgus stress to knee May have heard or felt "pop" Medial knee pain Localized swelling 1–4 hours	Tenderness to palpation Varying degree of joint laxity Small effusion
Lateral collateral ligament (LCL) injury	Adolescents and adults Contact sports	Direct blow to medial aspect of knee (varus stress) Similar to MCL injury but lateral	Tenderness over LCL Varying degree of joint laxity Small, if any, effusion
Anterior cruciate ligament (ACL) injury	Adolescents and adults Athletes	Pain and almost immediate swelling after sudden turning, deceleration, jumping May have heard or felt a "pop" Weight-bearing difficult due to feelings of instability	Effusion (hemarthrosis) Pain or tenderness in posterolateral joint Positive provocation tests (anterior drawer, Lachman's)
Posterior cruciate ligament (PCL) injury	Athletes Gymnasts	Forced hyperextension of knee Direct blow to anterior proximal tibia while knee is flexed and foot is planted	Mild to moderate effusion Positive posterior drawer, Godfrey's tests
Meniscus tear	Adolescents, adults Athletes Older adults with OA of knee	Pain, especially with twisting of knee (getting in and out of vehicles) Locking, catching or giving way Harder to descend stairs than climb them	Swelling Tenderness over tibial medial or lateral joint line Positive McMurray's test
Quadriceps rupture	Athletes Older adults with concomitant diseases (diabetes, peripheral vascular disease)	Often, fall on extended knee that forces joint into flexion Inability to straighten knee	Swelling Sometimes, palpable defect just superior to patella Inability to extend knee against resistance

TABLE 14–4
CLINICALLY RELEVANT PROVOCATIVE TESTS OF THE KNEE

TEST NAME	HOW TO PERFORM TEST
Valgus stress (tests MCL)	With patient's knee in 20°–30° of flexion, the examiner stabilizes the leg with one hand while applying inward-directed pressure to the joint. Test is repeated with knee in full extension.
Varus stress (tests LCL)	As above, but stress at joint is directed from medial to lateral direction.
Anterior drawer (tests ACL)	With patient supine, knee is flexed to 90° while examiner stabilizes patient's tibia (usually by sitting on foot and ankle). Examiner grasps proximal posterior tibia, pulling it forward. Anterior movement (translation) of tibia greater than uninvolved side is positive test.
Posterior drawer (tests PCL)	Patient and examiner in same position as for anterior drawer, but examiner pushes tibia posteriorly.
Lachman's test (more accurate than anterior drawer)	With patient supine, knee is flexed to 30°. Using one hand, examiner stabilizes patient's distal femur while using other hand to pull proximal tibia anteriorly.
McMurray's test (for meniscus injury)	Patient's knee maximally flexed, then internally rotated; as leg is passively extended, examiner simultaneously externally rotates leg while palpating tibial joint line. Repeat with leg externally rotated, internally rotating while extending. Positive test is palpable click or tibial joint line pain.

When to Consult, Refer, Hospitalize

► Consult for grade II, III sprains.

► Refer immediately for suspected fracture, inability to flex or extend joint, hemarthrosis, suspected septic joint or tumor.

Follow-up

► In 1–2 weeks and at 2–4-week intervals until resolved

Expected Course

► Except for fractures, meniscus tears, and complete ligamentous disruption, most knee injuries will heal in 4–8 weeks.

Complications

► Deformity, accelerated degenerative changes of joint, stiffness, or instability

CONDITIONS THAT CAUSE ANKLE PAIN

ANKLE SPRAIN

Description

- ▶ Stretching or tearing of ligaments around the ankle
- ▶ Standard grading indicates extent of damage
    - » Grade I: Stretching but no tearing of ligament; no joint instability (local tenderness, minimal edema, full ROM, can bear weight, discomfort)
    - » Grade II: Partial (incomplete) tearing of ligament; some joint instability but definite end-point to laxity (immediate pain, localized edema, ecchymoses, pain on weight-bearing, reduced ROM)
    - » Grade III: Complete ligamentous tearing; joint unstable with no definite endpoint to ligamentous stressing (acute pain with injury, significant edema of foot and ankle, profound and continuing development of ecchymoses, cannot bear weight, ankle ROM restricted)

Etiology

- ▶ Usually a forced inversion, affects lateral ankle, most common; or eversion injury affects medial ankle — second most common type

Incidence and Demographics

- ▶ Most common musculoskeletal injury
- ▶ Occurs at rate of 1 per 10,000 persons per day; males affected more often

Risk Factors

- ▶ Sports requiring sudden turns, jumping; foot in supinated, plantar-flexed position

Prevention and Screening

- ▶ Conditioning exercises for sports, avoidance of high-heeled shoes, ankle-strengthening exercises

Assessment

History

- ▶ Sudden, forced inversion or eversion of foot, often in plantar-flexed position
- ▶ Sudden onset of pain, rapid onset of swelling; often with inability to initially bear weight on affected ankle
- ▶ Possible bruising within 2–4 days
- ▶ Sensation of pop, snap, locking of joint

Physical Exam

▶ Edema, ecchymosis, tenderness over injured ligaments; pain aggravated by repeating motion that caused original injury

▶ Talar tilt test used to assess stability of calcaneofibular ligament (heel is grasped and supinated)

▶ Anterior drawer sign used to assess anterior talofibular ligament (while holding the lower leg steady, the heel is grasped and pulled forward)

▶ Consider use of Ottawa Ankle Rules.

Diagnostic Studies

▶ X-rays not indicated in adult population unless at least one of the following (Ottawa rules)

  » Unable to bear weight right after injury or when examined

  » Tenderness over posterior edge of distal 6 cm of the medial or lateral malleolus

  » Tenderness over tarsal navicular or fifth metatarsal

▶ If X-rays necessary, AP, lateral, and mortise views should be ordered

Differential Diagnosis

▶ Syndesmosis injury   ▶ Fracture   ▶ Tendon rupture

Management

Nonpharmacologic Treatment

▶ Remember the mnemonic—all grades respond to RICE protocol:

  » **R:** Rest (non–weight-bearing)

  » **I:** Ice (20 minutes q.i.d. until swelling has resolved)

  » **C:** Compression (elastic bandage)

  » **E:** Elevation for 48–72 hours

▶ Splinting, weight-bearing as tolerated, ankle ROM and strengthening exercises

▶ Grade III injuries may require casting, surgery

Pharmacologic Treatment

▶ NSAIDs taken with food or OTC analgesics

How Long to Treat

▶ Most Grade I or II sprains heal in 6–8 weeks.

Special Considerations

▶ Medial ankle sprains require greater force to cause injury; may have other associated injury

▶ Geriatric patients: Older patients may require longer healing time.

When to Consult, Refer, Hospitalize

▶ Consult for any degree of ankle instability; refer for positive anterior drawer or talar tilt test, or for suggestion of syndesmosis injury.

Follow-up

▶ In 1–2 weeks if not improving after initial diagnosis

Expected Course

▶ Most uncomplicated sprains show improvement in 3–4 weeks, heal within 6–8 weeks

Complications

▶ Syndesmosis injury, peroneal tendinitis, recurrent injury, chronic instability, avascular necrosis

SEVER'S DISEASE

Description

▶ Inflammatory condition causing a calcaneal apophysitis

Etiology

▶ Traction-induced microtrauma at insertion of Achilles tendon on the calcaneus, causing inflammation

Incidence and Demographics

▶ 8–13-year-olds
▶ Athletes

Risk Factors

▶ Accelerated growth
▶ Tight heel cords
▶ Soccer players or runners

Assessment

History

▶ Heel pain with activity
▶ Bilateral or unilateral

Physical Exam

▶ Tenderness at insertion of the Achilles tendon on the calcaneus

Diagnostic Studies

▶ X-rays may show partial fragmentation and increased density of the os calcis.

Differential Diagnosis

▶ Bone cyst   ▶ Stress fracture   ▶ Strain

Management

Nonpharmacologic Treatment

▶ Activity modification

▶ Stretching, ice

▶ Heel cups

Pharmacologic Treatment

▶ NSAIDs

How Long to Treat

▶ Until resolved, 4–6 weeks

Special Considerations

▶ May need to modify activity, exercise, or shoes until improved

When to Consult, Refer, Hospitalize

▶ Achilles tendon rupture or not improving with treatment

Follow-up

▶ In 2 weeks, to make sure it is resolving

Expected Course

▶ Improvement in 2–4 weeks with activity modification

Complications

▶ Rupture of the Achilles tendon

CONDITONS THAT CAUSE SHOULDER PAIN

FRACTURED CLAVICLE

Description

▶ Fracture of clavicle; most frequently fractured bone during delivery

Etiology

▶ Birth trauma due to delivery of shoulder in vertex position and extended arms in breech delivery

▶ Fall on out-stretched arm or on clavicle

Incidence and Demographics

▶ 3.5% of births

▶ 80% middle third of clavicle

▶ Occurs in all ages; more common in children; in adults, usually occurs after a fall

Risk Factors

▶ Large fetus, shoulder dystocia

▶ Breech position

▶ Fall on outstretched arm

Prevention and Screening

▶ Methods to reduce birth trauma

▶ Check for fractures at birth and 2-week well-child visits.

Assessment

History

▶ Difficult delivery or characteristic injury

▶ Pain, displacement, or bump on clavicle

Physical Exam

▶ Newborn or patient may not move arm on affected side (Erb's palsy)

▶ Absent Moro reflex on affected side in newborn

Diagnostic Studies

▶ X-rays not usually done in newborns

▶ X-rays done if history of fall or trauma

Differential Diagnosis

▶ Fractured humerus

▶ Brachial nerve palsy

Management

▶ Prognosis is excellent even with no treatment if fracture is not displaced.

▶ Callus formation occurs in 1–2 weeks.

Nonpharmacologic Treatment

▶ Consider immobilization of arm and shoulder on affected side, figure of eight sling or clavicular strap

Pharmacologic Treatment

▶ Analgesics as needed

How Long to Treat

▶ Until healed (4–6 weeks)

Special Considerations

▶ Check in babies with history of breech or difficult delivery, large size, mothers with gestational diabetes

When to Consult, Refer, Hospitalize

▶ Refer to orthopedist for any symptoms of neurovascular injury.

Follow-up

▶ If not improving in 3–4 weeks

Expected Course

▶ Heals in 3–4 weeks in children

▶ Heals in 6 weeks in adults

Complications

▶ 10% of infants will also have concomitant brachial plexus injuries.

▶ Permanent bump at site of callus formation in adults; rare in children < 10 years

▶ Neurovascular injury

OTHER SHOULDER INJURIES AND CONDITIONS

Description

▶ Pain in the shoulder girdle

Etiology

▶ Traumatic, arthritic, infectious, or degenerative conditions (Table 14–5)

TABLE 14–5
COMMON CAUSES OF ACUTE AND CHRONIC SHOULDER PAIN

ACUTE CONDITIONS	CHRONIC CONDITIONS
Trauma: Fracture (proximal humerus, greater tuberosity, clavicle, scapula)	Inflammatory conditions:
	Bursitis (subacromial and subdeltoid)
Rotator cuff strain, tear	Bicipital, rotator cuff tendinitis
Dislocation (anterior most common)	Impingement syndrome
Acromioclavicular separation ("separated shoulder")	Degenerative conditions:
	Osteoarthritis
	Subacromial spurring
Sternoclavicular injury	Other:
	Chronic instability
	Adhesive capsulitis (frozen shoulder)

Incidence and Demographics

▶ Acute injuries tend to occur in adolescents and younger adults; chronic shoulder pain and fracture due to falls are more often found in older adults.

Risk Factors

▶ Repetitive overhead activity (occupational, recreational)

▶ Rheumatoid or osteoarthritis

▶ Previous shoulder injury

Prevention and Screening

▶ Injury prevention

Assessment

▶ See Table 14–6.

Diagnostic Studies

▶ Plain X-ray: Useful for evaluating fracture, AC separation, presence of osteophytes, calcific tendinitis

▶ MRI: Can show tendinitis, rotator cuff tear, ligamentous or cartilage injury

▶ Arthrogram: Still used to identify extent of rotator cuff tear

TABLE 14-6
ASSESSMENT OF SHOULDER INJURIES

CONDITION	HISTORY	PHYSICAL FINDINGS
Fracture	Fall directly onto shoulder or outstretched arm Localized pain, swelling Decreased ROM Often, no bruising evident for first few days after injury	Patient holds arm close to body Point tenderness Varying degree of bony deformity (usually most pronounced with clavicle fracture) Decreased ROM
Rotator Cuff Tear	Age usually > 40 years Pain may radiate into deltoid area May have felt "pop" or "something give" in shoulder Inability to raise arm overhead Weakness or inability to externally rotate arm Inability to sleep on affected side	Weakness or inability to externally rotate shoulder Limited abduction, forward flexion of shoulder Inability to maintain resisted abduction at 90°
Dislocation	Direct blow to shoulder or trying to avoid fall by grabbing onto something; shoulder in abducted, externally rotated position Sensation of shoulder slipping out of joint "Popping" or clicking of joint May note swelling	Positive apprehension test: Shoulder abducted to 90° and elbow flexed to 90°; shoulder then passively externally rotated; resistance by patient is a positive test Palpable clicking with ROM Deformity may be visible
Separated Shoulder	Usually, direct blow or fall onto top of shoulder Pain, especially with adduction of arm Swelling Deformity depends on severity of injury	Tenderness over acromioclavicular (AC) joint Pain with adduction (across chest) Varying degree of AC deformity (more deformity with more severe injury) Bruising may be present
Inflammatory Conditions	Progressive pain with certain activities (usually overhead) that may progress to constant pain Pain often worse with lifting, pushing objects away Difficulty lying on affected side	Tenderness over inflamed tendon(s)—palpated in bicipital groove May have weak abduction Painful arc (i.e., pain at 70°-120° of abduction)
Adhesive Capsulitis	Middle-age women more likely to be afflicted May or may not have history of trauma Progressive loss of motion Pain varies from minimal to severe	Marked restriction in active and passive ROM Pain over anterior joint, rotator cuff Patient often uses scapular muscles to "increase" abduction

Differential Diagnosis

▶ Septic joint

▶ Gout

▶ Complex regional pain syndrome

▶ Chondroclavicular disease

▶ Acromegaly

Management

Nonpharmacologic Treatment

▶ Initially, short period of rest or immobilization (no more than 14 days) then begin passive ROM exercises; progress to active, resistive exercises as healing continues

▶ Surgical intervention indicated for complete rotator cuff tear, displaced fracture

▶ Manipulation under anesthesia may be necessary for severe adhesive capsulitis.

▶ Physical therapy to maintain, improve ROM; strengthen muscles

Pharmacologic Treatment

▶ NSAIDs, other analgesics

▶ Local corticosteroid injection

How Long to Treat

▶ As long as symptomatic

When to Consult, Refer, Hospitalize

▶ Refer for any fracture, suspected rotator cuff tear, rheumatoid arthritis, AC separation with deformity, dislocation or chronic instability, adhesive capsulitis, corticosteroid injection

Follow-up

▶ Visits are variable depending on condition and severity, may be 2–4 week intervals

Expected Course

▶ Varies according to pathology

▶ Tendinitis symptoms should improve within 3–4 weeks of conservative therapy but may not resolve for 6 or more weeks; follow up in 3–4 weeks if no improvement.

▶ AC separation (mild) should be re-evaluated in 2–3 weeks; resolution usually in about 6 weeks

▶ Osteoarthritis: Reevaluate 4–6 weeks after starting treatment.

Complications

▶ Permanently decreased ROM, muscular weakness

CONDITIONS THAT CAUSE ELBOW PAIN

EPICONDYLITIS

Description

▶ Inflammation of the lateral or medial epicondyle

» Lateral epicondylitis ("tennis elbow"): Involves extensor tendons of forearm; common

» Medial epicondylitis ("golfer's elbow"): Involves flexor tendons of forearm; less common

Etiology

▶ Overuse syndrome caused by damage to tendons, progressing to periostitis at origin on epicondyle

▶ Stress on tendons; may be due to repetitive motions, poor technique when playing racquet or throwing sports; most common in middle age

Risk Factors

▶ Weak shoulder and wrist muscles (extensors, flexors, or both)

▶ Repetitive motion of forearm with wrist extended or flexed against resistance

Prevention and Screening

▶ Strengthening of shoulder muscles, wrist extensors and flexors

▶ For sports, appropriate-sized grips on racquets, proper body mechanics when throwing

Assessment

History

▶ Pain on affected side of elbow that progresses down forearm, occasionally into wrist

▶ Difficulty lifting objects, even a cup of liquid

▶ Numbness and tingling are *not* usually associated

Physical Exam

▶ Lateral or medial epicondyle is tender to palpation

▶ Lateral epicondylitis: Pain upon grasping a weighted cup or resisted wrist extension

▶ Medial epicondylitis: Pain with pronation, flex wrist against resistance, or squeezing hard rubber ball

Diagnostic Studies

▶ None

Differential Diagnosis

- ▶ Carpal tunnel syndrome
- ▶ Ulnar nerve entrapment
- ▶ Septic arthritis
- ▶ Elbow fracture
- ▶ Collateral ligament injury

Management

Nonpharmacologic Treatment

- ▶ Rest, ice
- ▶ Avoid activities that exacerbate pain.
- ▶ Compression with counterforce bands—tennis elbow band
- ▶ Physical therapy, including ultrasound, stretching exercises after pain subsides
- ▶ Recalcitrant cases may require surgery (Bosworth procedure).

Pharmacologic Treatment

- ▶ NSAIDs
- ▶ Triamcinolone corticosteroid injection if not improving with rest and NSAIDs

How Long to Treat

- ▶ Symptoms should resolve in 3 months with conservative treatment or maximum of 3 injections at 6-week intervals.

Special Considerations

- ▶ More than 3 corticosteroid injections unlikely to improve chance of remission but more likely to cause adverse effects (tendon weakening, subcutaneous fat necrosis, hypopigmentation of skin)

When to Consult, Refer, Hospitalize

- ▶ Refer to orthopedist if no improvement after 3 months of conservative treatment.

Follow-up

- ▶ Provide patient education about removing underlying cause of the problem to avoid recurrence.

Expected Course

- ▶ Noticeable improvement should occur within 6 weeks of treatment.

Complications

- ▶ Not common but chronic, untreated epicondylitis can progress to epicondylar spur formation and damage to collateral ligament

SUBLUXATION OF RADIAL HEAD

Description

▶ Subluxation of the annular ligament into the radio humeral joint; also known as "nursemaid's elbow"

Etiology

▶ Sudden longitudinal pull on hand with elbow extended and forearm pronated

▶ Ligament becomes trapped when radius recoils

Incidence and Demographics

▶ Most common elbow injury in 2–4-year-olds

▶ Peak incidence 1–3-year-olds

Prevention

▶ Avoid pulling on child's arm, swinging child by hands, or lifting by one hand.

▶ Screening: No routine screening; with presenting symptoms only

Assessment

History

▶ Report of child's arm being suddenly and vigorously pulled immediately followed by crying and refusal to move arm

▶ May have heard or felt a "click"

Physical Exam

▶ Child holds arm close to body in flexed, pronated position

▶ Flexion and extension normal; limited supination

▶ No swelling, deformity, point tenderness, warmth, or erythema noted

Diagnostic Studies

▶ X-ray if reduction unsuccessful

Differential Diagnosis

▶ Fracture

▶ Sprain or strain

Management

Nonpharmacologic Treatment
▶ Reduce subluxation by gentle supination with arm in 90° flexion
▶ "Click" usually heard or felt with immediate pain relief

Special Considerations
▶ Observe child after reduction to ensure use of arm.
▶ Have child grasp a sticker with affected hand.

When to Consult, Refer, Hospitalize
▶ Refer to orthopedist if closed reduction unsuccessful or recurrent.

Follow-up

Expected Course
▶ Full use returns in 30 minutes.

Complications
▶ Can be recurrent in some children

CONDITONS THAT CAUSE WRIST PAIN

LIGAMENT AND TENDON INJURIES

Description
▶ Acute or chronic pain in the wrist due to inflammation of soft tissue

Etiology
▶ Trauma (radiocarpal sprain), developmental (ganglion cyst), overuse (De Quervain's tenosynovitis, tendinitis)

Incidence and Demographics
▶ Common problem that affects all ages, sexes, races

Risk Factors
▶ Repetitive use of hands, wrists
▶ Injury to wrist
▶ Osteoarthritis

Prevention and Screening

▶ Wear protective wrist guards for sports.

▶ Properly position computer, keyboard, or other equipment.

▶ Avoid overuse.

Assessment

▶ See Table 14–7.

TABLE 14–7
COMMON CAUSES OF WRIST PAIN

CONDITION	HISTORY	PHYSICAL FINDINGS
Radiocarpal sprain	Trauma: Usually forced hyperextension or flexion Pain with movement Decreased ROM	Varying degree of swelling Numbness and tingling are unusual more than a day or two after injury Pain with active and passive ROM Tenderness over radiocarpal joint, but no point bony tenderness
Ganglion cyst	Usually no history of trauma May have repetitive use of hands or wrists Progressive localized swelling that tends to fluctuate in size depending on activity Usually non-painful	Most common on dorsum of wrist, but also seen on volar surface Encapsulated, slightly fluctuant, mobile lesion Pain may occur with compression of mass
De Quervain's tenosynovitis	Insidious onset of burning, aching pain over radial aspect of wrist and base of thumb Common in nursing mothers (due to holding infant with thumb extended); pain often worse with grasping movements	Pain with passive or active thumb extension May have visible thickening of tendon Positive Finkelstein's test: Pain with ulnar deviation of clenched fist (with thumb tucked inside fist)

Diagnostic Studies

▶ Clinical examination usually sufficient to diagnose these problems

▶ X-rays should be obtained if any suggestion of fracture.

▶ MRI can be used to differentiate ganglion cyst from other soft tissue masses; look for more serious wrist injury (triangular fibrocartilage tear).

Differential Diagnosis

▶ Nerve entrapment

▶ Fracture

▶ Gout

▶ Rheumatoid arthritis

▶ Osteoarthritis

Management

Nonpharmacologic Treatment

▶ Splinting, moist heat, aspiration of ganglion (fairly high recurrence rate)

▶ Surgical release of tendon sheath, surgical excision of ganglion

Pharmacologic Treatment

▶ NSAIDs

▶ Corticosteroid injection into first dorsal tendon sheath for de Quervain's

Special Considerations

▶ Women more often affected by de Quervain's, ganglion cysts

When to Consult, Refer, Hospitalize

▶ Consult with orthopedist for wrist condition that doesn't improve within 3–4 weeks of conservative treatment; refer for corticosteroid injection, any suspicion of fracture.

Follow-up

▶ If not improving in expected timeline

Expected Course

▶ Most wrist pain resolves in 4–6 weeks; ganglion cysts tend to recur.

Complications

▶ Few but chronic wrist pain can occur

OTHER MUSCULOSKELETAL CONDITIONS AND INJURIES

FRACTURES

Description

▶ Complete or incomplete chip or break in bone

Etiology

▶ Usually some type of trauma, but tumor, osteoporosis, osteomyelitis, osteomalacia can also cause bone to break

Incidence and Demographics

▶ Common in children due to activity, and in advancing age

▶ Caucasian women over age 60 have higher incidence of fracture than men

» Vertebral fractures are most frequent, followed by wrist fracture

Risk Factors

▶ Trauma, falls

▶ Neoplasms

▶ Osteoporosis, osteomyelitis

▶ Smoking, malnutrition (vitamin D deficiency), malabsorption, chronic steroid use

▶ Renal osteodystrophy

▶ Osteogenesis imperfecta

Prevention and Screening

▶ Maximize bone density during adolescence and young adulthood

▶ Weight-bearing physical activity

▶ Adequate dietary intake of calcium and vitamin D

▶ Avoidance of smoking, excessive alcohol intake

Assessment

History

▶ Pain is predominant symptom (fall, direct or indirect violence are also common)

▶ Pain worse with movement

▶ Swelling occurs rapidly, may be associated with bruising, variable degree of deformity or asymmetry

Physical Exam

▶ Point tenderness over bone; muscle weakness or pain with movement; deformity

Diagnostic Studies

▶ X-ray: Most cost-effective; usually adequate for showing fracture

▶ Bone scan: Useful for identifying occult and stress fractures

▶ CT: For evaluating degree of displacement, compression of fracture

▶ MRI: Identifying lesions that may affect bone

▶ Laboratory studies not usually indicated

Differential Diagnosis

- ▶ Sprain
- ▶ Hematoma
- ▶ Abscess
- ▶ Tumor

Management

Nonpharmacologic Treatment

- ▶ Immobilization by splinting or casting of extremity
- ▶ Monitor and maintain neurovascular integrity.
- ▶ Surgery may be necessary for open reduction and internal fixation if fracture is displaced.

Pharmacologic Treatment

- ▶ Analgesics, narcotic analgesia common
- ▶ NSAIDs after first 24 hours (immediate administration may increase hematoma formation due to platelet inhibition)

How Long to Treat

- ▶ Primary care treatment is immobilization and referral to orthopedic surgeon.
- ▶ Most simple fractures heal in 4–6 weeks; longer immobilization should be expected in presence of displaced fractures, chronic disease (diabetes, cardiovascular disease), smoking, or malignancy.

Special Considerations

- ▶ In geriatric patients, consider X-ray even if no trauma to rule out compression fracture or tumor.
- ▶ Consider stress fracture if persistent bony tenderness and negative initial X-ray.
- ▶ Epiphyseal fractures (Salter I–V) in children may disrupt growth of the bone.

When to Consult, Refer, Hospitalize

- ▶ Refer all compound, displaced, or compression fractures immediately.
- ▶ Consult with orthopedist to determine need for specialty care.
- ▶ Need to hospitalize is determined by orthopedist.

Follow-up

- ▶ In 4–6 weeks if improving, sooner if pain persists

Expected Course

- ▶ Fracture healing should occur in 4–6 weeks; if casted, persistent but gradually decreasing swelling and improving strength may take another 4–6 weeks to resolve.

Complications

- ▶ Persistent deformity, arthritis, compression neuropathy, fibrous union

STRESS FRACTURE

Description

▶ Fracture resulting from indirect trauma to a bone, creating a very fine fracture line that cannot easily be seen on X-ray

Etiology

▶ Microtrauma to a normal bone that exceeds that bone's capability for repair

▶ Fracture of a bone without trauma

Incidence and Demographics

▶ More common in runners, athletes who participate in jumping activities, military recruits

▶ Metatarsal stress fractures most common but tibial shaft, calcaneus, patella, pubic ramus, pars interarticularis also affected

Risk Factors

▶ Training errors (sudden increase in intensity or duration)

▶ Overuse

▶ Metabolic disorders

Prevention and Screening

▶ Proper training, wearing appropriate footwear, using good body mechanics

Assessment

History

▶ Insidious onset of pain intensified by running, jogging; pain may persist for 2–3 weeks before patient seeks treatment

Physical Exam

▶ Mild erythema, diffuse swelling, and point tenderness over fracture site

Diagnostic Studies

▶ Bone scan most useful for early diagnosis since X-ray changes not usually apparent for 3–4 weeks

Differential Diagnosis

▶ Sprain

▶ Infection

Management

Nonpharmacologic Treatment

▶ Limit physical activity.

▶ Correct underlying biomechanical problem.

Pharmacologic Treatment

▶ NSAIDs

▶ Narcotic analgesics rarely necessary

How Long to Treat

▶ 4–6 weeks

Special Considerations

▶ Consider in athletes, postmenopausal women with persistent bone pain without trauma

When to Consult, Refer, Hospitalize

▶ Consult or refer to orthopedist if any question about diagnosis, treatment.

Follow-up

▶ In 4–6 weeks, sooner if not improving

▶ Stress fractures can progress to complete fractures.

Expected Course

▶ Once treated, normal activities can usually be resumed in 4–6 weeks.

Complications

▶ Left untreated, can progress to full fracture

MUSCLE STRAIN

Description

▶ Over-stretching or partial tearing of muscle fibers; graded I–III

    ▹ Grade I: Stretching, tearing of muscle fibers but fascia remains intact, no loss of muscle function; movement strong and painful

    ▹ Grade II: Tearing of muscle fibers resulting in significant hemorrhage, mild loss of muscle strength; movement fairly strong and painful

    ▹ Grade III: Rupture of muscle, damage to fascia; movement is weak and pain-free

Etiology

▶ Excessive stress placed on any muscle resulting in overstretching of fibers and resultant tearing and inflammation

Incidence and Demographics

▶ Common problem, many instances self-treated

Risk Factors

▶ Contact sports, running

▶ Lifting or moving heavy objects

Prevention and Screening

▶ Appropriate stretching, warm-up exercises before participating in running, sports; proper body mechanics

Assessment

History

▶ Sudden onset of muscle pain associated with activity; bruising, swelling, and loss of function may occur with more severe injury

▶ Gradually increasing muscle pain may occur with repetitive use of specific muscle or group

Physical Exam

▶ Localized tenderness, swelling, ecchymosis; pain with resisted muscle contraction and passive stretching of muscle; weakness with more severe injury

Diagnostic Studies

▶ Physical exam

▶ MRI may be useful to identify extent of muscle involvement, but usually not necessary

Differential Diagnosis

▶ Tendinitis   ▶ Tumor

Management

Nonpharmacologic Treatment

▶ Rest, ice, compression (if an extremity), elevation; physical therapy to regain strength, mobility

Pharmacologic Treatment

▶ NSAIDs are mainstay of treatment

▶ Narcotic analgesics may be necessary for first 2–3 days

How Long to Treat

▶ 10–14 days

Special Considerations

▶ More active patients should not return to contact sports until they are pain-free.

When to Consult, Refer, Hospitalize

▶ Consult with orthopedist for grade III injuries; refer for any injury involving muscle weakness.

Follow-up

▶ In 2 weeks if not improving

Expected Course

▶ Varies with degree of injury

▶ Mild strains resolve in 2–3 weeks; severe injuries may require > 8 weeks of treatment

Complications

▶ Permanent deformity, loss of strength

BURSITIS

Description

▶ Inflammation or infection of synovial membrane of the bursal sac overlying bony prominences

▶ Common sites are shoulder (subacromial or subdeltoid), elbow (olecranon), hip (trochanteric), knee (prepatellar, pes anserine, suprapatellar), heel (retrocalcaneal)

Etiology

▶ Trauma, overuse causing pressure and irritation of bursa lining

▶ Bacterial infection may cause inflammation.

Incidence and Demographics

▶ No accurate incidence available in research literature. Estimated to account for up to 0.4% of all primary care visits.

▶ Most commonly seen in athletes or as an overuse injury

Risk Factors

▶ Chronic pressure on bursa (kneeling, resting point of elbow on hard surface, overhead activity)

- Rheumatoid, gouty, or inflammatory arthritis
- Baker's cyst
- Chronic or acute overuse, particularly in middle age or older adults

Prevention and Screening

- Avoidance of activities that apply pressure to bursae
- Use of appropriate protective or padded equipment

Assessment

History

- Sudden or gradual onset of localized painful swelling
- Increased pain and discomfort with activity

Physical Exam

- Localized fluctuant swelling (swelling over greater trochanter difficult to evaluate), sometimes warm or painful to touch
- No loss of ROM
- If erythema or warmth, consider septic bursitis

Diagnostic Studies

- None needed unless redness or warmth
- If redness or warmth, fluid aspiration analysis to evaluate for infection or gout; CBC

Differential Diagnosis

- Septic joint
- Gout
- Joint effusion
- Trauma
- Rheumatoid arthritis
- Cellulitis

Management

Nonpharmacologic Treatment

- RICE protocol
- Aspiration of bursal sac to reduce pain from pressure

Pharmacologic Treatment

- If septic bursitis, oral antibiotics, often dicloxacillin (Dynapen) or cephalexin (Keftab)
- NSAIDs (ibuprofen, sodium naproxen)
- Local corticosteroid injection: Not performed unless infection is ruled out
- Retrocalcaneal injection not recommended, due to risk of Achilles tendon rupture

How Long to Treat

▶ NSAIDs for 1–3 weeks until swelling subsides

Special Considerations

▶ Surgical drainage or removal may be necessary if infection does not respond to antibiotics, local aspiration.

When to Consult, Refer, Hospitalize

▶ Refer to physician or other specialized healthcare provider for bursa aspiration as necessary.

▶ Consult with physician or other healthcare provider for local skin infection, marked cellulitis, or signs of systemic illness associated with bursitis for parenteral antibiotics, possible hospitalization.

Follow-up

▶ Provide patient education about need for rest for area.

Expected Course

▶ Symptoms usually improve within 2–3 days of aspirating or injecting bursa (if not infected).

▶ If infected, localized erythema should improve within 3–5 days.

Complications

▶ Chronic bursitis

CARPAL TUNNEL SYNDROME (CTS)

Description

▶ Entrapment neuropathy of median nerve at the wrist

Etiology

▶ Multiple causes, includes any process that encroaches on the carpal tunnel, compressing the median nerve, or causes enlargement of median nerve

▶ Mnemonic for causes is **PRAGMATIC**: **P**regnancy, **R**heumatoid Arthritis, **G**rowth hormone abnormalities, **M**etabolic disorders, **A**lcoholism, **T**umors, **I**diopathic, **C**onnective tissue disorders

　　» Work or hobby repetitive flexion and extension of wrist: Computer typists, cashiers, sorters, musicians, hairdressers, use of vibrating tools, painters

　　» History of trauma to wrist: Fracture, dislocations

Incidence and Demographics

► Affects approximately 1% of U.S. population

► Women affected more often than men; onset ages 30–50 years, incidence increases with age

► More common in people using forceful, repetitive wrist and hand movements or vibratory tools

Risk Factors

► Repetitive wrist flexion or extension movement; collagen vascular disease, history of Colles' fracture

Prevention and Screening

► Proper ergonomics for wrist

► Treatment of underlying problem

Assessment

History

► Initially burning or aching pain, numbness, tingling that wakes patient at night and resolves after shaking the affected hand ("wake-and-shake")

► As disorder progresses, symptoms affect thumb, index and middle finger; may radiate into arm

Physical Exam

► Tinel's sign: Positive if symptoms are reproduced by tapping the median nerve at the wrist

► Phalen's sign: Positive if pain within 60 seconds of bilateral wrist flexion with hands held in opposition (clinically, may be more useful than Tinel's)

► Carpal compression test: Positive if numbness and tingling develop with direct pressure over carpal tunnel

► Painless thenar muscle wasting is late finding; usually no visible abnormality; pain exacerbated by extreme volar flexion

► May have decreased grip strength, decreased sensation in first three digits

Diagnostic Studies

► Electromyography/nerve conduction studies: EMG/NCS

► Electromyography/nerve conduction velocity (EMG/NCV) studies are standard.

► Mild to moderate symptoms should be present for 6 months for EMG/NCV studies to be accurate.

► Plain X-rays if any history of trauma to rule out fracture

► If secondary cause suspected, order appropriate test, e.g., TSH, RF, HbgA1c

Differential Diagnosis

▶ Cervical radiculopathy (C6, C7)

▶ Brachial plexopathy

▶ Carpal navicular fracture

Management

Nonpharmacologic Treatment

▶ Splinting (cock-up wrist splint at night) to relieve compression on nerve, elevate extremity

▶ Ergonomic modification of work, hobby

▶ Surgical release if conservative methods fail

Pharmacologic Treatment

▶ NSAIDs in standard doses, on daily basis

▶ Acetaminophen up to 4000 mg/day in divided doses p.o.

▶ Corticosteroid injection into carpal tunnel (not nerve)

How Long to Treat

▶ Depends on severity of symptoms

▶ Generally, allow 6 weeks from onset of symptoms before obtaining EMG/NCS

Special Considerations

▶ Pregnancy: Increased incidence likely due to fluid retention

▶ Lactation: May be aggravated by wrist flexion while holding nursing infant

When to Consult, Refer, Hospitalize

▶ Consult with orthopedist or neurologist if patient's symptoms not improved with splinting, NSAIDs.

▶ Consider referral for corticosteroid injection.

Follow-up

Expected Course

▶ Mild cases usually respond to conservative measures.

▶ Patient may require surgical release of nerve if burning, numbness, or tingling persist or increase; loss of grip or pinch strength is persistent; or there is evidence of muscle atrophy.

Complications

▶ Irreversible nerve damage, thenar muscle atrophy

LOW BACK PAIN (LBP) AND HERNIATED NUCLEUS PULPOSUS (HNP)

Description

▶ Common problem; goal is to rule out serious causes

 » LBP: Pain in lower lumbar, lumbosacral, or sacroiliac area that may radiate down one or both buttocks or legs

 » HNP: Rupture of an intervertebral disc with herniation of nucleus pulposus into spinal canal; disk compresses spinal cord or irritates associated nerve root

 » *Spondylolysis* is an acquired condition with a bony defect of the pars interarticularis, usually at L5–S1.

 » *Spondylolisthesis* is a slip of the vertebral body in an adjacent vertebra with a bilateral pars defect at a single vertebral level.

 » Sciatica refers to pain and paresthesias extending down the leg in a dermatomal pattern.

Etiology

▶ LBP: Ligamentous (sprain) or muscular problems (strain), osteoarthritis, other diseases (fibromyalgia, osteoporosis, osteomyelitis), tumor

▶ HNP: Trauma, degenerative spine disease, spinal stenosis

▶ Spondylolysis and spondylolisthesis develop in children doing vigorous athletic activity.

▶ Spondylolisthesis can occur in adults with degenerative changes of the facet joints without spondylolysis of the pars.

▶ The most common cause of sciatica is a herniated disk at L4–5, L5–S1.

Incidence and Demographics

▶ Estimated that 80% of adults in U.S. have an episode of back pain, 10% HNP

▶ Most common at 20–40 years old, working adults

▶ Back pain not common in children

▶ Spondylolysis occurs in 5% pre-adolescent children, 12% in divers/gymnasts

Risk Factors

▶ Physical deconditioning, weak paraspinal or abdominal muscles

▶ Poor body mechanics, poor posture

▶ Occupational strain, poor body mechanics, heavy lifting

▶ Obesity, arthritis

▶ Mechanical disorders, e.g., scoliosis, leg-length discrepancy, kyphosis

▶ Tobacco use

Prevention and Screening

▶ Regular exercise program

▶ Maintaining ideal body weight

▶ Proper body mechanics

Assessment

▶ See Table 14–8.

TABLE 14–8
DIFFERENTIATING LOW BACK PAIN

CLINICAL PROBLEM	HISTORY	PHYSICAL EXAMINATION
Low back pain	Pain in back, buttocks, thigh Onset after exertion and with movement No history of trauma, infection, malignancy Pain relieved by lying supine	Paravertebral tenderness, muscle spasm Loss of normal lumbar lordosis common No neurologic deficit
Herniated nucleus pulposus	Initially, back pain severe Chronic herniation usually results in leg pain greater than back pain Often, + history of trauma, forced flexion Central herniation results in bilateral leg weakness, bowel or bladder dysfunction	L5–S1 (most common): Pain in posterior thigh, posterior or lateral calf, heel; weak plantar flexion of foot; diminished ankle reflex L4–5: Pain in lateral thigh, anterior calf and dorsum of foot; weak dorsiflexion of foot L3–4: Pain in anterior and lateral thigh, medial calf, and foot; weak quadriceps; diminished patellar reflex
Spinal stenosis	Gradual onset bilateral pain, neurogenic claudication: leg pain, paresthesias, weakness with walking, standing May have bowel and bladder dysfunction Usually relieved when flexes spine or rests	X-ray: Osteophytes Weakness: Foot, ankle Diminished reflexes: Ankle, knee May have atrophy in leg muscles
Spondylosis and spondylolisthesis	Vigorous athletic activity as child Positive family history Low back pain, may radiate into buttocks Wakens patient at night	Lumbosacral tenderness Accentuation of pain with hyperextension of spine, one leg raised off ground, flexed 90° at knee and hip Reduced side bending
Low back pain in children	More common in adolescence Red flag if: constant, under age 11, lasts several weeks, wakes child at night, limitation of motion, fever, neurologic signs	If spinal tenderness, fever, neurologic or systemic symptoms, X-ray and labs indicated

History

- ▶ Assess carefully: Duration of symptoms, any known precipitant, any associated symptoms

- ▶ Symptoms suggestions more serious problem: Bilateral leg weakness, bowel or bladder incontinence, saddle paresthesia, pain unrelieved by rest, pain worse at night, pain worsens with rest

- ▶ Symptoms suggesting strain: Pain, stiffness associated with identified activity; worsens with activity, improves with rest

- ▶ Ask if bowel or bladder dysfunction or saddle numbness or paresthesia; indicates cauda equina syndrome, a neurologic emergency

- ▶ Children: Ask if trauma, recent infection, athletics, inflammatory disease, or malignancy

- ▶ Adults and geriatric patients: Ask about occupation, sports, leisure activities, underlying medical problems

- ▶ Exclude urgent medical conditions with mnemonic **MICE** (**M**etastatic, **I**nfection, **C**ompression fracture, cauda **E**quina syndrome) or referred pain from pelvic or abdominal pathology.

- ▶ HNP is associated with pain radiating to buttock, leg, or foot.

Physical Exam

- ▶ Note gait, check for ability to walk on heels and toes

- ▶ Palpate spinal column, note abnormal curvature

- ▶ Perform ROM extension, flexion, hyperextension, lateral bend, rotation

- ▶ Palpate paraspinal muscle tenderness, spasm

- ▶ Check deep tendon reflexes bilaterally: Knee, Achilles, Babinski

- ▶ Check strength, vibratory, and proprioceptive sensation bilaterally

- ▶ Check weakness in dorsiflexion (ankle and great toe)

- ▶ Check light touch sensation of medial, dorsal, and lateral foot, peroneal area

- ▶ With the patient on his or her back, raise one leg with knee absolutely straight, until pain is experienced in the thigh, buttock, and calf. Record angle at which pain occurs. A normal (pain-free) value would be 70–90°, higher in people with lax ligaments.

- ▶ Then perform sciatic stretch test: Dorsiflex foot at point of discomfort. Test is positive if more pain results.

- ▶ Flexing the knee will relieve the buttock pain, but this is restored by pressing on the lateral popliteal nerve.

- ▶ Severe root irritation is indicated when straight raising of the leg on the unaffected side produces pain on the affected side.

Diagnostic Studies

- ▶ X-ray studies usually not necessary unless history of trauma, suspicion of systemic or structural changes

- ▶ Order diagnostic imaging and testing when severe or progressive neurologic deficits present, or serious underlying conditions suspected.

- ▶ MRI: Most useful for identifying HNP, diskitis, tumors

▶ CT: May help identify cord impingement (especially laterally), good for examination of osseous areas

▶ Bone scan: Helpful for identifying metabolically active processes such as tumor, occult fracture, infection, abscess

▶ Serum studies usually not helpful but ESR elevated in infection; HLA-B27 elevated in ankylosing spondylitis

Differential Diagnosis

Spinal Disorders

▶ Herniated disk

▶ Spondylolisthesis

▶ Spinal stenosis

Metabolic Disorders

▶ Osteoporosis

▶ Osteomalacia

▶ Paget's disease

Rheumatologic Disorders

▶ Rheumatoid arthritis

▶ Reiter syndrome

▶ Psoriatic arthritis

▶ Ankylosing spondylitis

Tumor

▶ Benign

▶ Malignant

▶ Metastatic

Infection

▶ Bacterial

▶ Tuberculous

Miscellaneous

▶ Peptic ulcer

▶ Sickle cell disease

▶ Pancreatic disease

▶ Renal stones

▶ Tumor

▶ Infection

▶ Peptic ulcer

▶ Abdominal aortic aneurysm

▶ Ovarian cysts, tumors

Management

▶ Most LBP responds to conservative treatment within 4–6 weeks; in the absence of acute neurologic deficit, 80% or more of patients with HNP also respond to conservative treatment.

Nonpharmacologic Treatment

▶ Short course of bedrest (1–2 days) then activity as tolerated; encourage patient to remain active

▶ Chiropractic manipulation may be helpful if no radiculopathy

▶ Patient education for proper body mechanics, back strengthening

▶ Physical therapy to learn muscle-conditioning exercises, proper body mechanics

▶ Behavioral management

Pharmacologic Treatment

▶ NSAIDs or acetaminophen are first-line treatment.

▶ Muscle relaxants may be helpful for first 48–72 hours if low back strain with spasm in those who fail to respond to NSAIDs

▶ Narcotic analgesics rarely necessary

How Long to Treat

▶ Most episodes resolve within 4–6 weeks of conservative treatment.

Special Considerations

▶ In jobs requiring heavy lifting or exertion, incidence is somewhat greater for women.

▶ Pregnancy: LBP common, as is sciatica; symptoms frequently resolve after delivery.

When to Consult, Refer, Hospitalize

▶ Refer to neurosurgeon or orthopedist for patients who do not respond to 4 weeks of conservative treatment, or with spinal instability, expanding pain that worsens at night, signs of infection, neurologic deficit, cauda equina syndrome.

▶ Hospitalize for abscess, tumor, signs suggestive of abdominal aneurysm.

Follow-up

▶ If patient in severe pain, reevaluate in 24–48 hours.

▶ Provide patient education about body mechanics, conservative therapy, use of medications and their side effects.

Expected Course

▶ Remitting and recurring symptoms are common; most LBP resolves in 4–6 weeks with conservative care; 90% resolves within 2 months.

Complications

▶ Without neurologic deficit, few complications if diagnosed and treated, though recurrence is common.

FIBROMYALGIA

Description

▶ Musculoskeletal syndrome characterized by generalized nonarticular pain, diffuse aching, stiffness, and fatigue with multiple tender points

Etiology

▶ Unknown

▶ Possible triggers are viral infections, stress, immunologic abnormalities, depression, heightened perception of physiologic stimuli

Incidence and Demographics

▶ Affects 2% of population

▶ Peak incidence at ages 20–40 years; 75% female

Risk Factors

▶ Unknown; possible genetic predisposition

▶ May be associated with rheumatoid arthritis, Lyme disease, osteoarthritis, sleep apnea, metastatic carcinoma, hypothyroidism

▶ Associated with sedentary childhood, although not sure if some problem produces more sedentary child or sedentary child is more likely to develop fibromyalgia

Assessment

History

▶ Diffuse, widespread myalgia pain and tender points

▶ Muscle weakness; stiffness after prolonged sitting or sleeping

▶ Fatigue disproportionate to exertion; nonrestorative sleep

▶ Headache, atypical chest pain, irritable bowel symptoms

Physical Exam

▶ Normal examination except for pain at trigger points; see diagnostic criteria (Box 14–1)

Diagnostic Studies

▶ No specific serum; radiographic, biopsy, radionucleotide abnormalities present

Differential Diagnosis

▶ Rheumatoid arthritis

▶ Hypothyroidism

▶ Myofascial pain syndrome

▶ Infections: HIV, hepatitis, Lyme disease

▶ Chronic fatigue syndrome

▶ Polymyalgia rheumatica

▶ Lupus

▶ Psychiatric disorder

▶ Multiple sclerosis

> **BOX 14–1**
> **CLASSIFICATION OF FIBROMYALGIA**
> **(American College of Rheumatology)**
>
> **History of widespread pain**
> *Description:* Pain is considered widespread when all of the following are present: pain in the left side of the body, pain in the right side of the body, pain above the waist, and pain below the waist. In addition, axial skeletal pain (cervical spine, anterior chest, thoracic spine, or low back) must be present. In this description, shoulder and buttock pain is considered as pain for each involved side. "Low back" pain is considered lower segment pain.
>
> **Pain in 11 of 18 tender point sites on digital palpation**
> *Description:* Pain on digital palpation, must be present bilaterally in at least 11 of the following 18 tender point sites:
>
> *Occiput:* At the suboccipital muscle insertions
>
> *Low cervical:* At the anterior aspects of the intertransverse spaces at C5–C7
>
> *Trapezius:* At the midpoint of the upper border
>
> *Supraspinatus:* At origins, above the scapula spine near the medial border
>
> *Second rib:* At the second costochondral junctions, just lateral to the junctions on upper surfaces
>
> *Lateral epicondyle:* 2 cm distal to the epicondyles
>
> *Gluteal:* In upper outer quadrants of buttocks in anterior fold of muscle
>
> *Greater trochanter:* Posterior to the trochanteric prominence
>
> *Knee:* At the medial fat pad proximal to the joint line
>
> Adapted from *Primer on the Rheumatic Diseases* (12th ed.). by J. H. Klippel, 2001, Atlanta: The Arthritis Foundation.

Management

Nonpharmacologic Treatment

▶ Behavior modification and patient education

▶ Gradual reconditioning program (low-impact aerobics, walking, swimming), biofeedback, heat, massage

Pharmacologic Treatment

▶ Cyclobenzaprine (Flexeril) 5–40 mg every night p.o.

▶ Amitriptyline (Elavil) 10–150 mg every night p.o.; if not tolerated, zolpidem (Ambien) 5–10 mg every night or an SSRI in low doses

▶ Tramadol (Ultram) 50–100 mg q4–6h p.r.n. may be helpful for pain

▶ Approved by FDA for fibromyalgia;

  ▸ Pregabalin (Lyrica): Initially 75 mg b.i.d., maximum dose 45 mg daily; requires tapering if discontinued

  ▸ Duloxetine (Cymbalta): Initially 30 mg p.o. for 1 week; maximum dose 60 mg daily; requires tapering if discontinued

  ▸ Milnacipran (Savella): Initially 12.5 mg daily with increasing doses as needed; maximum dose 200 mg daily; requires tapering if discontinued

▶ Selective serotonin reuptake inhibitors—fluoxetine (Prozac)

▶ Corticosteroids and opioids are ineffective.

How Long to Treat

▶ Chronic, may require years of medication

Special Considerations

▶ Psychogenic factors need consideration.

When to Consult, Refer, Hospitalize

▶ Hospitalization generally not indicated

▶ Patient-involved therapy seems to have better prognosis

▶ Consult or refer if differential diagnoses cannot be excluded or if there is suggestion of psychiatric component; rheumatology referral to assist with evaluation and management plan

Follow-up

Expected Course

▶ Only 5% have complete remission.

Complications

▶ Chronic pain, lack of "cure" may initiate depression.

CASE STUDIES

CASE 1. A 12-year-old White male presents with pain in right hip that has worsened over the past 2 weeks.

HPI: Prefers to play video games, does not play sports, denies trauma

PMH: Adenoidectomy and PETs at age 3, > 100% for weight on growth chart, BMI > 32

- ▶ What other history would you like to obtain—recent illness, description of pain, associated symptoms?
- ▶ What type of examination should be done?

Exam: Patient has local tenderness over hip with decreased flexion, abduction, and internal rotation.

- ▶ What diagnostic tests should be ordered?
- ▶ What is the diagnosis and plan for management?

CASE 2. 34-year-old man with complaint of left elbow pain for the last 2 weeks.

HPI: Played in two golf tournaments 2 weeks ago. Denies trauma. C/o dull ache in elbow joint that radiates down forearm. Denies numbness or tingling.

PMH: Overweight, history of "borderline hypertension"

- ▶ What other history would you like to obtain?
- ▶ What should be done on physical exam?

Exam: Medial epicondyle is tender to palpation, + pain with pronation, flexing wrist against resistance, or squeezing hard rubber ball.

- ▶ What diagnostic tests should be ordered?
- ▶ What is the diagnosis and plan for management?

CASE 3. A 15-year-old girl presents with complaint of bilateral knee pain during and after exercise.

HPI: Pain in anterior knee area, just below knee joints during and after exercise. Denies trauma, plays basketball on her high school team, currently practicing nightly for an upcoming tournament.

PMH: Well, no history of serious illness, accidents, or medical problems

- ▶ What other history would you like to obtain?
- ▶ What type of examination should be done?

Exam: No fever; no redness, edema, warmth, or effusion; ROM/ligaments all intact; bony tenderness, bilateral swelling at tibial tubercle.

- ▶ What diagnostic tests should be ordered?
- ▶ What is the diagnosis and plan for management?

REFERENCES

Agency for Healthcare Research and Quality. (2013). *Toward optimized practice. Guideline for the evidence-informed primary care management of low back pain.* Retrieved from www.guidelines.gov/content.aspx?id=37954&search=low+back+pain

American College of Rheumatology. (2012). *2012 American College of Rheumatology guidelines for management of gout part 1& part 2.* Retrieved from http://ww2.rheumatology.org/practice/clinical/guidelines/gout.asp

American College of Rheumatology Subcommittee on Rheumatoid Arthritis Guidelines. (2012). *Practice guidelines.* Retrieved from www.rheumatology.org/practice/clinical/guidelines/

Arcangeo, V. P., & Peterson, A. M. (2012). *Pharmacotherapeutics for advanced practice* (3rd ed.). Philadelphia: Lippincott Williams & Wilkins.

Domino, F. J., Baldor, R. A., Golding, J., Grimes, J. A., & Taylor, J. S. (2013). *The 5-minute clinical consult* (21st ed.). Philadelphia: Lippincott Williams & Wilkins.

Fitzcharles, M., & Yunus, M. B. (2012). The clinical concept of fibromyalgia as a changing paradigm in the past 20 years. *Pain Research and Treatment, 2012*, article 184835.

Goroll, A. H., & Mulley, A. G. (2009). *Primary care medicine: Office evaluation and management of the adult patient* (6th ed.). Philadelphia: Lippincott Williams & Wilkins.

Hay, W. W., Levin, M. J., Deterding, R. R., Abzug, M. J., & Sondheimer, J. M. (2012). *Current diagnosis and treatment pediatrics* (21st ed.). New York: McGraw-Hill Companies, Inc.

Papadakis, M. A., McPhee, S. J., Rabow, M. W. (2013). *Current medical diagnosis and treatment 2013.* New York: McGraw-Hill.

Salt, E., & Crofford, L. (2012). Rheumatoid arthritis: New treatments, better outcomes. *Nurse Practitioner, 37*(11), 16–22.

U.S. Preventive Services Task Force. (2013). *Guide to clinical preventive services,* Chapter 14.docx. Retrieved from www.guidelines.gov

NEUROLOGIC DISORDERS

Deborah Gilbert-Palmer, EdD, FNP-BC

GENERAL APPROACH

For All

▶ Neurologic problems range from chronic to acute to lethal.

▶ A screening neurologic exam should be done on all patients with symptoms suspicious for a neurologic disorder and would include: mental status (level of consciousness, orientation, memory, cognitive function, language), motor function (body position, involuntary movement, muscle tone, strength), sensory function (light touch, pain, position sense), reflexes (deep tendon reflexes [DTRs], abdominal, Babinski), cerebellar function (gait, rapid alternating movements, point-to-point movements, Romberg), cranial nerves (I–XII, motor and sensory components).

▶ Abnormalities should be further evaluated with additional assessment techniques (Mini Mental Status Examination [MMSE], discriminating sensory testing [stereognosis, two-point discrimination], and meningeal irritability testing), referred to a neurologic specialist and for diagnostic testing, or any combination of these.

Children

▶ The nervous system is more difficult to examine in the infant and younger child because it is less mature. Special attention is paid to head circumference and fontanels, general appearance and positioning, primitive reflexes, and developmental milestones.

▶ Knowledge of normal childhood developmental milestones and the patient's previous behavioral history is important to the diagnosis.

▶ Early recognition of problems is of utmost importance to future development and prevention of disability.

▶ Birth history of the patient, including gestational age, type of birth, complications, Apgar scores, incidence of trauma, congenital anomalies, birth weight, perinatal illness or drug use, is important.

▶ Consider a cardiac or metabolic etiology or an adverse medication reaction in the differential diagnosis whenever a neurologic problem is suspected.

▶ Neurologic "soft signs" (clumsiness, hyperkinesis, language disturbances, developmental delays, mirroring movements, echolalia, short attention spans) are more difficult to assess and diagnose but must be considered in the neurologic evaluation.

▶ In infants and toddlers, fontanels can provide information regarding increasing intracranial pressure (IICP) as well as hydration status and clues to development.

Older Adults

▶ 20% decrease in blood flow to the brain with changes in autoregulation; contributes to risk of orthostatic hypotension

▶ No changes in thinking, behavior, or intellectual function, although response time and processing of information is slower

▶ Greater incidence of sensory deficits with aging and chronic illness (decreased hearing, decreased visual acuity, decreased position sense) may contribute to or mimic neurologic problems.

▶ Consider cardiac or metabolic etiology, or adverse medication reactions, particularly for global complaints such as syncope, weakness, or change in cognition without focal (unilateral) neurologic symptoms; also consider dementia, delirium, or depression.

RED FLAGS

For All

▶ Refer to a neurologist if unusual presentation or no response to adequate trial of standard therapy.

Children

▶ Obtain timely consultation and referral for the following:

　» Any sudden loss of function or developmental milestone

　» Retention of normal newborn reflexes past the sixth month of life

　» A bulging fontanel, widening of suture lines, sunset eyes, frontal bossing, or head circumference growth inconsistent with percentiles in the newborn

　» Headache associated with early morning vomiting or awakening from sleep

　» Sudden onset of vomiting after head injury — *immediate referral*

　» Nuchal rigidity with fever — *immediate referral*

Adults and Older Adults

▶ If focal findings suggest a space-occupying lesion of the brain or spinal cord, or a peripheral compressive neuropathy, refer to neurologist or neurosurgeon.

▶ Acute or sudden onset of symptoms such as headache, unilateral weakness, aphasia, visual changes, or change in level of consciousness require immediate consult, referral, or hospitalization, as do deficits resulting from head or spinal trauma.

GENERAL NEUROLOGIC AND NEUROSURGICAL DISORDERS

SPINA BIFIDA OCCULTA

Description

▶ A midline defect of the vertebral bodies without protrusion of the spinal cord or meninges

▶ Occasionally accompanied by a dermoid sinus, which may have a hairy tuft, discoloration of the skin, or a lipoma

▶ Usually found at L5 and S1

▶ More benign than other variants of spina bifida (meningocele and myelomeningocele) and, with a normal physical and neuro exam, requires no treatment unless other symptoms occur

Etiology

▶ Neural tube defect (NTD) resulting from failure of the neural tube to close during the third and fourth week of fetal development

▶ Neural tube defects include anencephaly, encephalocele, myelomeningocele, and occult spinal dysraphism

Incidence and Demographics

▶ Incidence for all NTDs is 1 per 1,000 live births.

Risk Factors

▶ Poor prenatal care

▶ Maternal folic acid deficiency

▶ Previous delivery of an infant with NTD (2%–4%)

Prevention and Screening

▶ Addition of folic acid to the diets of women of child-bearing age, starting in adolescence

▶ Alpha-fetoprotein screen prenatally at 16–18 weeks' gestation

Assessment

History

▶ History of pregnancy, birth, and delivery as well as prenatal care and maternal risk factors, especially nutrition and folic acid deficiency, gestational diabetes, maternal use of anticonvulsants or alcohol, maternal hyperthermia during days 20–28 of gestation

▶ Patient history of back pain, bowel or bladder dysfunction, decreased motor strength or coordination

▶ Past history of meningitis or recurrent episodes of meningitis

Physical Exam

▶ Neurologic exam for strength, coordination, and reflexes, especially in the lower extremities

▶ Gait evaluation

▶ Back examination for small sinus tract in the lower midline region along the vertebrae, and skin integrity at the site

▶ Scoliosis

▶ Head circumference

▶ Presence of other dysmorphic features

▶ Rectal exam to assess sphincter tone

Diagnostic Studies

▶ Spinal X-ray will show defect in the closure of posterior vertebral arches and laminae, typically involving L5 and S1

▶ Ultrasound in the newborn period

▶ MRI to rule out tethered cord, if having motor symptoms or back pain, or other brain abnormalities

▶ Urodynamic studies to assess bladder function, if affected

Differential Diagnosis

▶ Spina bifida occulta complicated by tethered cord

▶ Syringomyelia, or diastematomyelia

▶ Dermal sinus tract

▶ Lipoma or other tumor

▶ Cysts

▶ Sacral agenesis

Management

Nonpharmacologic Treatment

▶ Usually no treatment, unless complications develop or associated defects become apparent

▶ Surgical release required for tethered cord

Pharmacologic Treatment

▶ None

Special Considerations

▶ Spina bifida occulta may be an incidental finding on X-ray in many children who have no dermal sinus.

When to Consult, Refer, Hospitalize

▶ With a normal physical and neurologic exam, no referrals are necessary.

▶ If a dermal sinus is found in the newborn or new symptoms (foot weakness, bowel or bladder dysfunction) develop in an older child, further evaluation is required; consult with a physician.

▶ Referral to a pediatric neurosurgeon is only necessary with associated defects, such as tethered cord.

Follow-up

▶ Patients with this deformity should have routine health assessments and immunizations.

▶ Pay special attention to the back evaluation, history of infections, bowel and bladder function, and lower limb motor strength at each assessment.

TOURETTE'S SYNDROME AND TICS

Description

▶ Tourette's syndrome is a lifelong chronic condition that has four components, not all of which have to be present in each case. They are: motor tics, vocal tics, obsessive–compulsive behavior, and attention-deficit hyperactivity disorder.

  ▸ Tics are sudden, rapid, recurrent, purposeless, nonrhythmic, stereotyped movements or vocalizations.

  ▸ Tics increase in intensity and frequency during any form of physical or mental stress.

  ▸ Tics tend to be unnoticed by the patient and even disappear during sleep.

  ▸ Tics develop over time from simple to complex.

  ▸ Tics begin midline and progress.

▶ Tourette syndrome differs from simple tic disorder in that tics are present for > 1 year, during which time no more than 3 consecutive months pass without tics.

Etiology

▶ Exact etiology unknown

▶ Suspected to be an abnormality along the circuits connecting the brain's cortex and subcortex, which leads to failure of the filtering mechanism along a neural pathway involving abnormal regulation of dopamine uptake and release and subsequent abnormal impulse in the involved muscle group

Incidence and Demographics

► 24% of all children experience tics; most are minor and do not lead to a clinical diagnosis.

► Lifetime prevalence of 5–10 per 10,000 (0.05%–0.1%)

► Motor tics typically present around age 6 or 7, the most common being eye blinking.

► Phonic tics present around age 8 or 9, usually as coughing, sniffing, or clearing the throat.

► Complex vocal tics include echolalia (repeating what is said by another or what is heard), palilalia (repetition of words and sounds made by the patient), and coprolalia (use of obscene language, but involuntarily so).

Risk Factors

► Genetic predisposition

► Low birthweight

► Maternal stress during pregnancy

► Obstetrical complications (e.g., use of forceps, vacuum delivery)

► Maternal use of coffee, cigarettes, or alcohol during pregnancy

► Androgenic hormones

► Autoimmune mechanisms or pediatric autoimmune neuropsychiatric disorders associated with streptococcal infections (PANDAS)

► Overuse of amphetamines

Assessment

History

► Medical and developmental history of the child

► Family history, including tics and other developmental and behavioral disorders

► Psychosocial adaptation

► Environmental supports and stresses

► Prior diagnosis of comorbid conditions, including attention-deficit hyperactivity disorder (ADHD) and use of amphetamines

► Child's impression of the tics, presence of aura, etc.

► Recent history of sore throat or throat infection, head trauma, or use of medications or drugs

Physical Exam

► The child may need to be observed from another room, via videotaping, etc., because the tics wax and wane.

► Assess for comorbid conditions through a general physical and screening neurologic exam.

Diagnostic Studies

► None unless to rule out comorbid conditions

▶ Head CT if onset of tics associated with head injury

▶ Throat culture and ASO titer if recent history of sore throat prior to onset of tics

▶ Urine or serum drug toxicology screen if history indicates

▶ Serum copper level if history of family hepatic and neurologic diseases

Differential Diagnosis

▶ Sydenham's chorea

▶ Drug-induced movements

▶ Wilson's disease

▶ Head injury

▶ Seizures

▶ Metal poisoning

Management

Nonpharmacologic Treatment

▶ Behavioral therapy and biofeedback

▶ Family support and counseling

▶ Individualized educational plans (IEPs), including classroom modifications

Pharmacologic Treatment

▶ Stimulants: Dextroamphetamine (Dexedrine) or methylphenidate (Ritalin) to treat comorbid ADHD

▶ Alpha-2 adrenergic agonists: Clonidine (Catapres) to treat tics alone or with comorbid ADHD

▶ Neuroleptic agents to treat tics alone: Risperidone (Risperdal), haloperidol, pimozide (Orap), and fluphenazine

How Long to Treat

▶ True Tourette's syndrome is a lifelong condition, requiring constant treatment.

Special Considerations

▶ For best outcome, need multimodal management plan, including the patient, family, and school

When to Consult, Refer, Hospitalize

▶ Consult with a physician for use of drug therapy when behavioral strategies are not working.

▶ Refer to neurologist if tics are hard to control or the diagnosis is not clear.

Follow-up

▶ Biannually to evaluate control of tics, school performance, need for further intervention

Expected Course

▶ At least one-third of children outgrow tics by adulthood, and another one-third have less severe tics by that time.

Complications

▶ Social problems

DOWN SYNDROME (TRISOMY 21)

Description

▶ A congenital syndrome consisting of mental retardation and multiple physical abnormalities, including hypotonia, flat facies, up-slanting palpebral fissures, and small ears.

▶ The defects are caused by trisomy of chromosome 21.

Etiology

▶ 95%–97% due to chromosomal nondisjunction in the maternal DNA

▶ 1% with trisomy 21 mosaicism occurring after conception; generally less severely affected

▶ Down syndrome is associated with many conditions, the most common of which are:

- Mental retardation (100%)
- Infant hypotonia
- Hearing loss (60%–90%)
- Visual problems: Refractive error (70%), strabismus (50%), nystagmus (35%), cataracts (3%)
- Obesity (50%)
- Congenital heart disease (40%)
- Hypothyroidism (10%–20%)
- Atlanto-occipital and atlanto-axial subluxation (15%)
- Gastrointestinal obstructions and atresias (12%)
- Seizures (6%–10%)
- Genitourinary problems, including hypospadias, cryptorchidism
- Blood dyscrasias, including leukemia, anemia
- Retinoblastoma and testicular germ cell tumors

Incidence and Demographics

▶ Incidence 1/600–800 live births

▶ Incidence increases with advancing maternal age — 1:100 by maternal age of 40–44

▶ Most recognized and frequent chromosomal syndrome in humans

Risk Factors

▶ Advanced maternal age

▶ Previous history of Down syndrome in sibling

Prevention and Screening

▶ Prenatal genetic testing via amniocentesis or chorionic villus sampling

Assessment

History

▶ History of previous infant in family with Down syndrome

▶ Review of genetic testing report

Physical Exam

▶ General: Hypotonia with an open mouth and protruding tongue

▶ Head: Brachycephaly with flattened occiput, microcephaly, false fontanel

▶ Eyes: Up-slanting palpebral fissures, inner epicanthal folds, Brushfield spots, strabismus, nystagmus

▶ Ears: Small, prominent, low-set ears, with overfolding of the upper helix; small ear canals

▶ Nose: Small, flat nasal bridge

▶ Tongue: Protruding tongue, which appears large for mouth

▶ Mouth: High-arched or abnormal palate

▶ Teeth: May have missing, irregular, or hypoplastic teeth

▶ Neck: Excessive skin at the nape (infants), short appearance

▶ Lungs: Assess for signs of infections or congestive heart failure.

▶ Heart: Assess for murmur, arrhythmia; cardiac defects are common.

▶ Abdomen: In neonate, observe for distention, which could indicate obstruction or atresia.

▶ Genital: Straight pubic hair, small penis, cryptorchidism (adolescents)

▶ Extremities: Hand is broad with simian palm crease, short metacarpals and phalanges; short fifth finger with clinodactyly; wide gap between second and third toes; hyperflexible joints

▶ Skin: Fine, soft, sparse hair; hyperkeratotic dry skin; may be cyanotic

Diagnostic Studies

▶ CBC as newborn

▶ ECG and echocardiogram within first month of life to detect associated cardiac defects

▶ Auditory brainstem response testing within the first 6 months of life

▶ Lateral cervical spine X-ray to rule out atlantoaxial instability by school age

▶ Diagnosis confirmed by karyotype testing, usually in utero or neonatal period

Differential Diagnosis

▶ Other genetic or chromosomal syndromes

Management

Nonpharmacologic Treatment

▶ Many infants require surgical repair of associated heart defects.

▶ Parents need ongoing emotional support.

▶ Genetic testing and counseling within family

Pharmacologic Treatment

▶ Specific to associated problems

How Long to Treat

▶ Down syndrome requires lifetime surveillance for management of the associated disabilities and emergence of new problems.

Special Considerations

▶ Parents need ongoing support, both emotional and financial; parents should apply for Supplemental Security Income (SSI) benefits for the child.

When to Consult, Refer, Hospitalize

▶ Almost always identified at birth and immediate referrals made for unstable newborn

▶ Otherwise, consult with physician or specialist for infant or child entering healthcare system

▶ If stable, referrals as follows:

  ▹ Cardiac consult within first month of life

  ▹ Ophthalmology consult by age 6 months and then every 1–2 years

  ▹ Audiologic evaluation, in first 3 years, than every 2 years; may need ENT referral to visualize tympanic membranes (TMs), due to small canals

  ▹ Orthopedic evaluation, as needed

  ▹ Endocrine consult, if thyroid screening abnormal

  ▹ Early language and learning intervention may prove helpful.

Follow-up

▶ Patients need routine health examinations, as well as routine immunizations, in the newborn period and at least every 2 years through childhood and adolescence.

▶ Encourage physical activity and review diet to prevent obesity.

Complications

▶ Wide variety of complications due to associated abnormalities, including recurrent otitis media, constipation, airway problems, joint problems

▶ Emergencies in the newborn period include intestinal obstruction and cardiac disease.

CEREBRAL PALSY

Description

▶ A group of nonprogressive disorders resulting from malfunction of the motor centers and pathways of the brain; a major cause of disability of children

▶ There are varying degrees and clinical manifestations.

▶ Symptoms generally include paralysis, weakness, incoordination, or ataxia.

Etiology

Prenatal Factors (most common)

▶ Infection, such as rubella, toxoplasmosis, herpes simplex, and cytomegalovirus

▶ Maternal anoxia, anemia, placental infarcts, abruptio placenta

▶ Prenatal cerebral hemorrhage, maternal bleeding, maternal toxemia, Rh or ABO incompatibility

▶ Prenatal anoxia, twisting or kinking of the cord

▶ Genetic factors

▶ Miscellaneous: Toxins, drugs

Perinatal Factors

▶ Anoxia from any cause, including anesthetic and analgesic drugs administered during labor, prolonged labor, placenta previa or abruptio placenta, respiratory obstruction, cerebral trauma during delivery, complications of birth

▶ "Small for date" babies, including prematurity and intrauterine growth retardation

▶ Hyperbilirubinemia

▶ Hemolytic disorders

▶ Respiratory distress

▶ Infections

▶ Serum chemistry disturbances (hypoglycemia, hypocalcemia)

Postnatal Factors

▶ Head trauma

▶ Infections, including meningitis, encephalitis, and brain abscesses

▶ Vascular accidents

▶ Anoxia

▶ Neoplastic and late neurodevelopmental defects

Incidence and Demographics

▶ Cerebral palsy occurs in approximately 2 per 1,000 live births.

Risk Factors

▶ Young or advanced maternal age

▶ Lack of prenatal care

▶ Birth trauma or anoxia

▶ Maternal infection

Prevention and Screening

▶ Prenatal care, including the provision of prenatal vitamins

▶ Prenatal screening for maternal illness and infection

▶ Management of maternal toxemia of pregnancy

▶ Developmental screening for well babies

▶ Immunization programs for well babies

Assessment

History

▶ A thorough history, including prenatal, perinatal, and postnatal risk factors

▶ Attention to birth trauma, prematurity, low birth weight, Apgar scores

▶ History of infant activity, feeding, crying, growth

Physical Exam

▶ Early signs

  » Asymmetric movements, hypertonia, scissoring of the lower extremities

  » Listlessness or irritability

  » Poor sucking with tongue thrust

  » Excessive, high-pitched, or feeble cry

  » Long, thin infants who are slow to gain weight

  » Poor head control

▶ Late signs

  » Failure to follow normal pattern of motor development — delayed gross motor development is universal manifestation

  » Persistence of infantile reflexes

  » Weakness

  » Preference for one hand before the infant is 12–15 months old

  » Abnormal postures

  » Delayed or defective speech

  » Evidence of mental retardation

- ► General health
    - » Functional assessment, including ability to perform normal daily activities
- ► Developmental assessment: Use Denver II developmental or other screening tool.
- ► Ability to protect airway: Gag reflex, swallowing
- ► Nutritional status: Growth, or weight loss
- ► Neuromuscular function and mobility: Range of motion, spasticity, coordination

Diagnostic Studies

- ► Computed tomography (CT) scan or magnetic resonance imaging (MRI) to rule out tumor
- ► Laboratory testing to include CBC, urinalysis, chemistry panel, toxicology screen to rule out other disorders
- ► Psychological testing to determine cognitive functioning in an older child
- ► Gait analysis
- ► EEG if seizures suspected

Differential Diagnosis

- ► Tumors and neoplasms
- ► Meningitis, encephalitis
- ► Metabolic diseases
- ► Connective tissue disorders

Management

Nonpharmacologic Treatment

- ► Orthopedic management of scoliosis, contractures, dislocations
- ► Selective surgical dorsal rhizotomy in an attempt to decrease spasticity
- ► Enrollment in a child-development program
- ► Physical, speech, and occupational therapy
- ► Assistive devices, such as braces, joint supports, walkers to assist with movement and prevent contractures
- ► Biofeedback (limited success)
- ► Family and individual counseling can be integral components of the management plan

Pharmacologic Treatment

- ► Administration of antispasticity medications, such as dantrolene (Dantrium) or diazepam (Valium)
- ► Administration of antireflux medications, metoclopramide (Reglan) or bethanechol
- ► Administration of seizure medications, as needed
- ► Injection of botulism toxin (Botox), can relax muscles up to 3–6 months
- ► Stool softeners as needed to help prevent constipation due to immobility

Special Considerations

▶ The best outcomes require a multimodal management plan, which includes the patient, family, neurology, orthopedics, nutrition, the school, and physical and occupational therapies.

▶ Parents need frequent support.

▶ Patients need to receive routine immunizations as scheduled.

When to Consult, Refer, Hospitalize

▶ Refer all cases to a pediatric neurologist; patient should be followed by a multidisciplinary team.

▶ Hospitalization is usually for amelioration of orthopedic problems.

Follow-up

▶ Routine health assessments and immunizations, biannual individualized education plan (IEP)

Complications

▶ Scoliosis, seizures, ADHD, behavioral problems

FRAGILE X SYNDROME

Description

▶ Congenital syndrome characterized by mental retardation or developmental delay, characteristic physical features, and abnormal behavioral patterns

Etiology

▶ The genetic defect is a discontinuous site on the long arm of the X chromosome.

Incidence and Demographics

▶ Frequency estimated at 1/2,500 to 1/1,250 in males and 1/5,000 to 1/1,650 in females

▶ Most common hereditary cause of mental retardation

Risk Factors

▶ Family history of the syndrome

Prevention and Screening

▶ Genetic testing and carrier detection for siblings and relatives of identified cases

Assessment

History

- ▶ Family history of mental retardation or fragile X syndrome
- ▶ Developmental history, speech or language delay
- ▶ Behavioral problems, such as hyperactivity, aversion of gaze, manneristic behavior, hand mannerisms or sterotypes, and perseverative speech
- ▶ School performance problems
- ▶ History of visual or hearing difficulties, motor or joint instability, or seizures

Physical Exam

- ▶ Appearance: Prominent forehead; a long, thin face and prominent jaw that appears late in childhood; large, protuberant, and slightly dysmorphic ears
- ▶ Strabismus, nystagmus, or ptosis
- ▶ Heart sounds for murmurs or clicks with associated mitral valve prolapse
- ▶ Musculoskeletal exam for flat feet, scoliosis, or loose joints; in infants, hypotonia
- ▶ Genitourinary exam for macroorchidism, inguinal hernias

Diagnostic Studies

- ▶ Echocardiogram to assess for mitral valve prolapse
- ▶ EEG if there is history of seizures or staring episodes

Differential Diagnosis

- ▶ Mental retardation
- ▶ Klinefelter's syndrome
- ▶ Autism

Management

Nonpharmacologic Treatment

- ▶ Behavioral, developmental, IQ testing
- ▶ Speech and language therapy as needed
- ▶ Orthotics for flat feet if a gait disturbance is present
- ▶ Corrective lenses or corrective surgery for strabismus
- ▶ Inguinal hernia repair
- ▶ Early intervention programs for education and learning

Pharmacologic Treatment

- ▶ Medications used only to treat symptoms of associated problems, such as hyperactivity or depression

Special Considerations

▶ Special classroom arrangements or learning situations

▶ Adolescents will need special counseling regarding sexuality and birth control.

▶ Patients may have trouble adjusting to social situations due to behavioral issues and may suffer from depression due to failure to fit in.

When to Consult, Refer, Hospitalize

▶ Refer all suspected cases to pediatric neurologist or developmental specialist.

▶ Refer to other specialties for associated problems (ophthalmology, orthopedics, psychology).

▶ Refer family for genetic counseling.

Follow-up

▶ Routine health assessments and immunizations according to the recommended schedule

Expected Course

▶ Life into adulthood with interdisciplinary support of the family, usually in group home situation

Complications

▶ School failure

▶ Behavioral dysfunction can be significant component

HEADACHE: TENSION, MIGRAINE, CLUSTER

Description

▶ Head pain may be a symptom of underlying disease or pathology or the disease process itself (cluster headache, migraine). Head pain arises from extracranial structures (muscles, skin, scalp arteries), or from the posterior fossa, the dura, intracranial arteries, and cranial nerves at the base of the brain.

▷ Brain tissue itself is not sensitive to pain.

▶ Tension, migraine, and cluster are primary headaches.

▶ It is unusual for new-onset primary headache syndromes to occur after age 50.

▶ Secondary headaches are a symptom of an underlying disorder.

▶ A sudden and severe headache is significant and warrants immediate attention.

▶ The pattern of a headache may suggest the etiology, such as acute recurrent headaches. A chronic nonprogressive pattern might suggest postconcussion syndrome. A chronic progressive headache is more concerning and would possibly indicate a brain tumor or other serious etiology.

▶ Tension headaches are described as squeezing, band-like pain; onset usually gradual and lasting days to years; present when awaking; and may be associated with anxiety or depression, no aura or associated neurologic symptoms

▶ Medication overuse headache (MOH), previously referred to as analgesic rebound headache, is a chronic headache that can develop from the frequent use of headache medications, including OTC analgesic, triptans, ergotamine, caffeine, opiates, or benzodiazepines.

▶ Cluster headaches have unilateral, excruciating pain lasting 20 minutes to 2 hours, with several attacks a day for 4–8 weeks, followed by a cluster-free interval for 6 months to years; or chronic form with little cluster-free interval.

▶ Migraines may be preceded by a prodromal or "warning" feeling; then some have an aura of visual or somatosensory disturbance immediately before headache; the headache may be unilateral or bilateral, lasting hours to several days, and associated with photophobia, phonophobia, and nausea and vomiting.

  ▹ Migraines are recurrent, throbbing headaches of vascular origin.

  ▹ The majority of primary pediatric headaches are migraines, MOH, and tension.

  ▹ Migraines may be classified as without aura (80%) or with aura (focal neurologic dysfunction begins and ends before onset of headache).

  ▹ Migraine variants include ophthalmoplegic; hemiplegic; basilar (vertigo, dysarthria, ataxia, tinnitus); persistent; and transformed (chronic).

Etiology

▶ Tension headache

  ▹ Essentially unknown cause

  ▹ Studies have not supported "muscle tension" or increased muscle contractions.

  ▹ Depression, anxiety, or stress may play a role.

▶ Migraines

  ▹ Believed to be caused by a genetically linked vascular disruption (constriction and dilation of extracranial and intracranial blood vessels), possibly triggered by neurochemical disruption

▶ Cluster

  ▹ Unknown; may be related to cyclic neurochemical imbalances causing an inflammatory response; tend to be seasonal, occurring in spring or fall

▶ Secondary headaches

  ▹ Most common in older adults, often due to disease outside the central nervous system (CNS)

  ▹ Causes include subarachnoid hemorrhage, head trauma, brain tumors, giant cell (temporal) arteritis, meningitis, encephalitis, cervical arthritis, visual acuity problems, fever, sinusitis, intoxication (drugs, chemicals, carbon monoxide), hypothyroidism

Incidence and Demographics

- ▶ 18 million outpatient visits a year are due to headache.
- ▶ Incidence declines in the 6th–10th decades.
- ▶ Tension
    - » 70%–90% of adults experience tension-type headache at some time.
    - » 5:4 ratio of women to men; 40% have family history
- ▶ Migraines
    - » Prevalence 16%–45% women, 10%–21% men
    - » Most common during ages of 30–45, unusual to begin after age 50; unmask earlier incidence of undiagnosed migraine via focused history; rule out other causes
    - » Migraine occurs in 3%–5% of children before puberty and increases to 10%–20% during the second decade of life.
    - » Female-to-male ratio is equal in childhood and rises to 2:1 after puberty.
    - » There is a strong genetic component; family history supports the diagnosis in the child.
- ▶ Cluster
    - » Rare, much more frequent in men > 30

Risk Factors

- ▶ Age, sex, stress, alcohol, caffeine (for all)
- ▶ Migraine triggers: Menstruation; foods such as chocolate and aged cheese; caffeine and nicotine or withdrawal; alcohol; sunlight; too much or too little sleep; missing meals; emotional stress or relief of stress; medications, including estrogen and vasodilators

Prevention and Screening

- ▶ Due to the many causes of headache, there is no primary prevention.
- ▶ Avoid identified individual triggers.
- ▶ Keeping a headache diary helps in the identification of triggers and also in the administration of prophylactic medications.

Assessment

History

- ▶ Evaluate every headache for chronology (most important item); location, duration quality; associated activity (exertion, sleep tension, relaxation); timing of menstrual cycle; presence of associated symptoms (focal neurologic deficits, vomiting, fever); and presence of triggers.
- ▶ Recent falls or head injuries, trauma, previous and current medical and nonpharmacologic management, diagnostic testing and referrals
- ▶ Activities using the trapezius muscles, such as wearing heavy backpacks
- ▶ Suspect tension headaches with gradual onset over months to years, with episodes lasting days without neurologic symptoms; may be associated with anxiety, depression, and stress.

▶ Suspect tension headache with constant, gradual onset, daily headaches; generalized, bilateral; and common around occiput, lasts for several hours, vague symptoms, no focal neurologic deficits.

▶ Suspect migraine with history of aura and neurologic symptoms that resolve, then actual headache accompanied by photophobia, nausea, or vomiting; usually follows the same pattern and precipitating events each episode.

▶ Suspect cluster headaches by cyclic nature of attacks.

▶ Headache described as the "first" or "worst" of the patient's life should be evaluated to rule out potentially serious etiology.

▶ Functional history: Headache interferes with work, school, functional activities of daily living (ADLs) and instrumental ADLs; headaches that do not interfere with ADLs tend to be tension type.

▶ Sudden onset, change in character, associated neurologic symptoms, fever, neck pain, and rash or weight loss suggest a serious headache and potential emergency; a brain tumor usually causes additional symptoms within 6 months of headache onset.

▶ If patient is febrile, consider meningitis, brain abscesses or other infection, encephalitis, or sinusitis.

▶ Family history of headache

▶ Review of systems

　» Neurologic: Aura, paresthesias, paralysis, vertigo, mood, sleep changes

　» Visual symptoms: Photophobia, diplopia, scotoma, tearing

　» Any ear, nose, or throat symptoms; may indicate sinusitis

　» Gastrointestinal: Nausea, vomiting, diarrhea, constipation

　» Constitutional symptoms: Fever, chills, weight changes, appetite changes

▶ Also see brain tumor, stroke, meningitis for pertinent history of these secondary causes

Physical Exam

▶ Screening neurologic exam is usually normal with primary headaches; neurologic deficits suggest a secondary cause, such as subarachnoid hemorrhage (SAH), cerebrovascular accident (CVA), tumor, or subdural hematoma.

▶ Funduscopic exam to rule out papilledema (signals increased intracranial pressure)

▶ Muscle tone, reflexes, gait, sensation, coordination, and strength for any abnormality

▶ Auscultate for bruits, a sign of cerebrovascular disease

▶ Measure head circumference and check the fontanels and sutures in the young child.

▶ Cervical and suboccipital tenderness, range of motion (decreased in cervical arthritis)

▶ Temporal artery tenderness and visual changes, particularly in patients > 50 years, suggests giant cell arteritis

▶ Focused physical exam, including vital signs, to rule out secondary causes or infectious process

▶ Rash over facial distribution of cranial nerve V with corresponding pain indicates herpes zoster.

▶ Examine the teeth for obvious cavities; include an assessment of jaw movement.

▶ ENT exam for signs of infection of the pharynx or sinuses

Diagnostic Studies

▶ History consistent with primary headache with normal physical exam usually does not require further diagnostic evaluation.

▶ For tension headaches with stress or psychogenic component, consider psychological testing.

▶ CBC if chronic anemia or infection is suspected

▶ Consider brain CT if:

    » Significant new type headache of few weeks' duration

    » New headache in patient over age 50

▶ Immediate CT if:

    » Sudden, severe headache

    » Progressive headache

    » Headache with exertion, straining, sexual activity, or coughing

    » Change in mental state, persistent focal neurologic deficits, or fever

▶ Lumbar puncture (if there is a negative CT but SAH suspected, or to rule out meningitis)

▶ Erythrocyte sedimentation rate (ESR) to rule out giant cell arteritis in those over age 50

▶ Sinus CT or X-rays if sinusitis without response to adequate antibiotics, recurrent sinus pain, vague symptoms without definite physical findings

▶ Cervical spine X-rays or MRI if cervical arthritis or radiculopathy is suspected

▶ Other diagnostic testing as directed by history and physical exam to rule out infectious, metabolic, or autoimmune process

▶ Evaluate for cardiovascular disease with ECG and risk factors before prescribing 5-HT agonists ("triptans") or dihydroergotamine (DHE 45 or Migranal).

▶ Electroencephalogram is not useful in screening or diagnosing headaches.

Differential Diagnosis

▶ Subarachnoid or intracranial hemorrhage or cerebral aneurysm

▶ Brain tumor

▶ Giant cell arteritis

▶ Subdural hematoma

▶ Posttraumatic headache

▶ Meningitis

▶ Encephalitis

▶ Brain abscess

▶ Hydrocephalus

▶ Sinusitis or other referred pain from ear, eyes, teeth, or temperomandibular joint (TMJ)

▶ Viral syndrome

▶ Drug-induced, caffeine withdrawal, or intoxication

▶ Depression and anxiety

▶ Postconcussive syndrome

▶ Stress

▶ Cervical radiculopathy

▶ Trigeminal neuralgia

▶ Pseudotumor cerebri or benign intracranial hypertension (cause unknown)

Management

Nonpharmacologic Treatment

▶ Tension

    » Relaxation techniques, biofeedback, stress reduction

    » Physical therapy: TENS, massage, ultrasound

    » Headache logs

▶ Migraine and cluster

    » Avoid food and drugs that trigger attacks

    » Rest and periods of exercise

    » During attack, rest in quiet, dark room with head elevated; use of cold compresses

    » 100% oxygen inhaled for 10–15 minutes

Pharmacologic Treatment

ABORTIVE THERAPY

▶ Tension

    » Analgesics: Acetaminophen 650–1,000 mg q.i.d. as needed, or NSAIDs taken with food

    » Under age 10, acetaminophen 15 mg/kg/dose q4h, or ibuprofen 10 mg/kg/dose q6h

    » Children under 10 with headaches more than once per week may benefit from daily prophylactic therapy with cyproheptadine (Periactin) 0.2–0.4 mg/kg/d in 2–3 divided doses, starting with 4 mg at bedtime.

    » Older children can be managed with analgesics, including acetaminophen and ibuprofen, to control pain.

    » Avoid opioids, including butalbital (Fiorinal and Fioricet), due to risk of habituation as well as rebound phenomenon.

    » If headache occurs more than once per week, preventive medications for adults and children include amitriptyline and propranolol (Inderal).

▶ Migraines and cluster headaches: Treatment very individualized

    » Analgesics: Acetaminophen, aspirin, or NSAIDs, often in combination with caffeine; taken as soon as possible at onset. Avoid opioids for reasons noted above.

    » 5-HT agonists (triptans) if nonnarcotic analgesics ineffective

    » Sumatriptan (Imitrex) — oral: 25 mg taken as soon as possible at onset, 25–100 mg every 2 hours up to 300 mg in 24 hours in adults; in children, maximum oral dose is 0.6 mg/kg

    » Injection: 6 mg SC adults; in children, maximum dose 0.6 mg/kg; may be repeated once after 1 h

    » Following initial injection, 25–50 mg tablets q2h up to 200 mg orally in 24 hours

    » Intranasal: Single dose of 5, 10, or 20 mg administered in one nostril, may repeat once after 2 hours, not to exceed 40 mg in 24 hours in adults; dosage based on body weight in children

- » Other 5-HT agonists include zolmitriptan (Zomig), naratriptan (Amerge), rizatriptan (Maxalt)
- » Ergotamine derivatives: Cafergot: 2 tablets taken as soon as possible at onset, may repeat at 30-minute intervals, do not exceed 6 tablets per day, 10 tablets per week; not recommended in children
- » Injectable triptans at migraine doses more effective than oral agents for individual attacks (*Note*: 1st dose of injectable preparations should be given under medical supervision and, possibly, accompanied by monitoring with ECG.)
- » Injectable or inhaled ergotamines and triptans are contraindicated in patients with history of uncontrolled hypertension, Prinzmetal's angina, myocardial infarction, or symptomatic ischemic heart disease.
- » Sumatriptan should not be used in conjunction with any vasoconstrictor medication, nor should it be used within 2 weeks of taking a monoamine oxidase inhibitor.

▶ Treat nausea or vomiting in adults and children with metoclopramide (Reglan) or phenothiazine 15–20 minutes before oral medication.

- » Prophylactic treatment for 2 or more migraine attacks per month that produce impairment lasting 3 or more days per month: Daily NSAIDs, beta-blockers, calcium channel blockers, tricyclic antidepressants (limited experience with SSRIs, especially in children; see Table 15–1)
- » Topiramate, lithium carbonate, methysergide, and valproate can also be effective. However, before initiating valproate, baseline liver enzyme levels must be drawn and then monitored thereafter approximately every 3–6 months.
- » Generally, prophylactic agent(s) should be tried for a minimum of 2–3 months before switching to another drug.
- » Neurology referral for headaches unresponsive to treatment or prophylaxis

PREVENTIVE THERAPY

▶ U.S. Headache Consortium Guidelines based on clinical efficacy, significant adverse events, safety profile, and clinical experience of the participants:

- » Group A—Medications with proven high efficacy and mild-to-moderate adverse events
- » Group B—Medications with lower efficacy (i.e., limited number of studies or studies reporting conflicting results) or efficacy suggesting only "modest" improvement, and mild-to-moderate adverse events
- » Group C—No dosing recommendations provided for treatments lacking relevant, randomized controlled trials

▶ Secondary headaches

- » Manage and treat the underlying cause.
- » Avoid opioids if the level of consciousness needs to be monitored.
- » Acetaminophen for pain and fever if not contraindicated

How Long to Treat

▶ Treat acute attacks until headache resolves or maximum daily dose is reached; narcotics can be used to treat intractable pain.

▶ Prophylaxis: Primary headache syndromes tend to decrease or resolve in late middle age or after menopause; attempt to wean periodically.

Special Considerations

▶ Consider cardiovascular, gastrointestinal, renal, and hepatic disease when prescribing therapy in geriatric patients.

▶ Increased risk of GI bleed, renal failure, edema, and elevated blood pressure (BP) with NSAIDs in older adults

▶ There are no randomized control studies for migraine treatment in older adults.

▶ Headaches are common in the first trimester of pregnancy.

▶ Migraines usually do not become worse during pregnancy.

▶ Counsel women of childbearing age regarding headache management and pregnancy.

▶ Ergotamine derivatives are strong uterine stimulants.

▶ Ergotamine is secreted in breast milk and may cause vomiting and diarrhea in infants.

TABLE 15-1
PHARMACOLOGIC TREATMENT: PREVENTIVE THERAPY FOR MIGRAINE

GROUP	MEDICATION	USUAL DAILY ADULT DOSE	USUAL DAILY PEDS DOSE	SIDE EFFECTS
A	Divalproex Na (Depakote)	Usual dose for age > 16: Start with 250 mg b.i.d.; usual max 1 g/day	20-40 mg/kg	GI upset, liver disease, thrombocytopenia; need to monitor closely
	Sodium Valproate (Depacon)	800-1500 mg/day	—	Alopecia, rash, abdominal pain, constipation, diarrhea, pancreatitis
	Propranolol (Inderal)	160-240 mg/day in divided doses	< 35 kg: 10-20 mg p.o. t.i.d. > 35 kg: 20-40 mg p.o. t.i.d.	Heart block, Raynaud's, SLE, fatigue, dizziness, constipation, hypotension
	Amitriptyline (indicated for relief of symptoms of depression only)	50-100 mg/day	—	HTN, syncope, QT prolongation, seizures, extrapyramidal symptoms, leukopenia, drowsiness, dizziness, dry mouth

CONTINUED

TABLE 15-1 CONTINUED

PHARMACOLOGIC TREATMENT: PREVENTIVE THERAPY FOR MIGRAINE

GROUP	MEDICATION	USUAL DAILY ADULT DOSE	USUAL DAILY PEDS DOSE	SIDE EFFECTS
B	Gabapentin (Neurontin)	900–2400 mg/day	—	Peripheral edema, myalgia, ataxia, dizziness, mood swings, fatigue
	Fluoxetine (Prozac)	20 mg q.o.d.–40 mg/day	—	Insomnia, fatigue, tremor, stomach pain, rash, sweating, xerostomia
	Atenolol (Tenomin)	100 mg/day	—	Arrhythmia, diarrhea, dizziness, fatigue, insomnia
	Verapamil	240 mg/day	—	Edema, hypotension, constipation, nausea, dizziness
	Clonidine	0.05–0.225 mg/day	—	Dizziness, drowsiness, sedation, hypotension, confusion
	NSAIDs:			
	Aspirin	325 mg/day	—	Gastritis, occult GI bleed, tinnitus, indigestion, nausea, vomiting
	Flurbiprofen (Ansaid)	200 mg/day		
	Ketoprofen (Orudis)	150 mg/day		
	Naproxen sodium (Naprosyn)	1,100 mg/day		
	Mefenamic acid (Ponstel)	1,500 mg/day		
	Fenoprofen (Nalfon)	1,800 mg/day		
	Asprin + dipyridamole (persantine)	975 to 1,300 + 75 mg/day		
	Ergotamine + caffeine + butalbital + belladonna	2 caps a day for 3 days before, during, and 2 days after menses	—	Pruritus, nausea, vomiting, muscle weakness, parasthesia, visual disturbances
	Estradiol (Estrogel)	1.5 mg/day for 7 days	—	Edema, pruritus, weight gain, nausea, amenorrhea, break-through bleeding
	Feverfew	50–82 mg/day	—	Eczema, edema, nausea, abdominal pain, diarrhea, tachycardia
	Magnesium	400–600 mg/day	—	Blurred vision, diarrhea, HTN, increased bleeding times
	Vitamin B_2	400 mg/day	—	Rare adverse events

HTN = hypertension

Adapted from *Evidence-Based Guidelines for Migraine Headache in the Primary Care Setting* by U.S. Headache Consortium, 2011, retrieved from www.americanheadachesociety.org/professional_resources/us_headache_consortium_guidelines/

When to Consult, Refer, Hospitalize

▶ Consult with physician as needed if narcotic analgesics needed.

▶ Refer to neurologist if unable to manage symptoms using typical therapy or if patient develops symptoms of increased intracranial pressure (ICP), or if tumor, aneurysm, or atriovenous malformation (AVM) suspected.

▶ Refer to neurologist if patient is experiencing multiple headaches per week, or is taking multiple doses of medication without benefit (e.g., rebound headaches due to medication effects).

▶ Refer to emergency department (ED) for severe unresponsive migraine or cluster headache with vomiting and need for IV hydration; or sudden, severe headache; or headache with change in level of consciousness.

▶ Refer to surgeon or ophthalmologist for temporal artery biopsy if temporal arteritis suspected.

▶ Refer to psychologist or therapist for relaxation therapy or psychotherapy, or when depression suspected that does not respond to trial of antidepressants.

▶ Refer to interdisciplinary pain center for chronic, intractable pain, or interference with daily life.

Follow-up

▶ Routine annual health assessments

▶ Weekly to monthly when adjusting or changing medications

Expected Course

▶ Tension headaches can be lifelong.

▶ Migraines get better in more than two thirds of all children, but the prognosis of remission diminishes after age 18.

▶ In adults, migraines and cluster headaches usually resolve during middle age, or following completion of menopause.

Complications

▶ Unrecognized or mistreated serious headaches from secondary causes

▶ Lost wages and productivity, troubled relationships from chronic pain

BRAIN TUMORS

Description

▶ Primary brain tumors are abnormal growth of cells arising from structures within the cranium.

▶ Classified by cell of origin (Table 15–2) and include gliomas, meningioma (rare in children), acoustic neuroma, ependymoma, craniopharyngioma, pediatric ganglioma (benign, may be accompanied by seizures)

▶ May be malignant or benign

▶ Secondary brain tumors most often metastasize from the lung, breast, kidney, or gastrointestinal tract.

TABLE 15-2
PRIMARY BRAIN TUMORS

TUMOR	STRUCTURE	TREATMENT AND PROGNOSIS
Astrocytoma (Grade I, II glioma)	Glial tissue	Total excision usually not possible May respond to radiation Variable prognosis
Glioblastoma multiforme (Grade III, IV glioma)	Glial tissues	Total excision not possible, reoccur Radiation and chemotherapy may slow growth Poor prognosis
Oligodendroglioma	Cerebral hemispheres	Slow-growing Successful surgical treatment
Ependymoma	Glioma usually of the fourth ventricle	Presents with signs of IIP Shunt, surgical resection if possible Radiation therapy
Craniopharyngioma	Sella tunica Depresses optic chiasm	Surgical resection usually incomplete Bitemporal visual field cuts Endocrine dysfunction
Meningioma	Dura or arachnoid mater	Surgical excision, difficult to completely remove posterior fossa tumors Cure with complete resection
Acoustic neuroma	Nerve sheath Vestibular branch of 8th cranial nerve at the cerebellopontine angle	Excision usually good outcome May have residual ipsilateral hearing loss, imbalance, facial weakness or numbness
Primary cerebral lymphoma	Reticuloendothelial system in immunocompromised patients	Shunt Prognosis depends on CD4 count

Etiology

▶ The exact cause of brain tumors is unknown.

▶ Gliomas of the supporting glial tissues account for 46% of all central nervous system tumors.

▶ Grades I, II (astrocytomas), III, IV (glioblastoma multiforme)

▶ Grade III and IV are more invasive, faster-growing, and have a poor prognosis.

▶ Meningiomas develop from the covering of the brain.

▶ Rarely malignant, usually cure is possible with complete excision, except for meningiomas of the posterior fossa where complete excision is difficult

▶ Presenting signs and symptoms depend on the location and size of the tumor.

Incidence and Demographics

▶ Second most common cause of cancer in children

▶ Occur in all age groups, but peak in the interval between ages 5 and 9 years

▶ Estimated incidence in children is 2.5 to 3/100, 000

▶ Incidence of primary brain tumor 8/100,000 in the U.S.

▶ Benign primary tumors (meningiomas) 10/100,000

▶ Malignant primary tumors (astrocytomas and glioblastoma multiforme) 5/100,000

▶ Greatest incidence in 60–70-year-olds; second most common cause of cancer in children; 20% of all malignant neoplasms; make up 50%–60% of all childhood brain tumors

Risk Factors

▶ Previous radiation therapy

▶ Neurofibromatosis

▶ Increase with age

▶ Primary cerebral lymphoma associated with AIDS

Assessment

▶ Classic triad: Morning headache, vomiting, papilledema

History

▶ Focused, complete neuro history including weakness, slurred speech or word-finding difficulty, visual changes including diplopia or field cuts, hearing loss, cognitive changes, drowsiness, seizures, headache

▶ Children: Changes in behavior or school performance; PMH, including birth history, recent illness or trauma; growth and development history, including delays; family history of neurologic disease or neurofibromatosis

▶ Tumors are suspected in patients with progressive deficits.

▶ The deficit may suggest the location of the tumor (Table 15–3).

▶ In children, presence of new-onset headache, especially for 1 week or intermittent for 1 month

▶ Headache associated with tumor is dull and aching, and increases over weeks.

▶ Headaches are usually secondary to hydrocephalus or posterior fossa tumors stretching pain-sensitive structures.

▶ New onset of seizures at any age suggests a tumor, possibly temporal lobe.

▶ Review of systems, including HEENT for loss of sense of smell or visual field cuts, suggest pituitary adenoma or craniopharyngioma; with unilateral hearing loss consider acoustic neuroma

▶ History of vomiting without nausea with deficits or headache in the morning suggests increased intracranial pressure.

▶ Assess for symptoms of Cushing's syndrome (see Chapter 17) if pituitary adenoma suspected.

TABLE 15–3
LOCATION AND SIGNS AND SYMPTOMS OF INTRACRANIAL LESIONS

LOCATION	SIGNS AND SYMPTOMS
Frontal lobe	Intellectual and cognitive decline
	Personality change
	Contralateral grasp reflex
	Expressive aphasia
	Focal motor seizures, contralateral weakness
	Anosmia
Temporal lobe	Seizures (may be partial without loss of consciousness)
	Emotional and behavioral change
	Auditory hallucinations
	Visual field cuts
	Receptive aphasia
Parietal lobe	Contralateral sensory loss
	Loss of tactile discrimination (astereognosis)
	Contralateral field cuts
	Alexia, agraphia, apraxia, acalculia
	Right-left confusion
Occipital	Homonymous hemianopsia
	Visual agnosia
	Cortical blindness
Cerebellum and brain stem	Ataxia and incoordination
	Cranial nerve palsies
	Nystagmus
	Motor and sensory deficits (unilateral or bilateral)
	Increased intracranial pressure

Physical Exam

▶ Attention to head circumference and fontanels in young children

▶ Complete neurologic exam may reveal focal cranial nerve or motor deficits.

▶ Other systems as indicated by history, including eye exam, eye movements, papilledema and, in children, skin for signs of neurocutaneous disease

▶ If pituitary adenoma suspected, will need complete endocrine assessment; elevated blood pressure may be present

▶ Metastatic brain tumor: If primary tumor site unknown, evaluate for lung, breast, kidney, or colon cancer.

▶ Gait abnormalities, incoordination, cranial nerve paralysis, optic atrophy, loss of visual fields, nystagmus, focal motor weakness and sensory abnormalities, hyperreflexia

Diagnostic Studies

▶ CT used as fast screening exam, but MRI gives better results.

▶ Magnetic resonance imaging for suspected posterior fossa lesions and intrasellar lesions

▶ Angiography of intrasellar lesion with normal hormone levels to differentiate pituitary adenoma from an aneurysm

▶ Pituitary adenoma: ACTH, thyroid function tests, serum glucose and electrolytes, prolactin

▶ Metastatic brain tumors: Chest X-ray, mammogram, colonoscopy as appropriate to locate primary tumor if unknown

▶ Open biopsy of the tumor

▶ EEGs are not helpful unless seizures are presenting symptoms.

▶ Skull X-rays many demonstrate nonspecific findings associated with increased ICP.

Differential Diagnosis

▶ Subdural hematoma

▶ Arteriovenous malformation, aneurysm

▶ Cerebrovascular accident

▶ Hydrocephalus

▶ Pseudotumor cerebri

▶ Epilepsy

▶ Primary headache syndrome

▶ Abscess

▶ Hamartoma (causing a brain gliosis)

▶ Neurofibromatosis with neuromas (when indicated by history)

▶ Viral infections

Management

▶ Surgery, radiation, chemotherapy as indicated

▶ Side effects of radiation therapy are hair loss and otitis externa.

▶ Patients must be monitored for panhypopituitarism, if radiation to the pituitary gland

▶ Side effects of chemotherapy are myelosuppression and infection, hair loss, and weight loss from nausea and vomiting.

▶ Patients and parents need continuous emotional support during therapy.

How Long to Treat

▶ Radiation therapy: 6 weeks

▶ Chemotherapy: 1–2 years

Special Considerations

▶ Patients who receive large-field radiation to the cerebrum are at high risk for cognitive deficits.

▶ All patients receiving radiation are at increased risk for recurrent tumors.

▶ Malignant brain tumors: Patients < 45 years old live 3 times longer than those > 65.

▶ Prognosis decreases with lower premorbid function based on the Karnofsky Performance Rating.

▶ Coordinate obstetrical and oncology care for pregnant or lactating patients

When to Consult, Refer, Hospitalize

▶ Consult with physician if unsure of symptoms or diagnosis.

▶ Refer to pediatric neurologist (for children and adolescents) or a neurologist (for adults) for further evaluation and treatment.

▶ Refer to social services, home health services, and counseling as needed.

Follow-up

» Patient will be closely followed by neurology, surgery, oncology team.

Complications

» Persistent neurologic deficits, seizures, increased intracranial pressure and death; refer to Table 15–3

TRIGEMINAL NEURALGIA

Description

▶ A pain syndrome, also called tic douloureux, consisting of paroxysmal lancinating pain of the face, usually unilateral; originates near mouth and shoots to nose, eye, or ear

▶ Can also occur in multiple sclerosis

Etiology

▶ Compression of the 5th cranial nerve root, usually by vascular structure or malformation

Incidence and Demographics

▶ Most common in middle age to older women

Risk Factors

▶ Pain triggers are touch, movement, cold air, chewing

Prevention and Screening

▶ None identified

Assessment

History

- ▶ Focused history if chief complaint is facial pain beginning near the side of the mouth, shooting up to ipsilateral eye, ear, or nostril; initially, episodes are separated by months of pain-free time

- ▶ Establish time frame, description of episode, any triggers and pain management

- ▶ Review of systems to identify any neurologic deficits such as weakness, numbness, diplopia, or other symptoms of a space-occupying lesion

- ▶ Any ear, nose, throat, or dental symptoms indicating sinusitis, dental abscess, or otitis

- ▶ History of 5th cranial nerve herpes zoster or multiple sclerosis

Physical Exam

- ▶ Examine head, eyes, ears, nose, throat, mouth, neck, and cranial nerves

- ▶ Neurologic exam if cranial nerve abnormalities

- ▶ No physical findings with classic trigeminal neuralgia except possibly poor dental hygiene or lack of shaving or makeup on affected side

Diagnostic Studies

- ▶ CT or MRI indicated if neurologic deficits present to rule out space-occupying lesion

- ▶ ESR if temporal (giant cell) arteritis suspected

Differential Diagnosis

- ▶ 5th cranial nerve tumor

- ▶ Post herpetic neuralgia

- ▶ Temporal arteritis

- ▶ Multiple sclerosis, particularly in the young or with bilateral pain

- ▶ Herpes zoster; pain may present before vesicular rash

- ▶ Sinusitis, otitis, dental abscess, TMJ

Management

Nonpharmacologic Treatment

- ▶ Avoid triggers.

- ▶ Surgical decompression, radiofrequency rhizotomy, gamma radiosurgery in severe cases

Pharmacologic Treatment

- ▶ Primary: Carbamazepine (Tegretol) 100 mg b.i.d., increase by 100–200 mg every 2–3 days up to 1,200 mg daily in divided doses; use lowest effective dose or oxcarbazepine 300 mg/day initially, maintenance dose is 600 mg for an adult given in 2 divided doses

▶ Secondary options: Oxcarbazepine *and* lamotrigine 25 mg p.o. initially, usual maintenance dose is 200–400 mg/day *or* topiramate 12.5 to 25 mg/day, increase gradually in relation to response, maximum dose will be 200 mg/day.

▶ Tertiary option: Gabapentin (Neurontin) 100 mg t.i.d.; titrate up to 1800 mg divided/day

How Long to Treat

▶ Attempt to decrease or discontinue dose every 3 months; decrease one drug at a time.

Special Considerations

▶ CNS side effects: Start with lowest possible dose of medications for older adults and titrate up slowly.

▶ Adjust gabapentin dose for renal insufficiency.

When to Consult, Refer, Hospitalize

▶ Refer to neurosurgeon for surgical decompression if intractable pain with adequate trials of medication or unable to tolerate medications.

▶ Surgery is inappropriate for trigeminal neuralgia secondary to multiple sclerosis.

Follow-up

▶ Follow every 3 months.

▶ Monitor CBC and liver function if on anticonvulsant medication.

Complications

▶ Generally none

BELL'S PALSY

Description

▶ An acute unilateral paralysis or paresis of the face in a pattern consistent with peripheral nerve dysfunction without a detectable cause; usually due to lower motor neuron facial weakness due to inflammation of the 7th cranial nerve

▶ Most patients have sudden onset of a unilateral facial droop, accompanied by drooling (especially in young children) and failure to completely close the affected eye; may also have discomfort behind ear or of jaw, change in hearing, loss of taste. Pain is usually transient.

▶ The paralysis may be difficult to assess when the patient is at rest, but evident with crying or talking.

Etiology

▶ Unknown, although reactivation of herpes simplex virus has been implicated

▶ Cases often preceded by an upper respiratory infection, Lyme disease

▶ Acute inflammatory response causing swelling of the facial nerve and entrapment in the foramen of the temporal bone

▶ Paresis typically progresses over 7–10 days; most patients fully recover in 6 months.

Incidence and Demographics

▶ 20–30 per 100,000 individuals a year; peak incidence is 10–40 years; no gender or race predilection

▶ 10% have familial association

Risk Factors

▶ Trauma, diabetes mellitus, hypothyroidism, AIDS, Lyme disease, syphilis, sarcoidosis, viral infection

▶ Pregnancy due to increased intravascular volume, particularly during the third trimester, increases the risk for facial nerve edema and subsequent compression.

Assessment

History

▶ In the newborn, history of birth trauma

▶ Abrupt onset facial paresis, face feels "pulled to side"

▶ Most important to establish time frame: Sudden onset over hours to a few days suggests Bell's palsy; progressive weakness over weeks indicates a tumor or other space-occupying lesion.

▶ Past medical history, including any recent upper respiratory infection; otitis; facial trauma; and history of chronic illness, including diabetes, thyroid disease, multiple sclerosis, sarcoidosis, HIV

▶ Review of systems of neuro and HEENT, including facial movements; visual changes, pain, or tearing; altered hearing or otalgia; altered taste; skin rash or possible tick bite

Physical Exam

▶ Vital signs, noting any increase in blood pressure or temperature

▶ Complete HEENT exam for decreased tone, signs of infection, lesions, or rashes

▶ Screening neuro exam, including all cranial nerves, paying attention to eye movement, jaw strength, symmetry of the face, hearing

▶ Bell's palsy indicated by complete unilateral peripheral 7th nerve paresis or paralysis, with flattening of forehead furrows, inability to raise eyebrow, inability to complete close ipsilateral eye, flattening of nasolabial fold, inability to puff out cheek, drooping of mouth, inability to smile or frown; rest of cranial nerves and neuro exam usually normal

▶ A central 7th nerve palsy, or only drooping of the mouth, indicates damage only to the lower branch of the facial nerve and an upper motor neuron lesion (stroke or tumor).

▶ Inspect eye for corneal abrasion and tearing.

▶ Inspect ear canal and TM for otitis or vesicular lesions, indicate cephalic herpes zoster.

- ▶ Palpate parotid glands for masses.
- ▶ Check for lymphadenopathy and thyroid enlargement.
- ▶ Inspect skin for rash, particularly target lesion or erythema migrans of Lyme disease (although rash may not still be present).

Diagnostic Studies

- ▶ No testing usually necessary unless diagnosis in question
- ▶ EMG and nerve conduction studies 5–10 days after onset of symptoms if complete paralysis or no improvement, to guide prognosis and treatment; if over 90% neural degeneration, surgical decompression may be indicated
- ▶ X-ray if temporal bone fracture suspected
- ▶ CT scan or MRI if tumor or space-occupying lesion suspected; also images facial nerve and temporal bone
- ▶ Complete blood count, chemistry panel, thyroid function tests, syphilis testing, HIV serology if indicated by history to rule out associated chronic diseases
- ▶ ESR if temporal (giant cell) arteritis suspected
- ▶ Lumbar puncture if meningitis suspected
- ▶ Lyme titer if exposure to ticks or rash suggestive of Lyme disease
- ▶ VDRL and HIV screen if history warrants
- ▶ Audiology testing if hearing affected > 1 week or acoustic neuroma suspected
- ▶ EMG testing occasionally used to predict prognosis and progression of disease (usually done if symptoms last longer than 6–12 months)

Differential Diagnosis

- ▶ Tumor
- ▶ Stroke or transient ischemic attack (TIA)
- ▶ Herpes zoster
- ▶ Temporal bone fracture or other trauma
- ▶ Giant cell arteritis
- ▶ Lyme disease
- ▶ HIV
- ▶ Guillain-Barré syndrome (typically symmetric bilateral weakness)
- ▶ Neurofibromatosis
- ▶ Möbius syndrome
- ▶ Infections (otitis media, mastoiditis, meningitis, mumps, rubella, syphilis)
- ▶ Parotid gland obstruction or mass
- ▶ Multiple sclerosis or other demyelinating conditions
- ▶ Diabetic neuropathy
- ▶ Hypothyroidism
- ▶ Pregnancy
- ▶ Sarcoidosis

Management

Nonpharmacologic Treatment

- ▶ Protect eye, artificial tears during the day, lubricant ointment and patch eye at bedtime
- ▶ No evidence that surgical decompression improves outcomes
- ▶ Physical therapy, including heat, electrical stimulation, or massage, may be beneficial.

Pharmacologic Treatment

▶ Medical treatment of Bell's palsy remains controversial.

▶ One study of prednisone and acyclovir demonstrated a statistically significant reduction in nerve degeneration compared to prednisone and placebo.

▶ Prednisone in children: 2 mg/kg/day for 1 week, with a slow taper, discontinue by day 14; in adults: 60–80 mg/day divided for 3–5 days, then taper over 10 days

▶ Acyclovir 400 mg 5 times/day for 10 days if evidence that herpes virus is the causative agent

▶ Artificial tears to keep affected eye moist during daytime and ointment at night

How Long to Treat

▶ Eye protection until patient can close and protect eye

▶ Steroid and antiviral therapy for 10–14 days

Special Considerations

▶ Incomplete recovery is associated with increased age.

▶ Poor prognosis is associated with complete paralysis, pain, or hyperacusis at presentation; these characteristics, combined with increased age and comorbidity, should guide decision to treat with steroids and antiviral agents.

When to Consult, Refer, Hospitalize

▶ Refer to ophthalmologist if corneal abrasion or significant prolonged decreased lacrimation.

▶ Refer to neurologist if other deficits present, recurrent paresis, or paresis lasting > 6 months.

▶ In patients > 6 years, refer to plastic surgeon for persistent cosmetic disfigurement.

Follow-up

▶ At 1-week intervals to ensure eye protection and recovery

Expected Course

▶ Most have spontaneous recovery in 2–3 weeks.

▶ 15% may have residual weakness for several months and some have permanent weakness.

Complications

▶ Incomplete recovery or recurrent paresis or paralysis

▶ Corneal abrasion

▶ Recurrent episodes

STROKE AND TRANSIENT ISCHEMIC ATTACK (TIA; "BRAIN ATTACK")

Description

▶ Strokes are ischemic or hemorrhagic.

▶ Interruption in blood flow to the brain causing neuronal death or infarction. Hemorrhage accounts for less than 10% of strokes; the bleed may be intraparenchymal or subarachnoid.

▶ Transient ischemic attack (TIA) is a temporary interruption in cerebral vascular blood flow; the deficit lasts less than 24 hours. There is no infarcted tissue.

Etiology

▶ Ischemic stroke
  ▹ Lack of blood flow to brain due to hypoxia, decreased cardiac output, thrombus, or embolus

▶ Thrombotic stroke
  ▹ Caused by progressive accumulation of atherosclerotic plaque that occludes an intracranial vessel
  ▹ Most common in the posterior cerebral circulation

▶ Embolic stroke
  ▹ Caused by atherosclerotic debris from the heart, aorta, or carotids that flow into the internal carotids and occlude the smaller vessels of the cerebral circulation
  ▹ Usually affects the anterior cerebral circulation

▶ Lacunar infarcts
  ▹ Less than 5 mm; occur in the internal capsule, basal ganglia, or thalamus
  ▹ Due to slow, progressive occlusion of the penetrating arterioles

▶ TIA: May be thrombotic, embolic, or lacunar in nature

▶ Hemorrhagic stroke
  ▹ Intracerebral hemorrhage:spontaneous bleeding into parenchyma from microaneurysm of perforating vessels; most commonly occurs in the basal ganglia; due to hypertension, hematologic disorders, or anticoagulation therapy

▶ Subarachnoid hemorrhage
  ▹ Bleeding from a ruptured aneurysm in the Circle of Willis or arteriovenous malformation

Incidence and Demographics

▶ Acute stroke afflicts 600,000 Americans per year; incidence increases with age.

▶ One-fourth will die, making stroke the third leading cause of death in the United States

▶ 50% of survivors will have some disability, 15%–30% will require nursing home placement.

Risk Factors

▶ Previous cerebrovascular disease, stroke, or TIA; 20%–40% of ischemic strokes preceded by TIA within days to months

▶ Aging

▶ Traditional risks for vascular disease: Hypertension, diabetes, hyperlipidemia, smoking

▶ Traditional risks for emboli: Atrial fibrillation, cardiomyopathy, coronary artery disease

Prevention and Screening

▶ Manage hypertension; screening for hypertension is recommended at least every 2 years in the normotensive; treatment is recommended per Joint National Commission 6 guidelines.

▶ Screening for asymptomatic carotid stenosis by auscultation of carotid bruits or carotid ultrasound remains controversial, with insufficient evidence to recommend for or against.

▶ High-risk patients over age 60 with other risk factors for vascular disease who have access to vascular surgery with morbidity and mortality rates of less than 3% may benefit from screening and subsequent endarterectomy.

▶ Antiplatelet therapy with aspirin, ticlopidine, or clopidogrel (Plavix) may decrease the risk of stroke in those with asymptomatic carotid artery stenosis.

▶ Anticoagulation is recommended for patients with atrial fibrillation, particularly those with additional risk factors.

▶ Evidence suggests improved glycemic control may decrease microvascular events in type 2 diabetes.

▶ Decreasing serum lipids may delay progression of carotid atherosclerosis and decrease cerebrovascular events.

▶ All patients will benefit from diet and exercise counseling and smoking cessation.

Assessment

History

▶ Onset, duration, and progression of symptoms are most important in determining etiology and management.

▶ Resolution of symptoms in minutes to hours is suggestive of a TIA.

▶ Onset during sleep with progression suggests thrombotic stroke.

▶ Sudden onset with activity suggests embolic or hemorrhagic stroke.

▶ Detailed description of symptoms or deficits, including visual changes, aphasia, motor weakness, or paresthesias, may give clue to location of stroke or lesion.

▶ Review of systems: Headache, seizure, loss of consciousness, syncope, vertigo, vomiting, cardiac symptoms:

  ▷ Lack of headache excludes hemorrhagic stroke.

  ▷ Vomiting is associated with increased intracranial pressure, usually due to hemorrhage.

  ▷ Loss of consciousness is associated with hemorrhage or posterior circulation thrombosis

    » Syncope is more often related to cardiac etiology than stroke.

    » Vertigo suggests vestibular disease, but may occur with vertebrobasilar insufficiency.

▶ Past medical history: Cardiac disease; peripheral vascular disease; diabetes; IV drug abuse; previous neurologic conditions such as seizure, head trauma, dementia, or brain tumors give clues to etiology and possible differential diagnosis.

▶ Review all medications, particularly those that can alter level of consciousness or cause bleeding.

Physical Exam

▶ Complete neurologic exam, including level of consciousness, cognitive ability (apraxia, agnosia, aphasia, agraphia), motor and sensory function (contralateral deficits), cranial nerve exam including funduscopic and visual deficits, reflexes (hyperreflexia or Babinski on affected side)

▶ Cardiovascular exam: Hypertension, orthostatic changes, atrial fibrillation, heart murmurs, carotid bruits, abdominal bruit from aneurysm

▶ Signs of carotid TIA: Weakness of contralateral arm, leg, or face, individually or in combination; numbness or paraesthesia may occur alone or in combination with motor deficit; dysphagia; monocular visual loss; carotid bruit; TRS may be hyperreflexic during attack; atherosclerotic changes on funduscopic exam. Signs and symptoms disappear as attack resolves.

▶ Signs of vertebrobasilar TIA: Vertigo, ataxia, diplopia, dysarthria, dimness or blurry vision, perioral numbness, weakness or sensory complaints on one or both sides of the body, drop attacks with bilateral leg weakness

▶ Lacunar infarction: Contralateral pure motor or sensory deficit, ipsilateral ataxia, dysarthria, with complete symptom resolution over 1–2 months

▶ Cerebral infarction: Deficit depends on vessel so any variety of focal neurologic deficits may develop.

▶ Cerebellar infarction: Vertigo, ataxia, nystagmus, nausea and vomiting

▶ Hemorrhagic CVA: Typically associated with hypertension, sudden onset, symptoms usually present during activity, initial loss of or impaired consciousness, rapidly evolving hemiplegia or paresis

Diagnostic Studies

▶ CT scan; MRI if posterior circulation involved

▶ Lumbar puncture if CT negative for hemorrhage and subarachnoid hemorrhage suspected

▶ Carotid duplex for evaluation of symptomatic carotid stenosis, if patient is surgical candidate for endarterectomy; carotid studies useless for evaluation of posterior circulation

▶ Angiography remains "gold standard" for assessing carotid stenosis, as well as identifying aneurysms, AVM, and vasculitis

▶ Electrocardiogram, chest radiograph, echocardiogram

▶ Transesophageal echocardiogram if intraventricular thrombus or patent foramen ovale is suspected

▶ Holter monitor to rule out paroxysmal arrhythmias

▶ CBC, ESR, coagulation studies, RPR, chemistry panel, and lipid profile to evaluate cause

Differential Diagnosis

▶ TIA, thrombotic, embolic or lacunar stroke

▶ Subarachnoid or intracerebral hemorrhage

▶ Cerebral aneurysm or AVM

▶ Intracranial tumor

▶ Seizure

▶ Migraine with aura

▶ Encephalopathy

▶ Intoxication

▶ Hypoglycemia

▶ Multiple sclerosis

▶ Syncope

▶ Vertigo

▶ Postural hypotension

Management

Nonpharmacologic Treatment

▶ Educate patients at risk and families about "brain attack," need for same immediate response as heart attack

▶ Diet and exercise counseling for primary and secondary prevention; smoking cessation

▶ Carotid endarterectomy for surgical candidates with carotid stenosis > 70%

▶ Care poststroke largely supportive: Physical therapy, occupational therapy, speech therapy

▶ Emotional support of patient and family

Pharmacologic Treatment

▶ Tissue plasminogen activator (TPA) must be administered in a hospital within 3 hours of onset of symptoms of ischemic stroke; contraindicated in hemorrhagic stroke. Patients awaking with focal deficits are not appropriate for TPA because duration of deficits is unknown.

▶ Medical management in the postacute phase involves anticoagulation or antiplatelet agents and treatment of underlying heart disease, hypertension, diabetes, and hyperlipidemia.

　▹ Aspirin 325 mg each day

　▹ Ticlopidine (Ticlid) 250 mg b.i.d., reduce dose to q.d. for renal patients, monitor for neutropenia, check CBC every 2 weeks for 3 months, then every 3 months

　▹ Clopidogrel (Plavix) 75 mg each day, does not cause neutropenia, but has been more effective at preventing peripheral vascular disease than stroke

　▹ Warfarin (Coumadin): Used for patients with symptoms on antiplatelet medication or those with atrial fibrillation or prosthetic heart valves. Dose is individualized due to small therapeutic window and interactions with food and other medications. International Normalized Ratio (INR) is stabilized at 2–3 for atrial fibrillation or antiplatelet failure and 2.5–3.5 for prosthetic valve.

How Long to Treat

▶ As long as antiplatelet or anticoagulation is not contraindicated (increase risk of GI or intracerebral bleeding)

Special Considerations

▶ Men are at greater risk than women, although more women die of stroke because of age and population dynamics.

▶ Increased risk with age and poorer prognosis, increased incidence of infection, myocardial infarction, renal failure, and delirium. Consider patient's risk of falls, ability to manage a complex medication regime, and INR monitoring when initiating warfarin therapy.

▶ Do not discount stroke in young people — may be hemorrhagic stroke secondary to AVM or embolic stroke secondary to unidentified patent foramen ovale (right-to-left shunt)

When to Consult, Refer, Hospitalize

▶ Send all patients with sudden onset of focal neurologic deficit to emergency facility; if TIA, may need urgent work-up and treatment to prevent stroke; if diagnosed as stroke and of less than 3 hours duration, may start TPA therapy.

▶ Send patients to emergency facility with sudden severe headache, decreasing level of consciousness, vomiting, or focal neurologic deficits.

▶ Consult with physician or neurologist for evaluation and management of patient with history of TIA or previous stroke.

Follow-up

▶ Patients with risk for cerebrovascular disease should be monitored every 3–6 months for symptoms of TIA and hypertension, and counseled regarding stroke prophylaxis, diet, exercise, and smoking cessation.

Expected Course

▶ Variable; most stroke recovery occurs early; the longer deficits last, the less likely they are to resolve, although improvement may be seen for 6 months

▶ 27% of stroke patients die within 1 year, and 53% within 5 years.

▶ Physical therapy improves functional recovery.

▶ Older age, coma, and early acute CT changes are associated with poor prognosis.

Complications

▶ Intracerebral hemorrhage from TPA therapy

▶ Myocardial infarction, infection, renal failure

▶ Falls, depression, dementia

▶ Intracerebral bleed or GI bleed from anticoagulation

ALZHEIMER'S DISEASE (AD)/ MULTI-INFARCT DEMENTIA (MID)

Description

▶ Dementia: Impairment of global intellectual and cognitive function characterized by memory loss, aphasia, agnosia, and apraxia with preservation of level of consciousness

▶ MID and Alzheimer's disease make up the majority of progressive, irreversible dementias.

▶ MID: Dementing process caused by strokes, characterized by step-wise decline

▶ AD: Gradual onset and progressive decline without focal neurologic deficits

  » 1st stage of AD manifested by short-term memory impairment. Activities of daily living become increasingly challenging. Social, occupational, and cognitive impairment manifest themselves.

  » 2nd stage of AD characterized by increasing loss of social and cognitive ability, with concomitant increasing behavioral changes. These can range from agitation and restlessness to outright combativeness. Eventually, the patient no longer recognizes friends and loved ones.

  » 3rd and last stage of AD brings the disease full cycle, as cognitive disability is eventually followed by physical decline.

Etiology

▶ AD: Not fully understood

▶ More neuritic plaques and neurofibrillary tangles are found on autopsy compared to nondemented patients.

▶ 3 genes on different chromosomes have been identified in families with history of AD, although not all cases may be inherited.

▶ MID: Multiple lacunar infarcts

▶ A correlation with sleep apnea and Alzhemier's increased mental deterioration

Incidence and Demographics

▶ Affects 5%–10% of people > 65 and increases with age

▶ AD and related dementias affect 2–4 million Americans.

▶ Often misdiagnosed or unrecognized, especially in early stages

▶ AD: 50%–60% of all dementias; MID: 10%–20% of all dementias

Risk Factors

▶ AD: Down syndrome

▶ Familial or inherited

▶ MID: Hypertension, previous stroke, TIA

Prevention and Screening

▶ Routine screening is not recommended because there is no definitive treatment, and it is difficult to recognize early dementia.

▶ People > 65 should have cognitive and functional evaluation at least every 3 years.

▶ Be aware of early symptoms to facilitate early assessment and recognition, and rule out age-related memory changes, unidentified conditions, or reversible forms of dementia (Table 15–4).

▶ Interpretation: Positive findings in any of these areas generally indicate the need for further assessment for the presence of dementia.

TABLE 15–4
GUIDE FOR RECOGNITION AND INITIAL ASSESSMENT OF DEMENTIA

Does the person have increased difficulty with any of the activities listed?	
Learning and retaining new information	Repeats information; has trouble remembering recent conversations, events, appointments; frequently misplaces objects
Handling complex tasks	Has trouble following a complex train of thought or performing tasks that require many steps such as balancing a checkbook or cooking a meal
Reasoning ability	Is unable to respond with a reasonable plan to problems at home or work, such as knowing what to do if the bathroom is flooded; shows uncharacteristic disregard for rules of social conduct
Spatial ability and orientation	Has trouble driving, organizing objects around the house, finding way around familiar places
Language	Has increasing difficulty with finding the words to express what he or she wants to say and with following conversations
Behavior	Appears more passive and less responsive; is more irritable than usual; is more suspicious than usual; misinterprets visual or auditory stimuli

Assessment

History

▶ Detailed history of present illness, including time frame and progression, any associated neurologic symptoms such as amaurosis fugax, aphasia, unilateral weakness

▶ Past medical history: Hypertension, strokes, head trauma

▶ Psychiatric history: Depression, anxiety, schizophrenia

▶ Social history: Present living situation, marital status, occupation, education, alcohol, tobacco, illicit drug use

▶ Medications, including over-the-counter, supplements, and home remedies

▶ Initial and periodic functional history and assessment

▶ Validate history with family member or caregiver, but also be aware of potential for self-serving motives; informants may exaggerate or deny symptoms.

Physical Exam

- ▶ Assess level of consciousness along a continuum from alert to drowsy, to stupor, to coma.

- ▶ Perform complete mental status evaluation using instrument such as Folstein Mini-Mental State Examination (MMSE), the Short Portable Mental Status Questionnaire, or Blessed Dementia Rating Scale; test results are not diagnostic, but serve as a baseline for assessing trends in cognitive impairment.

  - » Generally, a score of < 26 on the MMSE (which tests orientation, registration, attention and calculation, recall and language) indicates cognitive impairment, but this is only a crude indicator of functioning.

- ▶ Complete neurologic exam with attention to focal neurologic deficits, which may indicate MID or other neurologic problem

  - » MID: Focal motor weakness or impaired sensation, reflex asymmetry, positive Babinski

- ▶ Assess for sensory impairments (hearing, vision) that masquerade as or worsen dementia.

- ▶ Pulmonary and cardiac exams (murmurs, arrhythmias, heart enlargement, orthostatic hypotension)

- ▶ Any evidence of infectious processes

- ▶ Signs of physical and mental abuse

Diagnostic Studies

- ▶ CBC, chemistry profile, thyroid function tests, B_{12} level, folate level to rule out causes of delirium and reversible dementia; syphilis, HIV, and drug toxicity if indicated by history

- ▶ CT for early dementia of < 2 years' duration may show atrophy, infarcts, or unexpected lesions.

- ▶ Other testing based on presentation

- ▶ Neuropsychological testing is recommended under certain circumstances: to differentiate depression, stroke, or delirium in unusual presentations; or identify areas of preserved cognitive function to develop a care plan.

- ▶ Sleep study if sleep apnea is suspected

Differential Diagnosis

- ▶ Delirium
- ▶ Other dementias: Lewey bodies dementia, Pick's disease
- ▶ Depression and anxiety
- ▶ Normal pressure hydrocephalus
- ▶ Tumor
- ▶ Hearing loss
- ▶ B_{12} and folate deficiency

- ▶ Parkinson's disease
- ▶ Trauma—consider subdural hematoma, falls (whether witnessed or not)
- ▶ Alcohol intoxication
- ▶ Infectious process: Chronic infection, AIDS, tertiary syphilis
- ▶ Cardiovascular or cerebrovascular accidents
- ▶ Medications: Polypharmacy, interactions

Management

▶ Foremost, rule out or treat any conditions that may contribute to cognitive impairment

▶ Discontinue all unnecessary medications, especially sedatives and hypnotics

▶ MID: Nonpharmacologic and pharmacologic reduction of stroke risks (see management of TIA and stroke)

Nonpharmacologic Treatment

▶ Explain memory and cognition status assessment results to the patient, putting them within the context of overall patient status.

▶ Educate patient and family about the illness, treatment, and community resources.

▶ Assist with long-term planning, including financial, legal, and advance directives.

▶ Assess home and driving safety.

▶ Behavior therapy identifies causes of problem behaviors, and changes the environment to reduce the behavior.

▶ Recreational, art, and pet therapy create pleasurable experiences for the patient.

▶ Reminiscence therapy

▶ Incontinence care; supportive care

Pharmacologic Treatment

▶ Cognitive symptoms

» Cholinesterase inhibitors such as donepezil (Aricept) 5 mg initially, may increase to 10 mg/day, memantine 5 mg initially, may increase to 10 mg b.i.d., or rivastigmine 1.5 mg b.i.d.

» Common side effects: Headache, nausea, diarrhea

» LFT monitoring not required

▶ Psychosis and agitation

» Primary: Risperidone (Risperdal) 0.5–3 mg b.i.d., olanzapine (Zyprexa) 2.5 mg/day, quetiapine (Seroquel)12.5 mg b.i.d., or aripiprazole (Abilitify) 10 mg/day

» Secondary option: Haloperidol (Haldol) 0.5–3 mg at bedtime or divided up during day

» Lorazepam (Ativan) 0.5–4 mg a day in divided doses as needed for anxiety

▶ Depression

» Sertraline (Zoloft) HCl 25–200 mg/day

» Citalopram (Celexa) 10–40 mg/day

» Escitalopram (Lexapro) 10–20 mg/day

▶ Sleep disturbances

» Trazodone (Desyrel) 25–75 mg at bedtime

How Long to Treat

▶ Cholinesterase inhibitors: May be initiated for mild to moderate Alzheimer's disease and discontinued when significant cognitive decline is noted; ineffective for MID

▶ Use other medications p.r.n.; if needed regularly, use lowest effective dose and attempt to wean periodically

Special Considerations

▶ Consider language and education level when administering and interpreting mental status tests.

▶ Integrate cultural beliefs into the management of minority patients with dementia.

When to Consult, Refer, Hospitalize

▶ Consult with physician for diagnosis and long-term treatment planning.

▶ Refer to neurologist for unusual presentation.

▶ Refer to psychiatrist if unable to differentiate from depression or see intractable behaviors.

▶ Use social worker and multidisciplinary services for long-term care planning.

▶ Hospitalize with deteriorating conditions, such as exacerbation of chronic heart failure (CHF), chronic obstructive pulmonary disease (COPD), dehydration, pneumonia, or injury. Be aware that demented patients are likely to become more confused and delirious, and fall, when hospitalized.

Follow-up

▶ Generally every 60 days

Expected Course

▶ AD: Slowly progressive

▶ MID: Stepwise with gradual deterioration; associated with new focal deficits and decline with each additional stroke

Complications

▶ Depression and suicide

▶ Complications usually related to comorbidity or complications, due to immobility with severe end-stage dementia

DELIRIUM

Description

▶ Acute disorder of attention with onset of hours to days, characterized by confusion, disorientation, and fluctuation over the course of a day

Etiology

▶ Functional disorder of the brain caused by organic factors

▶ Any number of factors can cause: Polypharmacy, infections, metabolic and electrolyte abnormalities, dehydration, nutritional deficiencies, cardiopulmonary disease, urinary retention, fecal impaction, trauma, anesthesia, environmental change

Incidence and Demographics

▶ 10%–40% of hospitalized patients > 65 years old

Risk Factors

▶ Age, dementia, frailty, visual impairment, presence of many other chronic diseases

Prevention and Screening

▶ Eliminate unnecessary medications.

▶ Provide and ensure adequate hydration, nutrition, and oxygenation

▶ Correct visual and auditory deficits.

▶ Continuity of care and environment.

Assessment

History

▶ Detailed history of present illness, including cognition, time frame, and progression

▶ Comprehensive review of systems to identify underlying etiology

▶ Functional history and assessment

▶ Validate history with family member or caregiver

Physical Exam

▶ Complete neurologic exam with attention to level of consciousness, focal neurologic deficits

▶ Hearing and visual impairments

▶ Pulmonary and cardiac exams (murmurs, arrhythmias, heart enlargement)

▶ Any evidence of infectious processes

▶ Signs of trauma

▶ Evaluation for orthostatic hypotension, urinary retention, and fecal impaction

▶ Folstein Mini-Mental State Examination

▶ Geriatric Depression Scale

Diagnostic Studies

▶ CBC, chemistry profile, thyroid function tests, B_{12} level, folate level to identify a reversible cause for cognitive impairment or etiology

▶ Computed tomography to identify infarcts, space-occupying lesions

▶ Syphilis, HIV, and drug toxicity if indicated by history

▶ Urinalysis if urinary tract infection suspected

▶ Arterial oxygen or pulse oximetry if hypoxemia considered

▶ ECG and chest X-ray identify cardiopulmonary cause

▶ EEG to rule out seizure disorder

▶ Lumbar puncture for suspected encephalopathy or meningitis

Differential Diagnosis

▶ Dementia ▶ Depression ▶ See etiologies above

Management

▶ Identify and treat underlying cause.

Nonpharmacologic Treatment

▶ Provide continuity of care.

▶ Minimize environmental stimuli.

▶ Provide eyeglasses or hearing aids.

▶ Coordinate clocks and calendars to maintain orientation.

▶ Maintain hydration, nutrition, oxygenation.

▶ Ensure adequate bowel and bladder regimen.

Pharmacologic Treatment

▶ Haloperidol (Haldol) 0.5 mg p.o. or IM q2–6h for agitation

How Long to Treat

▶ Depends on etiology; often continue therapy until baseline cognitive function returns

Special Considerations

▶ Highest incidence in hospitalized older adults

When to Consult, Refer, Hospitalize

▶ Consult physician for any primary care patient with suspected delirium.

▶ Hospitalize to ensure patient safety, adequate hydration, and prescribed treatment unless underlying etiology such as urinary tract infection (UTI) without sepsis can be managed at home with supervision.

Follow-up

▶ Regularly to monitor for recurrence

Expected Course

▶ Usually reversible

Complications

▶ Injury due to falls

▶ Associated with increased morbidity and mortality

PARKINSON'S DISEASE

Description

▶ Neurodegenerative disease characterized by slow movement (bradykinesia), rigidity, flexed posture, loss of postural reflex, freezing, resting tremor

Etiology

▶ Unknown, although genetics, endogenous toxins, and exogenous toxins have been implicated

▶ In Parkinson's disease, destruction of the substantia nigra and nigrostriatal tract occur resulting in damage to dopaminergic neurons, leaving active unopposed acetylcholine neurons intact.

▶ Imbalance of dopamine and acetylcholine results in loss of refinement of voluntary movement.

▶ Parkinson's that is reversible can occur in patients receiving metoclopramide, neuroleptic agents, or reserpine.

Incidence and Demographics

▶ Prevalence 350 per 100,000 in U.S. with 50,000 new cases per year

▶ Greater in men than women at a 3:2 ratio; usual onset during ages 45–65

▶ Less prevalent in Africans and African Americans than in Asians, Europeans, and Caucasian Americans

▶ Affects 1% of people age > 50

Risk Factors

▶ Age, heredity

▶ Possible environmental factors

Prevention and Screening

▶ None, although older patients may benefit from periodic assessment of mobility, cognitive, and functional status

Assessment

History

▶ Focused, detailed history of chief complaint, including time frame and progression, aggravating and alleviating factors such as stress or rest; interview family, patient, and caregiver

▶ Complete review of neurologic symptoms, including weakness, paresthesia, tremor, diplopia, aphasia, mood, and cognitive changes

▶ Past medical history, including neurologic disorders, exposure to environmental toxins, illicit drugs

▶ Family history of Parkinson's disease, other movement disorders or dementia

▶ Medications, including over-the-counter anticholinergics, antihistamines, decongestants, or cough and cold preparations that worsen condition

▶ Functional assessment: Difficulty with functional and instrumental ADLs; mobility, including stair-climbing (patients with progressive supranuclear palsy will have problem descending stairs) and rising from chair

▶ Falls and injuries

▶ Review of systems for associated autonomic dysfunction, including perspiration, incontinence, constipation, and postural hypotension

▶ Assess for depression and mental status—may use Geriatric Depression Scale and MMSE or other tools

Physical Exam

▶ General: Manner, affect, dress and hygiene; speech may be soft and monotone

▶ Cranial nerve exam: Normal in Parkinson's, 4th cranial nerve palsy with progressive supranuclear palsy

▶ Motor exam: No weakness but cogwheel rigidity (rigidity to passive movement)

   ▸ Bradykinesia: Slowness of voluntary movement and difficulty initiating movement, difficulty rising from chair, shuffling gait, problems with turns and stopping movement

   ▸ Tremor: Slow (4–6 cycles per second) resting tremor present in one limb, limbs on one side, 4 limbs, or absent in 20% of Parkinson's patients; tremor may be obvious at rest and exaggerated with stress; some tremor of mouth and lips

   ▸ Tremor may increase with emotional stress, decrease with voluntary activity

▶ Gait and posture: Stooped posture with knees and hips flexed; hands held in front, close to body

▶ "Masked facies": Fixed facial expression, drooling, wide palpebral fissures, soft voice

▶ Meyerson's sign: Repetitive tapping on bridge of the nose produces sustained blink response.

▶ Incoordination of rapid alternating movements; decreased automatic movement, decreased blinking

▶ Deep tendon reflexes unaffected

▶ General examination: Seborrhea

▶ Vital signs: Orthostatic hypotension

Diagnostic Studies

▶ Consider head CT if diagnosis not clear and stroke or space-occupying lesion is suspected.

Differential Diagnosis

▶ Benign essential tremor

▶ Progressive supranuclear palsy

▶ Depression

▶ Dementia

▶ Cerebrovascular disease

▶ Brain tumor

▶ Adverse effects of anticholinergic medications, particularly antipsychotics

▶ Drug-induced Parkinson's

▶ Carbon monoxide poisoning

▶ Normal pressure hydrocephalus

▶ Huntington's disease

▶ Creutzfeldt-Jakob disease

Management

▶ There is no cure for Parkinson's. Current therapy is aimed at managing symptoms to preserve independence and mobility.

▶ The Hoehn and Young Scale can be helpful for staging the disease and guiding pharmacologic and supportive therapy.

  ▹ Stage I: Unilateral involvement

  ▹ Stage II: Bilateral involvement but no postural abnormalities

  ▹ Stage III: Bilateral involvement with mild postural instability; patient leads independent life

  ▹ Stage IV: Bilateral involvement with postural instability; patient requires substantial help

  ▹ Stage V: Severe, fully developed disease; patient is restricted to bed and chair

Nonpharmacologic Treatment

▶ Patient and family education regarding progressive nature of disease and complex pharmacologic treatments

▶ Nutritional counseling regarding low-protein diet and dietary management of constipation

▶ Compression stockings for postural hypotension

▶ Physical, occupational, speech therapy with appropriate assistive devices for ambulation and ADLs

▶ Fall precautions and home safety evaluation; installing rails, raised toilet seats, tub chairs

▶ Encouragement for walking, social activities, and interaction

▶ Emotional support

▶ Deep brain stimulation

▶ Surgical interventions: Unilateral stereotaxic thalamotomy or pallidotomy, implantable high-frequency thalamic stimulation to suppress resting tremor for difficult-to-control cases

Pharmacologic Treatment

▶ See Table 15–5.

TABLE 15–5
TREATMENT ALGORITHM FOR PARKINSON'S DISEASE

STAGE OR PROBLEM	THERAPEUTIC ALTERNATIVES
Mild disease (Stage I and II)	Selegiline for neuro protection Anticholinergics if tremor predominant Amantadine (best for rigidity and bradykinesia) Group support, exercise, education, nutrition
Functionally impaired (Stage III)	
Age ≤ 60 years	Tremor predominant: Anticholinergics Functional disability: Sustained-release carbidopa/levodopa (lowest dose possible); dopamine agonist
Age ≥ 60 years	Sustained-release carbidopa/levodopa
Stage IV or V	Immediate-release carbidopa/levodopa Dopamine agonists
Poor symptom control	Increase carbidopa/levodopa dose Add or increase dopamine agonist dose Add COMT inhibitor
Suboptimal peak response	Begin combination dopaminergic therapy Add levodopa (Larodopa) to dopamine agonist Add dopamine agonist to levodopa (Larodopa) Increase dose of levodopa/carbidopa or dopamine agonist Add COMT inhibitor as levodopa adjunct, switch dopamine agonists
Wearing off	Begin combination of dopaminergic therapy Add levodopa to dopamine agonist Add dopamine agonist to levodopa Increase frequency of levodopa dosing Increase dose of levodopa/carbidopa (sustained or immediate release) Add COMT inhibitor and decrease levodopa dose Change to sustained-release carbidopa/levodopa Add liquid levodopa/carbidopa Add selegiline if not already taking
On-off	Begin combination dopaminergic therapy. Add levodopa to dopamine agonist. Add dopamine agonist to levodopa. Add COMT inhibitor. Modify distribution of dietary protein.
Freezing	Increase or decrease carbidopa/levodopa dose. Add dopamine agonist. Increase or decrease dopamine agonist dose. Discontinue selegiline. Gait modification, assistance device
No "on" time	Manipulate time and dose of levodopa. Add COMT inhibitor. Avoid dietary protein. Increase GI transit time.

Adapted from "Antiparkinson Agents" by L. R. Young, 2004, in M. W. Edmunds & M. S. Mayhew (Eds.), *Pharmacology for the Primary Care Provider* (2nd ed., p. 512), St. Louis, MO: Mosby.

- ▶ Dopamine precursor
  - » 25 mg carbidopa/100 mg levodopa (Sinemet) t.i.d.–q.i.d.; or 10 mg carbidopa/100 mg levodopa t.i.d.–q.i.d., titrate up by 1 tablet every 2–7 days as needed and tolerated, not to exceed 200 mg carbidopa and 800 mg levodopa a day
  - » "On-off" phenomenon in 40%–50% of patients after 2–3 years — patients experience inconsistent effect from same dose
  - » "Wearing-off" symptoms appear before next dose is due
  - » Use lowest doses possible; consider addition of dopamine agonists.
- ▶ Dopamine agonists
  - » Pramipexole (Mirapex) 0.125 mg t.i.d., titrate up to 1.5 mg t.i.d. over 7 weeks
  - » Ropinirole (Requip) 0.25 mg t.i.d., titrate up weekly by 1.5 mg a day to a total dose of 24 mg a day. Maintenance dose is 3–24 mg a day. Discontinue slowly over 1 week.
- ▶ MAO-B inhibitor:
  - » Selegiline (Eldepryl) 5 mg b.i.d. (at low doses, is a selective MAO inhibitor and can be safely administered with levodopa)
  - » Nonselective MAO inhibitors contraindicated in combination with levodopa; use can precipitate hyperpyrexia and hypertensive crisis; must be discontinued at least 14 days before initiating levodopa
- ▶ Anticholinergic agent
  - » Benztropine (Cogentin) 1–2 mg q.d.
- ▶ Catechol O-methyltransferase (COMT) inhibitor
  - » Entacapone (Comtan) 200 mg b.i.dy up to q.i.d, max 1,600 mg/day
  - » Tolcapone (Tasmar) 100–200 mg t.i.d.

How Long to Treat

- ▶ Medication combinations and dosages must be individualized and adjusted during the course of the disease; disease is lifelong and progressive.

Special Considerations

- ▶ Prescribe Parkinson's medications with caution in older patients, particularly those with comorbidity of heart, renal, or liver disease.
- ▶ Avoid anticholinergics in older patients, tend to be poorly tolerated, and have increased risk of side effects including confusion, agitation, arrhythmias, urinary retention.
- ▶ Differentiate Parkinson's disease from essential tremor, which may occur at any age from childhood but increases with age and affects the distal upper extremities and head; may be familial.
  - » If mild, reassurance may be only intervention needed
  - » May be treated with beta-adrenergic blockers, such as propranolol (Inderal) and metoprolol (Lopressor); primidone (Mysoline); benzodiazepines
  - » May be disabling; refer for possible neurosurgery

When to Consult, Refer, Hospitalize

▶ Refer to neurologist for confirmation of diagnosis and guidance with medical management.

▶ Neurosurgical consultation for patients with severe symptoms refractory to medications, or unable to tolerate medications

Follow-up

▶ Every 3 months, as well as any time a change is made in medication or therapy regimens

▶ Episodic office visit if symptoms worsen

▶ Annual health assessment and physical examination

Expected Course

▶ Progressive; 30% develop coexisting dementia with poorer prognosis

Complications

▶ Related to immobility and falls; hip fractures common, pneumonia may occur in Stage 5

▶ Aspiration of food

▶ Depression and social isolation occur.

MULTIPLE SCLEROSIS (MS)

Description

▶ Progressive neurodegenerative disease characterized by demyelination and inflammation of the neuronal sheath in the brain and spinal cord that produces episodic neurologic symptoms such as sensory abnormalities, visual disturbances, sphincter disturbances, and weakness with or without spasticity

Etiology

▶ Autoimmune disease; possible causes may be genetic, viral, immunologic, or environmental; strong association with HLA-DR2 antigen

Incidence and Demographics

▶ Incidence 250,000–300,000 per year in the U.S.

▶ Prevalence is higher in temperate zones, ranging from only 5–10/100,000 in tropical zones to 50–175/100,000 in cooler environments.

▶ Women-to-men ratio 2–3:1;estrogen and progesterone may be implicated because symptoms often develop during the menstrual cycle and after pregnancy

▶ Age of onset 15–55 years; greatest incidence in young adults < 55 years

▶ Late onset of MS in the 6th – 7th decade usually severe and rapidly progressive

Risk Factors

- ▶ Familial 1%–3% increased risk in first-degree relatives (15 times greater than general population)

- ▶ Climate or place of residence, established by residence in the first 15 years of life

- ▶ Urban dwelling, upper socioeconomic status; Western European descent

Assessment

History

- ▶ Neurologic history: Paresthesias, weakness and spasticity, ataxia, fatigue, heat intolerance, visual changes, diplopia on lateral gaze, vestibular disturbances, trigeminal neuralgia, facial myokymia, optic neuritis, bowel and bladder dysfunction

- ▶ Time frame with exacerbations and remission

- ▶ Past medical history for differential diagnosis: Systemic lupus erythematosus, Lyme disease, cerebral and spinal tumors, HIV, seizures, peripheral neuropathy, head or spinal trauma

- ▶ Triggers may be infection, trauma, pregnancy

Physical Exam

- ▶ Complete neurologic exam

  - » Cranial nerve deficits

  - » Optic neuritis: Decreased visual acuity, abnormal pupillary response, hyperemia and edema of optic disk

  - » Internuclear ophthalmoplegia: Cranial nerve 6 palsy or weakness of the medial rectus muscle with lateral gaze, nystagmus

  - » Decreased strength, increased tone, clonus, positive Babinski; weakness, numbness, tingling or unsteadiness in a limb; disequilibrium; urinary urgency, hesitancy, incontinence

  - » Decreased proprioception and vibratory sensation, positive Romberg; pyramidal, sensory, or cerebellar deficits in some or all limbs

  - » Lhermitte's sign: Electrical sensation down the back into the legs is produced with neck flexion

Diagnostic Studies

- ▶ MRI may show characteristic multiple lesions of demyelinated areas with reactive gliosis

- ▶ Cerebrospinal fluid analysis for lymphocytosis, immunoglobulins, and oligoclonal bands

- ▶ Visual, auditory, and sensory evoked potentials

Differential Diagnosis

- ▶ Stroke
- ▶ Cerebral or spinal tumors
- ▶ Ischemic optic neuropathy
- ▶ Systemic lupus erythematosus
- ▶ Lyme disease
- ▶ Peripheral neuropathy
- ▶ Seizure disorder
- ▶ AIDS
- ▶ Intoxication
- ▶ Amyotrophic lateral sclerosis

Management

▶ Aimed at delaying progress, managing chronic symptoms, treating acute exacerbations

Nonpharmacologic Treatment

▶ Physical and occupational therapy

▶ Mental health services for assistance with coping strategies

Pharmacologic Treatment

▶ Complex; treatment regimen *must* be coordinated with a neurologist.

▶ Immunosuppressive therapy may arrest progression.

   ▸ Interferon beta (Avonex) 30 mcg IM once a week

   ▸ Glatiramer acetate (Copaxone) 20 mg SQ q.d.

   ▸ Azathioprine (Imuran) unlabeled use

▶ Acute exacerbations: Prednisone 60–80 mg/day for 1 week, taper over 2–3 weeks

▶ Spasticity: Baclofen (Baclosan) 40–80 mg/day in divided doses; start with 5 mg t.i.d., titrate up every 3 days

   ▸ Clonazepam (Klonopin) unlabeled use

▶ Fatigue

   ▸ Amantadine 100 mg b.i.d.

   ▸ Consider tricyclic antidepressants or selective serotonin reuptake inhibitors.

   ▸ Treat underlying spastic bladder, depression.

How Long to Treat

▶ Use corticosteroids only for acute exacerbations, not for maintenance.

▶ Antibodies to interferon may develop.

▶ Stop interferon if progression of disabilities continues after 6 months of treatment.

Special Considerations

▶ New onset or exacerbations with menstrual cycle and post-partum

▶ Family planning and fertility should be discussed with women of childbearing age — menses may be irregular and fertility impaired due to demyelination, but pregnancy not contraindicated.

▶ Oral contraceptives are not contraindicated except with impaired mobility.

▶ Consult with obstetrician regarding medications for pregnancy and lactation.

When to Consult, Refer, Hospitalize

▶ Refer all patients with suspected MS to neurologist for confirmation of diagnosis and development of management plan.

▶ Ophthalmology referral

▶ Continence specialist or urologist for bladder dysfunction

▶ Mental health referral for coping or depression

Follow-up

▶ Followed closely by neurology; primary care for routine health visits

Expected Course

▶ Progressive, with exacerbations and remissions

Complications

▶ Hydronephrosis and renal failure secondary to urinary retention

▶ Falls

▶ Depression

VERTIGO

Description

▶ Sensation of motion of the body or environment when there is no movement

▶ Not a disorder, but a symptom of an underlying condition

Etiology

▶ Peripheral vestibular dysfunction

  ▸ Benign positional vertigo: Believed to be caused by free-floating debris in the semicircular canal

  ▸ Occurs with change in position with delay between movement and symptoms; symptoms fatigue or disappear with repeated movement

  ▸ Labyrinthitis: Infection of the inner ear, most likely viral, often follows an upper respiratory infection

  ▸ Ménière's disease: Swelling of the endolymphatic system of the inner ear; may be caused by syphilis or head trauma, or viral

▶ Traumatic vertigo is due to labyrinth concussion or basilar skull fracture.

▶ Central vestibular dysfunction is due to vertebrobasilar insufficiency, acoustic neuroma, or compression of the 8th cranial nerve by blood vessel loops, similar to trigeminal neuralgia.

Incidence and Demographics

▶ Benign positional vertigo most common in those over 60

▶ Labyrinthitis: Affects any age, usually after upper respiratory infection

▶ Ménière's occurs at 40–70 years

▶ Central lesions less common

Risk Factors

▶ Age: Increasing incidence with increasing age

▶ Upper respiratory infection

▶ Trauma

Assessment

History

▶ Detailed description of sensation without using terms "dizzy" or "vertigo"; include time frame, duration, association with movement, alleviating and precipitating factors

  ▹ Vertigo is associated with a sensation of movement.

  ▹ Dizziness or lightheadedness is associated with presyncope due to cardiac cause.

  ▹ Imbalance or gait instability is associated with cerebellar disease or peripheral neuropathy.

▶ Associated symptoms of hearing loss, tinnitus, nausea, vomiting with Ménière's

▶ History of upper respiratory infection or trauma

▶ Timeframe

  ▹ Positional vertigo and vertebrobasilar insufficiency occur in seconds

  ▹ Ménière's, vestibular migraine over hours

  ▹ Labyrinthitis, traumatic vertigo, and vestibular neuritis over days

  ▹ Acoustic neuroma, multiple sclerosis, cerebellar disease over months, progressive

Physical Exam

▶ Screening neurologic exam with attention to cranial nerves.

▶ Sustained nystagmus is indicative of vertigo but may be central or peripheral.

▶ Facial palsy may or may not be present with acoustic neuroma.

▶ Assess gait and balance.

▶ Dix-Hallpike maneuver: Lay patient flat with head to one side and hanging over edge of table, sit patient up quickly with head held to side, repeat with other ear down; reproduction of symptoms and nystagmus is positive for positional vertigo. Nystagmus that is purely vertical and not fatigueable with subsequent trials may be due to central vestibular dysfunction.

▶ Otologic exam

Diagnostic Studies

▶ MRI if central lesion suspected

▶ Audiogram to evaluate sustained hearing loss, which may occur with Ménière's

▶ Depending on clinical findings and suspected underlying etiology, may consider CBC, chemistry panel, lipid panel, thyroid function studies, ESR, RPR

Differential Diagnosis

- ▶ Benign positional vertigo
- ▶ Labyrinthitis
- ▶ Ménière's disease
- ▶ Cerumen impaction
- ▶ Otitis media or externa
- ▶ Sinusitis
- ▶ Vertebrobasilar insufficiency

- ▶ Vestibular migraine
- ▶ Acoustic neuroma
- ▶ Presyncope with probable cardiac etiology
- ▶ Multiple sclerosis
- ▶ Cerebellar disease
- ▶ Peripheral neuropathy

Management

Nonpharmacologic Treatment

- ▶ Remove cerumen if present.
- ▶ Rest in quiet, darkened room.
- ▶ Safety precautions to change positions slowly, may need walker for support
- ▶ Bland diet with small portions, fluids if nausea and vomiting present
- ▶ Ménière's disease: Low-sodium diet
- ▶ Benign positional vertigo: Vestibular rehabilitation to reduce symptoms

Pharmacologic Treatment

- ▶ Meclizine (Antivert) 25–100 mg in divided doses may reduce vertigo
- ▶ Hydrochlorothiazide 25–50 mg or triamterene 50 mg a day for Ménière's
- ▶ Antibiotics may be helpful in labyrinthitis if bacterial infection suspected.

How Long to Treat

- ▶ Taper and stop meclizine when symptoms resolve, generally within 1–2 weeks; do not use prophylactically or as maintenance.

Special Considerations

- ▶ Older adults are more sensitive to antihistamines; use only if necessary for severe debilitating symptoms; may cause drowsiness, confusion, anticholinergic symptoms.

When to Consult, Refer, Hospitalize

- ▶ Hospitalize for dehydration and inability to take oral rehydration secondary to severe nausea and vomiting.
- ▶ Neurosurgical referral for acoustic neuroma or other space-occupying lesions
- ▶ Neurology referral if focal neurologic deficits, severe headaches, seizures, or other suggestions of central nervous system problem, or symptoms do not resolve with treatment

Follow-up

- ▶ As needed for recurrence or worsening symptoms

Expected Course

▶ Benign positional vertigo episodes last several days; may reoccur.

▶ Labyrinthitis resolves in several days.

▶ Ménière's may have multiple episodes with remissions.

Complications

▶ Hearing loss with Ménière's

▶ Falls

▶ Dehydration with associated nausea and vomiting

MENINGITIS

Description

▶ Central nervous system infection of the covering of the brain and spinal cord by any infectious agent, including bacteria, virus, mycobacteria, spirochetes, fungi, protozoa, and parasites

Etiology

▶ Caused by virulent infectious organism in a susceptible host; local host defenses overcome

▶ Bacteria causing meningitis varies by the age of the patient:

  ▹ < 1 month: Group B streptococci, *E. coli, Listeria monocytogenes*

  ▹ 4–6 weeks: *H. influenzae* type b, *E. coli, S. pneumoniae,* Group B streptococci

  ▹ 6 weeks – 6 years: *S. pneumoniae, N. meningitides, H. influenzae* type b

  ▹ > 6 years: *S. pneumoniae, N. meningitides*

▶ Viral meningitis can be caused by any of more than 70 different strains of viruses; most common are the enteroviruses (85%) and herpes simplex; less serious, resolves spontaneously

▶ Most common fungal causes *Candida* sp., *Aspergillus, Cryptococcus neoformans*

▶ Candidal meningitis occurs mostly in ill premature infants and immunocompromised patients, but 30% of all patients with fungal meningitis have no underlying immunodeficiency.

▶ Aseptic meningitis can be caused by *Borrelia burgdorferi* (Lyme disease) or *Treponema pallidum* (syphilis).

▶ Meningitis can also be caused by tuberculosis.

▶ *H. influenzae, N. meningitides,* and *S. pneumoniae* cause 80% of bacterial meningitis in adults.

▶ *S. aureus, S. pneumoniae,* and Gram-negative bacilli are common causes of postsurgical or posttraumatic meningitis.

▶ Possible Gram-negative bacilli in geriatric patients

Incidence and Demographics

▶ In children, 80% of bacterial meningitis occurs before 24 months of age.

▶ Incidence approximately 1/100,000 people a year

▶ More prevalent in lower socioeconomic groups, crowded housing, urban areas

▶ 3 times more prevalent in college students residing on campus than those living off campus and the general population

Risk Factors

▶ Poverty and lack of childhood immunizations

▶ Crowded living conditions

▶ Immunodeficiency

▶ College students living in campus housing and soldiers in barracks

▶ Infectious disease close to meninges: Pneumonia, pharyngitis, otitis media, sinusitis, endocarditis

▶ Penetrating head trauma

▶ Syphilis infection

▶ Lyme disease

Prevention and Screening

▶ Routine administration of the *H. influenzae* type b (Hib) vaccine has significantly reduced the incidence of meningitis.

▶ Administration of the Prevnar vaccine

▶ Adolescents planning to attend college and reside in dormitories should receive meningococcal vaccine.

▶ Post-exposure prophylaxis for bacterial meningitis with oral rifampin (Rifadin) for household and daycare contacts, and anyone with direct exposure to oral secretions (kissing) of infected patient

  ▸ *H. influenzae:* Rifampin (Rafidin) 20 mg/kg/dose q.d. for 4 days

  ▸ *N. meningitides:* Rifampin (Rafidin) 10 mg/kg/dose b.i.d. for 2 days

▶ The American Academy of Pediatrics recommends prophylaxis to daycare or nursery school contacts if 2 or more index cases occur in a unit within 60 days of each other.

Assessment

History

▶ Rapid onset within 24–36 hours

▶ Progressive, severe headache accompanied by neck and back pain with flexion

▶ Neurologic symptoms: Drowsiness, irritability, confusion, photophobia, hearing loss, focal neurologic deficits, seizures, nuchal rigidity, photophobia

▶ Associated symptoms: Fever, nausea, vomiting, rash

▶ In infants, complaints of sleep disturbances, irritability, or vomiting

▶ Recent history of respiratory infection, head trauma, invasive neurosurgical procedures, or dental procedures

▶ Past medical history: Meningitis, polio, immunodeficiency

▶ Social history: Living in crowded environment, IV drug use, foreign travel

▶ Environmental exposure to bird or pigeon droppings (fungal) or tick bite (Lyme)

▶ Medications: Immunosuppressants

Physical Exam

▶ General: Fever, tachycardia, hypotension, rash

▶ Assess fontanels in infants for bulging, hydration status.

▶ Complete neurologic exam: Decreased level of consciousness (drowsiness or agitation), papilledema, cranial nerve III, IV, VI, VII, VIII deficits, focal motor deficits, seizure, mental status

▶ Meningeal irritation: Nuchal rigidity, positive Brudzinski's sign (adduction and flexion of legs with neck flexion), positive Kernig's sign (after flexing thighs, extension met with resistance and pain in hamstring muscles)

▶ Complete physical exam for sites of primary infections:

  » Head trauma or surgery, dental abscess or caries, otitis media, sinusitis, pneumonia, pancreatitis, genital lesions, skin rashes

Diagnostic Studies

▶ Cerebrospinal fluid analysis, culture (diagnosis usually made on Gram stain): Gold standard

  » Viral infection: Some lymphocytes, normal glucose, moderately hig protein content, normal or mildly elevated opening pressure

  » Bacterial infection: Increased lymphocytes, decreased glucose, high protein content, markedly elevated opening pressure

▶ Brain CT before lumbar puncture (LP) if space-occupying lesion (brain abscess, subdural empyema, tumor, subdural hematoma) suspected with papilledema or focal neurologic findings; LP contraindicated with increased intracranial pressure

▶ CBC, platelet count, PT/PTT, electrolytes, BUN, creatinine, glucose, arterial blood gases (as indicated), blood cultures

▶ Chest or sinus X-ray, or both, if exam indicates source of infection

Differential Diagnosis

▶ Bacterial meningitis

▶ Aseptic meningitis

▶ Encephalitis (herpes, rabies)

▶ Brain abscess

▶ Noninfectious meningeal irritation (sarcoidosis, systemic lupus erythematosus, cancer, medications and chemical irritants)

▶ Bacterial sinusitis or mastoiditis

▶ Vertebral osteomyelitis

▶ Amebic meningoencephalitis

Management

Nonpharmacologic Treatment

▶ Medical emergency; immediate transport to hospital for IV antibiotics and supportive care

▶ Assurance of adequate airway, cardiac function, fluid support

▶ Educate family and significant others regarding illness, treatment, and prognosis.

▶ Inform family and contacts of postexposure prophylaxis.

Pharmacologic Treatment

▶ IV antimicrobials in acute-care setting; usually cefotaxime, ceftriaxone, or vancomycin

▶ Acyclovir has been used in the neonate with viral meningitis.

▶ Administration of dexamethasone (Decadron) before or with antibiotics appears to reduce the incidence of sensorineural hearing loss without increasing mortality or complications.

How Long to Treat

▶ *H. influenzae* and *N. meningitidis:* 7 days

▶ *S. pneumoniae*: 10–14 days

▶ Gram-negative bacteria: 21 days

Special Considerations

▶ Antibiotics given in smaller doses than usually used to treat meningitis for the 3–4 days before lumbar puncture will not significantly alter the cerebrospinal fluid (CSF) findings.

▶ Rifampin is contraindicated for post-exposure prophylaxis in pregnant patients — it is secreted in breast milk.

When to Consult, Refer, Hospitalize

▶ Medical emergency: Immediately transfer all suspected meningitis cases to an acute care facility.

▶ Most patients with viral meningitis can be managed at home, if stable, after physician consultation.

Follow-up

▶ Patients should be seen a few days after hospital discharge.

▶ Parents and patients should be instructed to follow up if any new neurologic sequelae present, include hearing and vision problems.

Expected Course

▶ 90% survival with early diagnosis, treatment, and supportive care

Complications

▶ Mortality rate is over 50% in patients who are not diagnosed early and referred; 10% for patients who receive prompt diagnosis, appropriate IV antibiotics, and supportive care. Mortality of bacterial meningitis in neonates is 10%–20%; in infant and children patients is 3%–10%.

▶ Complications of meningitis include seizures (2%–8%), hearing defects (10%), mental retardation (10%), visual abnormalities (3%–7%), language delay (15%), motor abnormalities (3%–7%), inappropriate ADH secretion (SIADH), and sixth cranial nerve palsy. Occurrence of sequelae is estimated at 25%–50% of meningitis survivors.

SEIZURES AND EPILEPSY

GENERAL INFORMATION

▶ A seizure is a transient, sudden, paroxysmal electrical discharge of a group of neurons in the brain that causes an alteration in neurologic function.

▶ May involve abnormal motor activity, sensory symptoms, change in the level of alertness, an alteration in autonomic function, or combination of these

▶ A seizure is not a diagnosis, but rather a clinical symptom of an underlying neurologic dysfunction.

▶ Seizures classified by etiology: Genetic (25%), symptomatic (50%), and idiopathic (25%)

▶ Neonatal seizures are rarely idiopathic and immediate attention must be paid to identifying the underlying disorder.

▶ Febrile seizures occur in infants and children as a result of fever, not underlying neurologic disorder.

▶ Epilepsy, or recurrent, spontaneous seizures unrelated to fever, may occur in children and adults:

　▸ Rolandic epilepsy, associated with a typical EEG pattern, is the most common type in children.

　▸ Infantile spasms are myoclonic seizures occurring in the first year of life, usually in clusters, associated with a typical EEG pattern.

NEONATAL SEIZURES

Description

▶ Seizures in a newborn almost always reflect a significant nervous system pathology.

▶ Seizures in this age group may present in several ways:

　▸ Focal-rhythmic twitching of muscle groups, including the face

　▸ Multifocal clonic: Similar to focal, but involving multiple muscle groups

　▸ Tonic: Rigid posturing of the extremities and trunk

» Myoclonic: Focal or generalized jerking of the extremities, generally involve the distal parts of the body

» Subtle: Chewing motions, excessive salivation, or autonomic changes such as apnea, blinking, nystagmus, pedaling motions, and skin color changes

Etiology

▶ Time of onset and characteristics of seizure may suggest most probable cause.

▶ Rarely idiopathic; typical causes of neonatal seizures include trauma from birth or from congenital malformations, including hypoxia, intracranial hemorrhage, infection, drug withdrawal, metabolic disorders, inborn errors of metabolism, neurocutaneous disorders, pyridoxine dependency, and cerebral dysgenesis

▶ Focal seizures may be caused by metabolic disturbances and do not necessarily imply a focal lesion.

Incidence and Demographics

▶ Thought to occur in 0.5% of all term infants and 20% of preterm infants

Risk Factors

▶ Complicated labor or delivery, prematurity

▶ Infants of mothers with diabetes

▶ Family history of metabolic disorder associated with seizures; maternal drug use

Prevention and Screening

▶ Neonatal seizures are not preventable, but the incidence of prematurity and birth trauma may be decreased with good prenatal care and maternal education.

Assessment

History

▶ Prenatal and perinatal history including maternal risk factors and complications of pregnancy, labor, and delivery

▶ Family history of seizure disorders or metabolic disease, congenital syndromes

▶ Exact description of the event, movements, or reactions that has triggered the concern

Physical Exam

▶ Complete physical, focusing on dysmorphic features, atypical or rhythmic movements.

▶ Assess growth, vital signs.

▶ Neurologic exam, presence or absence of newborn reflexes, head size and shape

▶ Eye exam to look for chorioretinitis (inflammation that destroys superficial tissue areas visible on funduscopic exam and causes a well-defined but irregular area of white sclera that has smaller areas of dark pigment); or coloboma (developmental abnormality in which a moderate-to-large sized area of sclera with well-demarcated borders is seen below the disc)

▶ Any unusual skin pigmentation or body odors for metabolic disorder

▶ Presence of hepatosplenomegaly, signs of drug withdrawal

Diagnostic Studies

▶ Laboratory testing to include CBC, electrolytes, calcium, magnesium, pH, sodium bicarbonate, bilirubin, BUN, and ammonia

▶ Urinalysis and urine toxicology screen

▶ Lumbar puncture, if presence or suspicion of infection or intracranial hemorrhage

▶ Neuroimaging to rule out brain injury or mass

▶ Chromosomal analysis if presence of dysmorphic features

▶ Metabolic screen, including amino acids, lactate, and urine organic acids

▶ Toxoplasmosis, rubella, cytomegalovirus, herpes simplex, HIV (TORCH) screen

▶ Drug screen

▶ EEG: Changes may not always be present.

Differential Diagnosis

▶ Jitteriness

▶ Gastroesophageal reflux disease (GERD)

▶ Apnea

▶ Benign idiopathic neonatal convulsions: "fifth-day fits"

▶ Benign familial neonatal convulsions: Days 2–4 of life, with familial history

Management

▶ Treatment is guided by correcting the underlying abnormality.

Nonpharmacologic Treatment

▶ Ensure adequate ventilation and perfusion.

Pharmacologic Treatment

▶ For metabolic disorders, consider calcium gluconate, magnesium sulfate, pyridoxine (vitamin B_6).

▶ Antibiotics if infection is present

▶ Seizure management includes the use of phenobarbital, phenytoin (Dilantin), or lorazepam (Ativan).

How Long to Treat

▶ Duration of therapy is based on the underlying etiology.

When to Consult, Refer, Hospitalize

▶ Any newborn with suspected seizures should receive prompt evaluation and admission for work-up.

▶ An infant with a history of neonatal seizures should be followed in conjunction with a physician and a neurologist.

Follow-up

▶ Infants should be followed by neurology at regular intervals until seizure-free and off medications; follow-up may be extended if neurologic sequelae ensue.

▶ Infants need routine health assessments to monitor growth and development and should receive routine immunizations.

▶ Infants with cognitive or motor deficits should be referred to early intervention programs.

Expected Course

▶ Highly individual; child may develop normally following seizure period

Complications

▶ Mortality rate is approximately 15%, but is much higher in preterm infants.

▶ Mental retardation and motor deficits are more common sequelae, occurring in about 29% of affected infants.

▶ Prognosis is dependent upon the underlying etiology, with cerebral dysgenesis having the worst outcomes.

▶ The likelihood of recurrent seizures is 15%–20% overall.

FEBRILE SEIZURES

Description

▶ A seizure event in infancy or early childhood, associated with fever, but without evidence of intracranial infection or defined cause

▶ Febrile seizures classified as

  » Simple: Isolated, brief, generalized seizure lasting < 15 minutes

  » Complex: Prolonged (> 10 minutes), multiple seizures within a 24-hour period, or focal in nature

Etiology

▶ Febrile seizures are caused or brought on by a fever.

▶ The most common causes are normal childhood illnesses, such as tonsillitis, upper respiratory infections, and otitis media.

▶ Genetic predisposition occurred in approximately 10% of parents; there is a 20% chance of occurrence in sibling.

Incidence and Demographics

▶ Occur in approximately 2%–4% of all children; more common in males

▶ Usual onset in the second year of life, but can occur at any time from 6 months to 5 years of age

▶ Usually occurs within the first 24 hours of fever

▶ Approximately 30% of children will experience one or more recurrences.

▶ Risk of recurrence is related to the age of the child, family history, and complexity of first seizure

Risk Factors

▶ Very high fever, > 38.8° C (101.8° F)

▶ Family history of febrile seizures

▶ Neonatal discharge from hospital ≥ 28 days

▶ Delayed development

▶ Daycare attendance (increased rate of febrile illness)

▶ Low serum sodium

Prevention and Screening

▶ Subsequent febrile seizures may be prevented by early and adequate fever control.

Assessment

History

▶ Family history of febrile seizures

▶ Complete description of the seizure, duration, recovery, motor involvement, etc.

▶ Any history of recent illness or exposure to illness, onset of headaches, vomiting, or unusual symptoms

▶ Recent trauma, medication exposure

▶ Prenatal and perinatal history, including developmental history

▶ Exposure to toxins, such as lead

Physical Exam

▶ Document presence of fever

▶ Complete physical exam: Identify underlying illness or infection requiring treatment.

▶ Complete neurologic exam, including level of consciousness, presence of meningismus, or a tense bulging fontanel; head circumference

▶ Signs of physical abuse

▶ Neurocutaneous skin lesions

Diagnostic Studies

▶ Lumbar puncture: If suspicion of meningitis or for children < 18 months with first seizure

▶ Routine lab studies *not* indicated, unless no source of fever can be elicited on physical examination

▶ EEG not warranted

▶ MRI limited to children with focal seizures

▶ Serum lead level, if indicated

Differential Diagnosis

▶ Meningitis or encephalitis

▶ Anoxia

▶ Trauma

▶ Stroke or hemorrhage

▶ Metabolic encephalopathy

▶ Neurodegenerative disorder

▶ Neurocutaneous syndromes

▶ Brain tumor

▶ Lead poisoning or other toxins

▶ Epilepsy

Management

Nonpharmacologic Treatment

▶ Because febrile seizures are very frightening to the parents, parental reassurance and education are vitally important.

▶ An active search for the underlying cause of the fever and appropriate treatment with each incidence

Pharmacologic Treatment

▶ Vigorous control of fevers by antipyretics and sponging with tepid water

  ▹ Acetaminophen 10–15 mg/kg per dose either orally or per rectum

  ▹ Ibuprofen 10 mg/kg per dose orally

▶ Prophylaxis is controversial, but may be used. Consider if 3–5 febrile seizures in 1 year.

  ▹ Diazepam (Valium) orally or rectally to prevent recurrences only during a febrile illness (1 mg/kg/day divided into 3 doses over the first 3 days of illness or 0.5 mg/kg rectally at onset of seizure)

  ▹ Phenobarbital has had limited results.

  ▹ Side effects of prophylaxis include ataxia, behavior problems, and lethargy.

How Long to Treat

▶ During febrile episodes

Special Considerations

▶ Seizure(s) occurring late in the course of a febrile illness raise serious concern about meningitis or encephalitis.

▶ Relieving parental anxiety should be the focus of management.

▶ Small risk of developing epilepsy later in life if:

  ▹ Abnormal development before the seizure

  ▹ Family history of afebrile seizures

  ▹ Complex first febrile seizure

When to Consult, Refer, Hospitalize

▶ Due to parental anxiety, the first febrile seizure may be evaluated at the emergency department.

▶ Consult with physician; however, no referrals or consultations are necessary in simple febrile seizures.

▶ Consult or refer to neurologist if seizures become more focal or complex.

▶ If the seizure is generalized, lasts longer than 20 minutes, or is focal, or the suspected disease process is complex, the child should be hospitalized.

▶ Continued seizures past age 6 are not compatible with febrile seizures and require a neurology referral.

Follow-up

▶ Patients with febrile seizures should receive the routine childhood immunizations and health assessments at regular intervals.

Expected Course

▶ Full return of function following resolution of fever; child will outgrow

Complications

▶ Permanent cognitive or motor damage or both can occur if febrile seizures are not treated in a timely and effective manner.

▶ Lacerated tongue, broken teeth, bones, etc., can occur if the child's seizure is not safely contained.

ROLANDIC EPILEPSY OF CHILDHOOD

Description

▶ Benign partial epilepsy of childhood with centrotemporal or rolandic spikes (EPEC) is the most common variant of epilepsy seen in children of school age. It is a syndrome consisting of unilateral tonic-clonic contractions of the face, paresthesias of the tongue and cheek, and occasional clonic seizures of the ipsilateral upper extremity.

Etiology

▶ The etiology of most seizures is unknown.

▶ Seizures are typically focal (e.g., twitching of the mouth).

Incidence and Demographics

▶ The prevalence of epilepsy in the pediatric population is 4–6 per 1,000 cases; the male-to-female ratio is 3:2.

▶ Rolandic epilepsy occurs at 2–14 years, with the peak incidence at age 9–10 years; the majority resolve or "outgrow" by age 16 years.

▶ Approximately 75% occur during sleep, but can occur during daytime with a brief 2–5-minute sleep seizure, an average of fewer than 4 episodes per year in most cases.

Risk Factors

▶ History of previous seizures (febrile or afebrile)

▶ Recent withdrawal of anticonvulsant medications

▶ History of remote neurologic insult such as head trauma

▶ Family history of seizures

Assessment

History

▶ Complete description of the seizures, including duration, aura, signs of infection, motor involvement, timing, or stimulus

▶ Family history of seizure disorders or previous history in this child

▶ History of any head trauma or insult

▶ Any recent use of medications or drugs

▶ Health history of the patient

▶ Any recent onset of headaches, weakness, or sensory deficits

Physical Exam

▶ Physical exam with attention to screening neurologic exam (usually normal)

▶ Parents may need to videorecord an event for the provider to view.

▶ Signs of systemic infection; signs of physical abuse

▶ Skin evaluation for neurocutaneous disorders

Diagnostic Studies

▶ EEG, either routine or 24-hour recording: Characteristic spike focus in the centrotemporal or rolandic area with normal background activity

▶ CT/MRI to rule out intracranial abnormality, especially if anticonvulsant therapy is not effective

Differential Diagnosis

▶ Night terrors

▶ Complex partial seizures

▶ Simple partial seizures

▶ Tics

▶ Migraine

▶ Breath-holding spells

Management

Nonpharmacologic Treatment

▶ Occasional seizures require no therapy, just careful monitoring.

Pharmacologic Treatment

▶ Carbamazepine (Tegretol) initial dose 10 mg/kg/day, increasing to 20–30 mg/kg/day as maintenance

▶ Phenytoin (Dilantin) 5–10 mg/kg/day in 3 divided doses

▶ Valproate (Depakene) 15–30 mg/kg/day in 2–3 divided doses

How Long to Treat

▶ If seizure-free for at least 2 years with a normal EEG, consider weaning from medication over a period of 4–6 months and supervise closely.

▶ Higher risk for seizure recurrence in children with developmental delay, age > 12 years at onset, neonatal seizures, and multiple seizures before control attained

Special Considerations

▶ In children with poor seizure control despite appropriate medication, consider drug compliance, growth spurts, and possible other epileptic etiologies.

▶ People with seizures should not swim alone or play sports that are conducive to head injuries (e.g., football, lacrosse).

When to Consult, Refer, Hospitalize

▶ If epilepsy is suspected, the patient should be referred and managed by a pediatric neurologist.

▶ Patients with rolandic epilepsy rarely need hospitalization.

Follow-up

▶ At least annual with pediatric neurologist

▶ Routine health maintenance

Expected Course

▶ Most — nearly 100% — remit by adolescence.

Complications

▶ Essentially none; response to anticonvulsant agents is excellent

SEIZURES AND EPILEPSY IN ADULTS

Description

▶ A transient alteration in behavior, function, consciousness, or combination of these that results from an abnormal electrical discharge of neurons in the brain

▶ Epilepsy refers to chronic recurrent seizures.

▶ Most older adults have partial seizures that may quickly generalize to tonic-clonic.

▶ The International League Against Epilepsy has classified seizures based on clinical presentation and EEG findings (Table 15–6).

Etiology

▶ A seizure is a symptom of an underlying disorder; the most frequent cause of repetitive seizures is failure to take antiseizure medications.

▶ Cause is unknown for most epilepsy, including primary epilepsy, but is believed to be related to abnormalities of neurotransmission.

▶ Patients with primary epilepsy can continue to have seizures into old age.

▶ Secondary epilepsy is due to injury to cerebral cortex.

▶ Most new-onset epilepsy in older adults is secondary due to tumors, hematomas, or stroke.

▶ Space-occupying lesions, stroke, metabolic disorders, and alcohol withdrawal can also cause seizures.

▶ Vascular disease is the most common cause of onset > age 60.

Incidence and Demographics

▶ 10% of Americans will have a seizure at some time during their lives; 1%–2% have epilepsy.

▶ New-onset epilepsy is highest among those < 20 years of age.

Risk Factors

▶ Intracranial lesions, head trauma, hypoglycemia, chronic illness that predisposes metabolic abnormality; medications that lower seizure threshold (e.g., selective serotonin reuptake inhibitors, certain atypical antidepressants, ciprofloxacin, metronidazole, theophylline)

▶ Certain triggers: Sleep deprivation, menses, flashing lights/television; emotional stress, fever, hormonal imbalance

▶ Alcohol intoxication or alcohol withdrawal

Prevention and Screening

▶ Head trauma prevention: Seat belt use, bicycle and motorcycle helmets

▶ Fall prevention for the elderly; home safety counseling

Assessment

History

▶ Interview witness to seizure if possible. This information is most important in making diagnosis.

▶ Detailed history of event; include description of seizure activity, loss of consciousness, duration, incontinence, possible triggers

▶ Prodromal symptoms such as aura, confusion, or focal neurologic symptoms

▶ Postictal state: Antegrade amnesia, level of consciousness

▶ Prior seizure history, including type, frequency, duration

► Seizure medications: Any changes, missed doses, levels

► Past medical history: Previous intracranial lesions or trauma, diabetes, HIV, stroke, migraines, dementia, psychiatric illness

► Medications: Ciprofloxacin (Cipro), metronidazole (Flagyl), theophylline, stimulants, antipsychotics can lower seizure threshold

► Diuretic, antihypertensives, diabetes medicines can cause metabolic disturbances that can cause seizure

► Family history of seizure

Physical Exam

► Assess for head trauma.

► Screening neurologic exam may be normal even with structural lesions.

► Focal deficits may be worse immediately after seizure.

► Evaluate cardiovascular and pulmonary status.

► Blood pressure and pulse will be elevated during and immediately after a seizure.

Diagnostic Studies

► First-time seizure: Metabolic panel, toxicology if appropriate

► Brain CT scan even with a metabolic etiology because the metabolic abnormality could lower the seizure threshold in the presence of a structural lesion

► EEG for first-time patient who has seizure with identified etiology; need not be repeated

► EEG for first-time seizure without etiology, may determine seizure type and guide treatment and prognosis; if seizures continue and EEG nondiagnostic, may consider closed-circuit video EEG

► Lumbar puncture if new neurologic findings are not explained by imaging, or if fever or continued unexplained headache present

Differential Diagnosis

Causes for Seizure

► Head trauma

► Brain tumor

► Stroke

► Metabolic disorders

► Alcohol withdrawal

► Withdrawal from some medications can also cause seizure

Disorders That May Appear to Be Seizures

► Syncope

► Transient ischemic attack

► Pseudo-seizures

► Panic attacks or psychosis

► Drug intoxication

► Migraine

► Multiple sclerosis

► Postural hypotension

Management

Nonpharmacologic Treatment

▶ Educate patient and family about seizure disorder and cause.

▶ Educate patient and family about safety management, including using any aura period to prepare for a seizure.

▶ Stress the importance of keeping an extra supply of medication readily available at all times.

▶ First episodes of seizures without known cause do not have to be treated with anticonvulsants.

▶ Educate family about acute seizure management such as protecting patient from injury by placing on left side to maintain airway if possible.

▶ Patients with known recurrent seizures do not need to go to the emergency department for every seizure — only if seizure lasts more than 2 minutes or breathing is impaired (aspiration).

▶ Advise regarding state driving regulations.

▶ Advise regarding swimming alone or operating dangerous equipment.

▶ Teach about side effects and toxic effects of medications, and not to discontinue seizure medicines abruptly, which may precipitate seizure.

▶ Discuss seizure triggers: Sleep deprivation, alcohol, menses, stress, low-grade fever, and infection.

▶ Wear medic alert bracelet.

Pharmacologic Treatment

▶ Anticonvulsants first initiated by a neurologist: Phenytoin (Dilantin), phenobarbital (Luminal), carbamazepine (Tegretol), and valproic acid (Depakene) are first-line choices (Table 15–6)

▶ 40%–50% of patients can be maintained seizure-free on a single agent.

▶ Phenytoin initially 100 mg 3 times a day, maintenance dose 300–600 mg/day divided

▶ Phenobarbital 60–100 mg/day

▶ Carbamazepine initially 200 mg twice a day, increase by < 200 mg/day in divided doses 3–4 times a day up to 1,200 mg

▶ Valproic acid initially 15 mg/kg/day, increase at 1-week intervals by 5–10 mg/kg/day until seizures are controlled or side effects prevent further increase in dose, maximum dose 60 mg/kg/day, divide totally daily doses over 250 mg. Before initiating, baseline liver enzyme levels (specifically ALT and AST) must be drawn and then monitored thereafter. approximately every 3–6 months, to determine safe serum levels.

How Long to Treat

▶ Consider discontinuing seizure medications in those without seizures for more than 2 years.

▶ Obtain an EEG before stopping medication.

▶ 40% will have a reoccurrence, most within the first year.

▶ Must consider risk factors of seizure reoccurrence and medications for each individual patient; consult with neurologist

TABLE 15-6
SEIZURE CLASSIFICATION AND RECOMMENDED MEDICATION

SEIZURE TYPE	DESCRIPTION	MEDICATION
Simple partial	Focal motor or sensory symptoms, reflect area of brain affected; no change in consciousness	Phenytoin, carbamazepine valproic acid, phenobarbital
Complex partial	Characterized by an aura, followed by impaired consciousness with automatisms, usually originating from temporal lobe	Carbamazepine, phenytoin, phenobarbital, valproic acid
Secondarily generalized	Simple or complex partial seizures that progress to generalized tonic-clonic seizures	Phenytoin, carbamazepine, phenobarbital, valproic acid
Generalized tonic-clonic	Formerly "grand mal," sudden loss of consciousness with tonic-clonic motor activity, postictal state of confusion, drowsiness, and headache	Phenytoin, carbamazepine, phenobarbital, valproic acid
Absence	Formerly "petit mal," brief (< 30 seconds) episodes of unresponsiveness characterized by staring, blinking, or facial twitching	Ethosuximide, valproic acid, clonazepam

Special Considerations

▶ With first-time seizures in patients > 50, must consider an underlying intracranial lesion or metabolic etiology

▶ Anticonvulsants are metabolized in the liver and involve the cytochrome P450 enzyme system; care must be used when administering these medications with any other medications.

▶ Patients must be counseled about the signs and symptoms of liver disease, including nausea and vomiting that seem protracted, abdominal pain, anorexia, fatigue, and dark urine or stools.

▶ Lower, less-frequent doses may be needed for those with hepatic and renal dysfunction.

▶ All anticonvulsants have been associated with increased birth defects.

▶ Babies of mothers with epilepsy have 2–3 times the normal risk of birth defects.

▶ Must counsel all women of child-bearing age regarding risks of medications during pregnancy

▶ Seizures may increase, decrease, or remain the same during pregnancy.

▶ A neurologist should be consulted before pregnancy for medical management.

▶ Anticonvulsants, except valproic acid, alter the effectiveness of birth control pills.

▶ Some anticonvulsants are excreted in breast milk and may have serious adverse effects for the nursing infant

▶ There is no evidence that prophylactic anticonvulsant therapy prevents epilepsy following head trauma or brain surgery; therefore it is not necessary to maintain these patients on long-term anticonvulsants.

▶ Educate patients about specifics of state laws limiting driving for seizure patients.

When to Consult, Refer, Hospitalize

▶ Referral to neurologist for first-time seizures, when considering discontinuing therapy, seizures refractory to adequate trials of monotherapy, pregnancy

▶ Neurosurgeon for stereotaxic procedures for intractable seizures

▶ Status epilepticus is a medical emergency defined as 2 or more seizures without complete recovery or a seizure lasting > 30 minutes; the primary care provider witnessing a seizure lasting > 2 minutes must activate 911 and be prepared to initiate emergency procedures. IV access and administration of IV benzodiazepines (lorazepam) should be initiated as protocols permit.

Follow-up

▶ Most patients should be seen every 3 months by their primary care provider and at least annually by their neurologist; more frequent visits are needed if medications or seizures change.

▶ Anticonvulsants have small therapeutic ranges; levels should be drawn when adjusting therapy, and with change in seizure frequency.

▶ Liver enzymes must be monitored.

Expected Course

▶ Variable, one seizure to intractable seizures

Complications

▶ Status epilepticus, airway obstruction, injury during seizure activity

CASE STUDIES

CASE 1. 49-year-old Black female presents with new onset headache over the last 2 months.

HPI: She states that, before these episodes, she never thought of herself as a "headachey" person. She relates that the headaches are "nearly always" occipital, and are often accompanied by pain so severe that she feels like the top of her head will come off. When questioned, it is clear that she is both photo- and phonophobic and also experiences lightheadedness associated with the headache.

PMH: Healthy female; perimenopausal. Medications: Monthly Advil for menstrual cramps. Has tried Excedrin migraine with these headaches to no avail.

▶ What other history is needed?

▶ What type of physical exam would you do?

▶ What screening tests would you do?

▶ What is the most likely diagnosis?

▶ How would you manage this patient?

CASE 2. A 3-year-old Asian male is brought in for follow-up after management in the emergency department for multiple febrile seizures.

PMH: No prior history of virus-induced high fevers associated with seizing. No medications except over-the-counter acetaminophen liquid for fevers.

▶ What other history do you want to obtain?

▶ What physical examination would you perform?

▶ What further diagnostic tests would you want to order?

▶ How would you initially manage this patient?

CASE 3. A 78-year-old male presents with his wife and daughter complaining of an episode over the weekend of sudden-onset right-sided weakness that resolved completely in about 2 hours. He did not seek medical attention at the time because it resolved.

PMH: Smoker, 64 pack-year history. Mild hypertension diagnosed in 1985. Was told he had elevated lipids "a few years back" but refused to take medication or change his lifestyle at that time. Has not been back to see a provider since.

Medication: Hydrochlorothiazide 50 mg/day "for a year or so," 1985–1986. Occasional acetaminophen.

▶ What other history is important?

▶ What systems would you examine?

▶ What is the most likely diagnosis?

▶ What is your plan?

REFERENCES

American Heart Association. (2013). Executive summary: Heart disease and stroke statistics — 2013 update: A report from the American Heart Association. *Circulation, 127,* 143–152.

Bauman, R. J. (2012). *Pediatric febrile seizures.* Retrieved from http:emedicine.medscape.com/article/1176205

Cordell, C. B., Borson, S., Boustani, M., Chodosh, J., Reuben, D. ... Fried, L. B. (2013). Alzheimer's Association recommendations for operationalizing the detection of cognitive impairment during the Medicare annual wellness visit in primary care setting. *Alzheimer's & Dementia, 9*(2), 141–150.

Domino, F. J. (2012). *The 5-minute clinical consult.* Philadelphia: Lippincott Williams & Wilkins.

Downey, D. (2008). Pharmacologic management of Alzheimer disease. *Journal of Neuroscience Nursing. 40*(1), 55–59.

Facts and Comparisons. (2013). *Drug facts and comparisons 2013.* St. Louis, MO: Wolters Kluwer Health.

Goroll, A. H., & Mulley, A. G. (2009). *Primary care medicine* (6th ed.). Philadelphia: Lippincott Williams & Wilkins.

Hauser, R. A. (2013). *Parkinson disease.* Retrieved from http://emedicine.medscape.com/article/1831191

Hay, W. W., Levin, M. J., Deterding, R. R., Abzug, M. J., & Sondheimer, J. M. (2012). *Current pediatric diagnosis & treatment.* New York: McGraw-Hill.

Luzzio, C. (2013). *Multiple sclerosis.* Retrieved from http://emedicine.medscape.com/article/1146199

Post, R. E., & Dickerson, L.M. (2010). Dizziness: A diagnostic approach. *American Academy of Family Physicians, 82*(4), 361–368, 369.

Robertson, W. C. (2011). *Tourette syndrome and other tic disorders.* Retrieved from www.medscape.com/article/1182258

Scorza, K. A., Raleigh, M. F., & O'Conner, F. G. (2012). Current concepts in concussion: Evaluation and management. *American Academy of Family Physicians, 85*(2), 123–132.

U.S. Headache Consortium Guidelines. (2012). *Evidence-based guidelines for migraine headache in the primary care setting.* Retrieved from www.americanheadachesociety.org/professional_resources/us_headache_consortium_guidelines/

HEMATOLOGIC DISORDERS

Colleen Stellabotte, RN, CCRN, MSN, FNP-BC

GENERAL APPROACH

Description

► Most common blood or hematologic disorder in all age groups is iron deficiency anemia

► Do not assume that anemia in patient with chronic inflammatory disease is "anemia of chronic disease."

► Do not begin treatment for B_{12} deficiency without assessing for and treating folate deficiency.

► *Physiologic anemia* of the newborn occurs at 10–12 weeks due to rapid growth, increase in blood volume, and shortened red cell survival time; hemoglobin (Hgb) level may reach a low of 10 g/dL in full-term infants; this is followed by a gradual increase in red blood cells (RBCs), with correspondingly slower hemoglobin rise; healthy term infants do not require therapy.

► Hematopoiesis is slowed in older adults when the presence and number of progenitor cells decline; 60% of all anemias are seen in people over age 65.

Definitions

► Anemia: Hematocrit (Hct) < 36% for females, < 40% for males; or Hgb < 12 for females, < 13.5 for males. In children, specific values defining anemia vary depending on age.

► Mean corpuscular (cell) volume (MCV): Represents the size of the red blood cell (RBC) and is calculated from the hemoglobin, hematocrit, or RBC count; used in differentiation of types of anemia

▶ Ferritin: Represents iron storage in the serum; may be elevated during infection or chronic inflammation and decreased in iron deficiency

▶ Hypochromic: Erythrocytes containing decreased level of Hgb, causing the cells to appear "paler" on smear

▶ Hyperchromic: Erythrocytes containing increased level of Hgb, causing cells to appear "darker" on smear

▶ Macrocytic anemia: Decreased Hct/Hgb/RBC with associated MCV > 100

▶ Megaloblastic anemia: Anemia characterized by a large, nucleated, embryonic type of cell that is a precursor of erythrocytes in an abnormal erythropoietic process seen almost exclusively in pernicious anemia

▶ Microcytic anemia: Decreased Hct/Hgb/RBC with associated MCV < 80

▶ Normocytic anemia: Decreased Hct/Hgb/RBC with associated MCV 80–100

▶ RDW: Red blood cell distribution width, a statistical index of the variation in red cell widths

▶ Total iron binding capacity (TIBC): Amount of iron in serum plus amount of transferrin available in serum (transferrin is a transport protein that regulates iron absorption); decreased in anemia of chronic disease

▶ Normal ranges for RBC studies can be found in Table 16–1.

TABLE 16-1
NORMAL RANGES FOR RBC STUDIES

TEST	FEMALES	MALES
Hematocrit	36%–48%	40–53%
Hemoglobin	12–16 g/dL	13.5–17.7 g/dL
RBC (10^6/µL)	4.0–5.4	4.5–6.0
MCV	80–100 fL	80–100 fL
MCH	26–34 pg	26–34 pg
MCHC	31%–37% g/dL	31%–37% g/dL
Reticulocyte Count	0.5%–1.5% of RBC	0.5%–1.5% of RBC
Serum Iron	50–170 mcg/dL	65–175 mcg/dL
TIBC	250–450 mcg/dL	250–450 mcg/dL
Ferritin	10–120 ng/mL (avg. 55)	20–250 ng/mL (avg. 125)

Note: MCH = mean corpuscular hemoglobin; MCHC = mean corpuscular hemoglobin concentration; RBC = red blood cells; TIBC = total iron binding capacity; fL = femtoliter (10^{-15} L); pg = pictogram (10^{-12} g); ng = nanogram (10^{-9} g); µL = microliter (10^{-6}).

RED FLAGS

▶ Blood values helpful in identifying anemias can be found in Table 16–2

TABLE 16–2
BLOOD VALUES HELPFUL IN DIFFERENTIATING ANEMIAS

ANEMIA	MCV	APPEARANCE OF RED CELL
Iron deficiency	< 80 fL	Normocytic or microcytic, hypochromic
Folate deficiency	> 100 fL	Macrocytic, hyperchromic
Vitamin B_{12}	> 100 fL	Macrocytic, hyperchromic
Chronic disease	Normal	Normochromic, normocytic or microcytic
Sideroblastic	< 80 fL	Hypochromic
Sickle cell	< 80 fL	Sickle cells, normochromic
G6PD	Normal	Heinz bodies, bite cells, blister cells
Thalassemia	< 80 fL	Microcytic
Drug-induced	Normal	Normocytic, normochromic
Aplastic	Normal	Normocytic, normochromic
Post-hemorrhagic	Normal	Normocytic, normochromic

▶ Anemia in the presence of splenomegaly requires further diagnostic evaluation.

▶ Anemia of prematurity manifests at 4–8 weeks of age and is more severe than physiologic anemia.

   » Influencing factors include birth weight, perinatal complications, blood transfusion history, and presence of vitamin E deficiency. Nadir Hgb values reach 6 g/dL.

   » Asymptomatic, growing preterm infants require no therapy; however, signs of hypoxia (apneic episodes, tachycardia, irritability, poor feeding) indicate need for evaluation and more aggressive intervention.

▶ Hemolytic anemia during the newborn period is due to physiologically immature liver incapable of rapidly conjugating bilirubin created by normally rapid turnover of relatively excessive RBC.

   » Hemolysis in the neonate is accompanied by reticulocytosis, nucleated RBC, and sometimes spherocytosis on peripheral blood smear.

   » Most common cause of hemolytic anemia in the newborn is ABO incompatibility with hyperbilirubinemia or jaundice, usually within 24 hours of birth.

   » All cases of suspected hemolytic anemia in the newborn should be evaluated in the hospital.

▶ Multiple myeloma is a malignant disease of the plasma cells with peak incidence during the 7th decade. It may present with bone pain of the back, chest, or extremities; weakness and fatigue; pathologic fractures; abnormal bleeding; palpable liver and spleen; Bence-Jones protein in the urine; elevated creatinine and calcium; and increased sedimentation rate. Refer for bone marrow biopsy.

▶ Hodgkin's lymphoma is a malignant disease with lymphoreticular proliferation and presence of Reed-Sternberg cells; there is a bimodal age distribution: 15–34 (peak at 20) and > 50 (peak at 70) with male-to-female ratio of 8:1.

  ▸ Presents with persistent fever, night sweats, persistent dry cough, unexplained pruritus, substernal discomfort, persistent painless lymphadenopathy, weight loss > 10%, anorexia, immediate pain after alcohol ingestion; increased incidence in persons with AIDS

  ▸ Diagnostic tests may show mediastinal adenopathy on chest X-ray, elevated erythrocyte sedimentation rate (ESR), increased serum alkaline phosphatase and lactate dehydrogenase (LDH), lymphocytopenia, mild leukocytosis, thrombocytosis, Reed-Sternberg cells on smear

  ▸ Refer suspected cases to hematologist for diagnosis and management with chemotherapy and radiation; prognosis is good depending on classification at diagnosis.

▶ Non-Hodgkin's lymphoma is a malignant disease of the lymphoreticular system differentiated from Hodgkin's lymphoma by absence of giant Reed-Sternberg cells; increased incidence in persons with AIDS

  ▸ Presents similar to Hodgkin's lymphoma; prognosis not as good

  ▸ Refer all suspected cases to hematologist for diagnosis and management.

▶ Deficiency of coagulant factor VIII (hemophilia A) or factor IX (hemophilia B) is rare and presents in males during first few years of life as excessive bruising, bleeding after circumcision, bleeding hours or days after injury, hematuria, or hemorrhage or hematoma after minor injury. Laboratory results include normal platelet count, greatly prolonged partial thromboplastin time (PTT), factor VIII low in hemophilia A, factor IX low in hemoglobin-B. Refer to hematologist for management.

NORMOCYTIC ANEMIAS

ANEMIA OF CHRONIC DISEASE

Description

▶ A mild hypoproliferative anemia associated with chronic disease, infections, and malignancies that has persisted for > 1–2 months; probably a consequence of long-term disease with inflammatory process

▶ Diagnosis of exclusion from active blood loss or production abnormalities associated with iron or folate intake

Etiology

▶ The pathophysiology of anemia of chronic disease is not well understood, but may be due to decreased RBC lifespan, erythropoietin reduction, and problems of iron transfer.

▶ Occurs as a result of renal disease, liver disease, endocrine disorders, rheumatoid arthritis, infections, some forms of cancer

Incidence and Demographics

▶ The second most common anemia in the world; incidence parallels the rate of chronic inflammatory disease

▶ The most common anemia in older adults

Risk Factors

▶ Chronic diseases: Renal, liver, endocrine disease; rheumatoid arthritis; infection; and some cancers

Prevention and Screening

▶ Attention to good nutrition

▶ CBC screening for patients with chronic disease

Assessment

History

▶ Chronic disease

▶ Fatigue, dyspnea on exertion, irritability, listlessness, easy fatigability

Physical Exam

▶ Perform a complete physical exam for signs of the underlying disease.

▶ Signs of anemia, depending on severity: Pallor, tachycardia, tachypnea on exertion

Diagnostic Studies

▶ See Table 16–2.

▶ CBC, reticulocyte count, iron studies (serum iron, TIBC, ferritin); studies pertinent to underlying disorder; repeat iron studies important for diagnosis and management

▶ Characteristic labs: Hgb usually 8–12 g/dL, Hct 25%–35%, MCV 75–85 as Hgb falls < 10, often low serum iron and TIBC, and normal or increased ferritin (TIBC is increased and ferritin decreased in iron deficiency); serum erythropoietin normal, but not generally assessed

Differential Diagnosis

▶ Iron deficiency anemia

▶ Multifactorial anemia

▶ Chronic renal insufficiency

▶ Liver disease (usually alcohol-related)

▶ Posthemorrhagic anemia

▶ Endocrine disorders: Hypothyroidism

▶ AIDS

▶ Aplastic anemia

Management

Nonpharmacologic Treatment

▶ Treat underlying disease.

▶ Ensure appropriate nutrition.

▶ Transfusion only in severe, symptomatic cases.

Pharmacologic Treatment

▶ Recombinant erythropoietin (Epogen, Procrit) in selected patients. Black box warnings for patients with certain types of cancers and patients with chronic kidney disease.

How Long to Treat

▶ Required as long as underlying disease and anemia persist

Special Considerations

▶ A similar profile as iron deficiency may eventually develop, with patient becoming mildly microcytic and hypochromic as Hgb falls < 10 g/dL.

▶ Patients with AIDS often have anemia of chronic disease. As disease progresses, pancytopenia may occur due to marrow damage. At that point, checking serum erythropoietin level may help determine if patient will benefit from recombinant erythropoietin injections.

▶ Anemia of renal disease relates to severity of renal failure, due to decreased erythropoietin production, may benefit from erythropoietin

▶ In patients with diabetes mellitus, anemia is frequently severe early in the disease process.

When to Consult, Refer, Hospitalize

▶ Refer if diagnosis is questionable.

▶ Refer to confirm underlying cause (e.g., rheumatologist for collagen or vascular problem, oncologist for cancer, nephrologist for renal disease, infectious disease specialist for infections).

Follow-up

▶ Frequent monitoring of blood pressure, CBC, iron studies with recombinant erythropoietin therapy

Expected Course

▶ Anemia will improve or worsen as the underlying disease improves or progress.

▶ A patient can often tolerate fairly low Hct and Hgb, as low as 30/10, as these develop gradually.

Complications

▶ Possible exacerbation of cardiopulmonary disease, particularly in older adults (anemia results in less oxygen delivered to tissues, heart rate and cardiac output increase to compensate, heart may begin to fail)

APLASTIC ANEMIA

Description

▶ Aplastic anemia is characterized by intrinsic bone marrow dysfunction or failure; pluripotent stem cell expression is impaired so pancytopenia with hypercellularity of the bone marrow is seen.

▶ Intrinsic marrow dysfunction produces defective RBC synthesis and produces anemia, neutropenia, thrombocytopenia, and pancytopenia.

Etiology

▶ Autoimmune suppression of hematopoiesis is most common cause, but may be precipitated by viral illness, autoimmune suppression, drug or chemical exposure, tumor, radiation, or inherited disorder

▶ Inherited: Fanconi's anemia, Schwachman-Diamond syndrome

Incidence and Demographics

▶ Not common in U.S.

▶ 50% idiopathic; 20% drug or chemical exposure (chloramphenicol [Chloromycetin] — rare); 10% viral

Risk Factors

▶ Family history, some medications (anticonvulsants, antibiotics, gold), radiation, exposure to some toxic chemicals such as insecticides, herbicides, organic solvents, paint removers, and others.

Prevention and Screening

▶ Most cases cannot be prevented.

▶ There are no recommended general screening methods.

▶ Avoid contact exposure to certain chemicals, such as insecticides, herbicides, organic solvents, paint removers, and other toxic chemicals. This is especially important if patient already has had aplastic anemia caused by toxic chemicals. Recurrent exposure may increase the risk of a reoccurrence of the disease.

▶ People who have had exposure to toxic chemicals or have had aplastic anemia in the past should have regular physical examinations.

▶ Patients should report the following signs and symptoms early: fever, fatigue, weight loss, weakness, sore throat, dyspnea, palpitations, and bleeding.

Assessment

History

▶ Insidious onset of fever, fatigue, weight loss, weakness, sore throat, dyspnea, palpitations

▶ Bleeding problems such as menorrhagia, rectal bleed, epistaxis

► History of potential sources of exposure to toxic agents: Medications, chemical exposure at work, hobbies, etc.

► History of associated anomalies: Kidney, hypospadias, short stature

Physical Exam

► General: Pallor, petechiae, bruises

► Thorough physical for tumors, signs of infection, signs of bleeding

  ▹ Cardiac exam: Systolic ejection murmur may be present

  ▹ Eyes: Retinal flame hemorrhage

  ▹ Rectal: Occult or rectal bleeding

Diagnostic Studies

► Pancytopenia is pathognomonic.

► Severe anemia, decreased reticulocytes

► CBC with differential, peripheral smear, bleeding studies, TIBC, urinalysis, bone marrow, liver function, CT of thymus as indicated

► Lab results: Normochromic, normocytic anemia; TIBC normal; hematuria

► Bone marrow shows hypoplasia, fatty infiltration

Differential Diagnosis

► Leukemia

► Hypersplenism

► Systemic lupus erythematosus (SLE)

► Myelodysplasia

► Sepsis

Management

Nonpharmacologic Treatment

► Perform education and supportive care.

► A well-balanced diet decreases risk of infection.

► Manage underlying cause.

► Perform human leukocyte antigen (HLA) testing on patients and immediate families for inherited conditions.

Pharmacologic Treatment

► Immunosuppression therapy, oxygen

► All cases: RBC and platelet transfusions, parenteral antibiotics for infection due to severe neutropenia

► Severe cases: Bone marrow transplant is considered (may be age-dependent)

How Long to Treat

► Lifelong treatment may be required unless effective bone marrow transplant is curative.

Special Considerations

▶ Must avoid further exposure to etiologic agents

When to Consult, Refer, Hospitalize

▶ Refer immediately to hematologist when diagnosis is suspected; work with hematologist throughout therapy.

Follow-up

Expected Course

▶ Often favorable outcome, depending on age and treatment response
▶ Untreated cases are fatal; successful bone marrow transplant is curative.

Complications

▶ Infection, leukemia, heart failure, hemorrhage

HYPOCHROMIC ANEMIAS

IRON DEFICIENCY ANEMIA

Description

▶ Microcytic, hypochromic anemia due to decreased iron stores, poor iron utilization, or poor iron reutilization

Etiology

▶ Hemorrhage, occult malignancy, increased need (pregnancy and growth spurts), impaired absorption, inadequate dietary intake

Incidence and Demographics

▶ Prevalent in all ages and populations in the U.S.
▶ Seen in 7%–10% of adult population; 10%–20% of infants and toddlers; 15%–45% of pregnant women; 20% women overall
▶ More common in women than men because of menstruation, pregnancy

Risk Factors

▶ Low iron stores; occurs in premature and low birth weight infants and when Hgb is lower than normal at birth (e.g., hemorrhage, smaller of twins)
▶ Increased need for iron; demands for iron higher than normal such as low birth weight infants experiencing rapid catch-up growth or normal rapid growth of infancy and adolescence; pregnancy and lactation; athletes

▶ Insufficient intake of iron from low dietary intake, poor bioavailability of the dietary iron, or malabsorption. Low intake is most common etiologic factor seen in infants, toddlers, teens, older adults, institutionalization.

▶ Increased loss of iron due to disease process, including Meckel's diverticulum, peptic ulcer disease, polyps, hemangiomas, parasitic infections, or cow's milk enteropathy. Losses may also occur from menorrhagia, chronic use of NSAIDs, uncommonly recurrent epistaxis, and possibly strenuous exercise.

▶ Conditions such as achlorhydria, gastric surgery, celiac disease, pica that cause impaired absorption

▶ Conditions such as neoplasm, duodenal or gastric ulcers, diverticulosis, ulcerative colitis

▶ Repeated blood donations

Prevention and Screening

▶ Encourage breastfeeding of all infants for the first 12 months of life; after 1 year of age, limit cow and soy milk consumption to < 24 ounces/day. Adequate diet; consume orange juice with meals to enhance iron absorption.

▶ Dietary supplements if patient has risk factors

▶ Selective screening for at-risk populations such as menstruating women and some older adults

Assessment

History

▶ Preterm and low birth weight (LBW) infants

▶ Initially asymptomatic; insidious onset of gradually progressing fatigue, dyspnea on exertion, irritable, listless, easy fatigability, dysphagia, postural hypotension

▶ Possible palpitations, shortness of breath, impaired muscular performance

▶ Diet history: Low in iron, pica

▶ Drug or chemical exposure

▶ Family history of iron deficiency anemia

▶ Review of systems (ROS) for blood loss, symptoms of gastrointestinal problems, neoplasms

Physical Exam

▶ Obtain height, weight for infants and children; plot on growth chart

▶ Observe for pallor or chlorosis (peculiar greenish pallor).

▶ Angular stomatitis, ulcerations or fissure of the mouth

▶ Ozena: Chronic atrophy of the nasal mucosa

▶ Dry skin and mucous membranes

▶ Koilonychia: Thinning and flattening of the nails, then spooning

▶ Auscultate heart for systolic flow murmurs

▶ Splenomegaly

▶ Brittle hair, tachycardia, tachypnea

Diagnostic Studies

▶ CBC with differential and smear, TIBC, serum iron, ferritin, special tests to determine underlying bleed

▶ Laboratory findings (see Table 16–3): Hgb < 12 g/dL in adults and older children, variable in younger children; serum ferritin level < 10 nanograms/mL in women and < 20 nanograms/mL in men; low Hct; "pencil cells" on smear, MCV and MCH decrease, RDW > 15, increased TIBC > 400 mcg/dL, low serum iron < 30 mcg/dL; transferrin saturation < 15%; MCV < 80 mcg/dL; reticulocyte count elevated in cases of blood loss, decreased in iron deficiency; increased platelet count > 400,000; bone marrow absent for iron staining

▶ Bone marrow aspiration if severe, questionable diagnosis, or resistant to treatment

TABLE 16–3
COMPARISON OF DIFFERENTIAL LABORATORY FINDINGS IN MICROCYTIC ANEMIAS

LABORATORY FINDING	THALASSEMIA TRAIT	LEAD POISONING	IRON DEFICIENCY	ANEMIA OF CHRONIC DISEASE
Hgb	Decreased	Decreased	Decreased	Decreased
MCV	Decreased	Decreased	Decreased	Normal
Ferritin	Normal	Normal	Decreased	Increased
FEP (free erythrocyte porphyrins)	Normal	Very High	High	Mild Increase

Differential Diagnosis

▶ Thalassemia

▶ G6PD deficiency

▶ Infection

▶ Cancer

▶ Chronic diseases

▶ Lead poisoning

▶ Hypothyroidism

▶ Renal failure

Management

Nonpharmacologic Treatment

▶ Diagnose and treat underlying cause.

▶ Normal dietary intake meets only daily losses, not therapeutic; RDA iron = 10 mg/day for men and up to15 mg/day for women and children; must increase iron intake

▶ No dairy product or antacid within 2 hours of oral iron

▶ Symptomatic care of treatment side effects (constipation, nausea, cramps, diarrhea)

Pharmacologic Treatment

▶ Oral iron supplements: Up to 300 mg of elemental iron divided 3–4 times a day for adolescents and adults

  ▹ 325 mg of ferrous sulfate contains 65 mg of elemental iron.

  ▹ Liquid preparation 2–3 mg/kg/day for children

  ▹ Oral iron therapy is safer and less costly than IM or IV iron.

  ▹ Reduce dose to decrease GI side effects; no real benefit to more expensive preparations

  ▹ Vitamin C will help increase absorption; meals will decrease absorption by up to 50%.

▶ Parenteral iron if poor absorption or inability to tolerate oral iron

▶ Blood transfusion is not recommended for iron supplementation.

How Long to Treat

▶ Until deficiency corrected; expect to see improvement within 4 weeks; return to baseline blood levels in 8 weeks; continue therapy 3–6 months to replace iron stores

Special Considerations

▶ If unresponsive to therapy, reevaluate underlying cause and compliance.

When to Consult, Refer, Hospitalize

▶ Refer to hematologist if patient is not responsive to treatment or underlying cause cannot be determined.

Follow-up

▶ Recommended after 1 month and every 6 months if stable until resolved

Expected Course

▶ Cure expected; increase in Hgb of 1 g/week expected

▶ Prolonged course of treatment may be required because of noncompliance

Complications

▶ May have unidentified underlying source of bleeding

▶ Growth delay, learning difficulty, heart failure (late, untreated)

MEGALOBLASTIC ANEMIAS

VITAMIN B$_{12}$ DEFICIENCY

Description

▶ A megaloblastic anemia in which MCV is > 100 resulting from a deficiency of intrinsic factor, which leads to inadequate vitamin B$_{12}$ absorption (< 200 picograms/mL) and impaired red blood cell synthesis

Etiology

▶ Pernicious anemia: Caused by congenital enzyme deficiency so B$_{12}$ cannot be absorbed; overgrowth of intestinal organisms, autoimmune reaction involving gastric parietal cells, gastrectomy

▶ Malabsorption: GI parasites, GI surgery, Crohn's, chronic alcoholism, strict vegetarians (rare)

▶ Older adult stomach is less acidic, B$_{12}$ needs acid to be absorbed

Incidence and Demographics

▶ Onset at age 50–60; median age at diagnosis = 60

▶ Women slightly > men

Risk Factors

▶ Age (commonly presents around age 60), family history of pernicious anemia

▶ Chronic alcoholism

▶ GI surgery, Crohn's disease, immunologic diseases

Prevention and Screening

▶ Adequate dietary intake: Meat and dairy products

▶ Routine screening for B$_{12}$ level in dementia and malnutrition

Assessment

History

▶ Insidious onset of peripheral numbness, personality changes, memory loss, anorexia, diarrhea, glossitis, distal paresthesias, ataxia

▶ Assess for risk factors, underlying causes

▶ Should be considered in differential diagnosis of dementia

Physical Exam

▶ Characteristic beefy-red, shiny tongue

▶ Abdominal tenderness, organomegaly, tachycardia, tachypnea, pallor, hepatosplenomegaly

▶ Neurologic signs: Numbness, sensory ataxia, limb weakness, spasticity, changes in deep tendon reflexes, decreased vibratory sense, impaired proprioception, impaired fine motor movement, positive Romberg test, progressive mental status impairment

Diagnostic Studies

▶ CBC with differential, peripheral smear, LDH, serum folate, and serum B_{12} levels; consider Schilling test with and without intrinsic factor to test B_{12} absorption; consider bone marrow aspiration

▶ Laboratory results: Serum B_{12} levels < 200 picograms/mL; Hct decreased; MCV markedly elevated; decreased reticulocyte count; WBC and platelet count reduced, elevated LDH

▶ On smear: A large, nucleated, embryonic type of cell that is a precursor of erythrocytes in an abnormal erythropoietic process

▶ Schilling's test documents decreased oral B_{12} absorption.

Differential Diagnosis

▶ Folic acid deficiency

▶ Myelodysplasia

▶ Liver dysfunction

▶ Side effects of medications

▶ Alcoholism

▶ Bleeding or hemorrhage

▶ Hypothyroidism

Management

Nonpharmacologic Treatment

▶ Education and supportive therapy; maintain balanced diet, good health and hygiene

Pharmacologic Treatment

▶ Initial: 800–1,000 mcg of vitamin B_{12} IM daily for 4–8 weeks

▶ Maintenance: 100–1,000 mcg monthly

▶ Oral cobalamin (vitamin B_{12}) 1,000 mcg daily is alternative replacement

▶ May require iron supplementation for the first month of therapy during rapid regeneration of RBCs

How Long to Treat

▶ Lifelong

Special Considerations

▶ If patient presents with abnormal neurologic signs, the symptoms might be irreversible.

▶ Might have hypokalemia in first week of treatment

▶ Do not begin treatment for B_{12} deficiency without also assessing for and treating folate deficiency.

▶ Check serum B_{12} levels in patients with distal polyneuropathies (even if no anemia or macrocytosis seen).

▶ Oral B-complex vitamin only valuable when B_{12} deficiency is nutritional

When to Consult, Refer, Hospitalize

▶ Refer as needed for underlying cause; refer for follow-up endoscopy q 5 years to rule out malignancy.

Follow-up

Expected Course

▶ Response rapid; good prognosis if treatment within 6 months of neurologic signs

Complications

▶ Stomach cancer

▶ Permanent central nervous system (CNS) signs/symptoms

FOLIC ACID DEFICIENCY

Description

▶ Anemia as a result of inadequate folic acid present for DNA synthesis and RBC maturation. Lack of folic acid (folate) causes macrocytic, normochromic, and megaloblastic anemia.

▶ Also associated with increased incidence of embryonic neural tube defects

Etiology

▶ Folic acid–deficient diet, malabsorption syndromes, or increased demand for folic acid (pregnancy)

Incidence and Demographics

▶ All races and age groups

▶ Most common at ages 60–70 years

Risk Factors

▶ Pregnancy, older adults, alcoholics

▶ Malnourished or malabsorption syndromes; hemodialysis patients

▶ Medications that interfere with folic acid absorption (e.g., trimethoprim, phenytoin, oral birth control pills, phenobarbital, sulfamethoxazole/trimethoprim, sulfasalazine)

Prevention and Screening

▶ Adequate intake of folic acid: 400 mcg for pregnant women, 400 mcg for all others

Assessment

History

▶ Indigestion, constipation, diarrhea, anorexia, lethargy

▶ Fatigue, weakness, headache, dizziness, dyspnea on exertion, depression, apathy

Physical Exam

▶ Pallor, atrophic glossitis (red, shiny tongue), stomatitis

▶ Change in mental status, confusion but no focal neurologic deficits

▶ Tachycardia, wide pulse pressure, heart murmur

▶ Peripheral neuropathy

Diagnostic Studies

▶ CBC, RBC folate more reliable for diagnosis than serum folate; serum B_{12}, TIBC, LDH, RDW

▶ Laboratory results: Serum folate < 3 nanograms/mL, RBC folate < 150 nanograms/mL, Hct decreased, Hgb normal, RDW elevated, TIBC normal, LDH and MCV elevated > 100 mcg/mL; MCHC normal, Schilling test normal, serum B_{12} normal

Differential Diagnosis

▶ Vitamin B_{12} deficiency

▶ Pernicious anemia

▶ Myelodysplastic syndromes

▶ Hypothyroidism

Management

Nonpharmacologic Treatment

▶ Education and supportive therapy; good oral hygiene

▶ Folate-rich diet: Green leafy vegetables, red beans, wheat bran, fish, bananas, asparagus

▶ Need for frequent rest

Pharmacologic Treatment

▶ Folic acid replacement 400 mcg for pregnant women, 200 mcg for all others

  » Prescription supplements usually contain 1 mg folic acid, but be aware that supplementation of greater than 400 mcg may mask B_{12} deficiency.

How Long to Treat

▶ Until anemia corrected, usually about 2 months until folic acid stores replenished

▶ Depends on elimination of underlying cause

Special Considerations

▶ Folate body stores can be depleted in about 4 months.

▶ Women on birth control who are potentially child-bearing should routinely take folic acid preparations to decrease incidence of embryonic neural tube defects.

When to Consult, Refer, Hospitalize

▶ Not usually needed; refer patients who do not improve with therapy.

Follow-up

▶ In 2 months and periodically thereafter

Expected Course

▶ Good prognosis

Complications

▶ Failure to thrive

▶ Neural tube defects of infants born to deficient women

HEMOLYTIC ANEMIAS

Description

Hemolytic conditions produce anemias in which accelerated RBC destruction occurs as a result of an intrinsic genetic RBC defect as seen in hemoglobinopathies (sickle cell and thalassemia), metabolic enzyme deficiencies (G6PD), or cytoskeleton disorders (spherocytosis or elliptocytosis). The intrinsic destruction could also be acquired as seen in paroxysmal nocturnal hemoglobinuria or alcoholic cirrhosis. Extrinsic causes of hemolysis include antibody-mediated processes such as autoimmune reactions, drug-related reactions, transfusion reactions, and reactions to infections.

Important Features

▶ Peripheral blood smear shows spherocytosis and may be hyperchromic.

▶ Coombs test will be positive in immune hemolysis.

▶ An elevated reticulocyte count in the patient with anemia is the most useful indicator of hemolysis.

▶ Other laboratory findings include increased unconjugated bilirubin (indirect), decreased heptoglobin, possible increase in LDH, increased urine hemoglobin, or increased urine bilirubin. Hemosiderin is a delayed sign and may represent chronic hemolysis.

▶ Bone marrow shows normoblastic erythroid hyperplasia.

SICKLE CELL ANEMIA AND TRAIT

Description

▶ Sickle cell disease (SSD) is a group of hemoglobin disorders characterized by production of hemoglobin S (HbS); the most common of which is sickle cell anemia (HbSS). Other common genotypes are sickle-cell C (HbSC) and sickle beta thalassemia (HbS beta thalassemia). Severe hemolytic anemia may be produced in which abnormal hemoglobin (due to DNA point mutation in the B-globin chain) leads to chronic hemolytic anemia, with recurrent painful crises in individuals who are homozygous for hemoglobin S.

▶ Sickle cell disorders are characterized by chronic hemolytic anemia.

Etiology

▶ Hemoglobin S readily deforms the RBC into a sickle shape, the sickle cells hemolyze, and clusters of sickle cells occlude small blood vessels.

▶ Autosomal recessive gene (hemoglobin S gene from each parent)

▶ Sickle cell trait (Hgb AS) is seen when one normal Hgb gene and one sickle hemoglobin–producing gene are inherited from the parents; this will not cause sickle cell disease.

Incidence and Demographics

▶ Present in about 1 in 400–500 Blacks; 8%–10% of Blacks carry hemoglobin S gene

▶ No gender predominance; onset in first year of life

Risk Factors

▶ Precipitate sickle cell crisis

    » Deoxygenation of Hgb molecule, as in high altitude

    » Infection

    » Dehydration

    » Overexertion, stress

    » Exposure to extreme temperatures, hot or cold

Prevention and Screening

▶ Screening for sickle cell trait and genetic counseling for couples at risk; prenatal diagnosis via chorionic villus sampling or amniocentesis

▶ Universal newborn screening

▶ Good health maintenance with anticipatory guidance for potential complications

▶ All regular immunizations, as well as pneumococcal and influenza (yearly) vaccinations

▶ Recognition and avoidance of known pain-precipitating factors

Assessment

History

▶ Hemolytic anemia starting in first year of life

▶ Family history of sickle cell anemia or trait

▶ Trait may be asymptomatic unless provoked by exertion at high altitudes or dehydration

▶ Sickle cell anemia: Acute, sudden, excruciating episodes with pain in long bones, back, chest, abdomen; priapism; chronic leg ulcers; delayed puberty

Physical Exam

▶ May include chronically ill appearance, jaundice

▶ Splenomegaly (primarily in children)

▶ Hot, tender, swollen joints

▶ Retinopathy

▶ Cardiomegaly (laterally displaced point of maximum impulse [PMI]), systolic murmur

▶ Chronic lower leg ulcers, blood loss

Diagnostic Studies

▶ Hgb electrophoresis: Definitive diagnostic test

▶ CBC: Classic findings (by age 1 year) include Hct in the 20s, reticulocyte count in the 20s, normal MCV, slightly elevated WBC count, and elevated platelet count.

▶ Peripheral blood smear: Fragmented cells, long crescent-shaped irreversible sickled cells, target cells, Howell-Jolly bodies, and occasional nucleated red blood cells

▶ Elevated LDH and indirect bilirubin during increased hemolysis

▶ Laboratory results: Hgb decreased, MCV might be elevated slightly, chronic neutrophilia, increased platelet count, erythrocytes with classic sickle shape on peripheral smear, Hgb S predominates

Differential Diagnosis

▶ Other hemoglobinopathies (e.g., hemoglobin C, D, or E)

▶ Compound hemoglobinopathies (e.g., hemoglobin SC disease, hemoglobin S beta thalassemia)

Management

Nonpharmacologic Treatment

▶ Hydration, nonpharmacologic pain modalities, patient and family education and supportive care, genetic counseling

Pharmacologic Treatment

▶ Do not give iron (increases Hgb S production).

▶ Manage pain (often narcotic analgesia will be needed).

▶ Folic acid 1 to 2 mg p.o. daily

▶ Oxygen for hypoxia

▶ Consider transfusion.

▶ Pencillin prophalaxis in childhood

How Long to Treat

▶ Lifelong

Special Considerations

▶ In some patients, hydroxyurea 500–750 mg daily may decrease number of painful crises (long-term safety unknown).

▶ Individuals have different patterns of crisis.

▶ Crises might increase during pregnancy.

When to Consult, Refer, Hospitalize

▶ Refer all suspected cases to a hematologist; hospitalize for acute episodes of sickling.

▶ Consult with physician for specialized care in the primary care setting.

▶ Any temperature of > 38.5° C (101.3° F) must be considered a medical emergency and hospitalized immediately.

Follow-up

Expected Course

▶ Number of crises decrease in young adulthood but complications increase.

▶ Life expectancy is 60 years.

Complications

▶ Anemia, bone infarct, cerebrovascular accident (CVA), cardiac enlargement, priapism, retinopathy, acute chest syndrome, infections, gallstones, hemosiderosis (secondary to multiple transfusions), increased fetal loss during pregnancy, sepsis

THALASSEMIA

Description

▶ A group of hereditary disorders with hypochromic microcytic anemia because of gene deletion or point mutation; causes abnormal synthesis of alpha and beta globin chains, resulting in abnormal hemoglobin synthesis and displacement of hemoglobin A1 with abnormal types—microcytosis is out of proportion to the degree of anemia

Etiology

▶ Autosomal recessive genetic disorder producing defective hemoglobinization of red blood cells. Normal adult hemoglobin, Hgb A, has 4 chains or globins, 2 alpha and 2 beta. Delta and gamma chains are similar to beta and are found in Hemoglobin A2 (2 gamma, 2 delta chains), and Hemoglobin F (fetal Hgb, 2 delta and 2 gamma chains). Hemoglobin cannot be formed without the α chains; unaffected individuals have 4 copies of gene for α globin.

▶ Alpha thalassemia is a result of a gene deletion with the result that not enough alpha chains can be synthesized.

▶ Beta thalassemia results when point mutation causes decreased or no synthesis of beta chains.

▶ Thalassemia major (beta) occurs when unbalanced hemoglobin chain synthesis results in severe anemia (usually presents in infants or young children).

▶ Thalassemia intermedia is a more minor form of beta thalassemia; may or may not need transfusions.

▶ Thalassemia trait (alpha or beta) is a milder form of anemia, not requiring aggressive therapy.

Incidence and Demographics

▶ Alpha thalassemia: People originating from Southeast Asia, China, occasionally Africa

▶ Beta thalassemia: People originating from the Mediterranean; less commonly, Asia and Africa; about 1,000 patients with severe thalassemia in the United States

▶ Trait present in 3%–5% of at-risk populations

Risk Factors

▶ One or both parents with any combination of alpha or beta thalassemia syndromes

Prevention and Screening

▶ Screening of prospective parents at risk (ideally before pregnancy), genetic counseling

▶ Prenatal diagnosis (fetal blood sampling or chorionic villus sampling) if desired

Assessment

History

▶ Alpha trait (one of four alpha genes affected) usually asymptomatic; alpha thalassemia minor (two of four alpha genes affected) and beta thalassemia (heterozygous form) are mild forms, usually asymptomatic; beta thalassemia major (Cooley's anemia—both genes affected): easy fatigueability, palpitations, shortness of breath with exertion, headaches

▶ Family or personal history of lifelong anemia

▶ Infants and children with thalassemia major will have symptoms of severe and chronic anemia: pallor, shortness of breath, and lethargy.

▶ Children and adults with thalassemia trait may present with history of unresponsive anemia or signs of iron toxicity.

Physical Exam

▶ Normal exam in thalassemia minor syndromes

▶ Pallor and enlarged spleen in alpha thalassemia with 1 alpha globin gene (also called hemoglobin H disease)

▶ Multiple abnormalities in thalassemia major (homozygous beta thalassemia) starting in infancy: bony deformities, jaundice, enlarged spleen, and enlarged liver

Diagnostic Studies

▶ See Table 16–4.

▶ CBC with attention to RBC morphology and hemoglobin electrophoresis, iron studies

▶ Laboratory results: Microcytic, hypochromic, acanthocytes, target cells, serum iron and TIBC normal to increased, serum ferritin > 100

Differential Diagnosis

▶ Iron deficiency anemia

▶ Combined hemoglobinopathies

Management

▶ No treatment needed for beta thalassemia minor or alpha thalassemia trait

Nonpharmacologic Treatment

▶ Severe thalassemia major: Regular transfusions; bone marrow transplants in children; splenectomy if needed; patient and family education and supportive care

Pharmacologic Treatment

▶ Folic acid supplementation

▶ Iron chelation therapy with deferoxamine (Desferal)

▶ Appropriate immunizations (especially if splenectomy contemplated)

▶ Avoid iron supplements and iron-fortified foods; avoid oxidative drugs (e.g., sulfonamides)

TABLE 16-4
DIAGNOSTIC STUDIES USED IN THALASSEMIA

DIAGNOSTIC STUDIES	FINDINGS
Alpha Thalassemia Trait	Hematocrit 28%–40% Very low MCV (60–75 mcg/mL) Reticulocyte count normal Iron parameters normal Mild anemia; significant microcytosis
Alpha Thalassemia Minor and Beta Thalassemia Minor	Hematocrit 28%–40% MCV 55–75 mcg/mL Reticulocyte count normal or slightly elevated Iron parameters normal Hemoglobin electrophoresis shows elevation HgB A2 to 4%–8% and occasional Hgb F to 1%–5%
Beta Thalassemia Major	Hematocrit 10% MCV < 75 mcg/mL Peripheral blood smear: Severe poikilocytoses, hypochromia, basophilic stippling, and nucleated red blood cells; virtually no Hgb A present; major hemoglobin present in Hgb F
Hemoglobin H Disease	Hematocrit 22%–32% MCV < 7 mcg/mL Peripheral blood smear markedly abnormal: Hypochromia, microcytosis, poikilocytosis Reticulocyte count elevated Hemoglobin electrophoresis shows HgbH as 10%–40% of Hgb

How Long to Treat

▶ Lifelong

Special Considerations

▶ Support for family; coping with guilt is a major problem for parents

When to Consult, Refer, Hospitalize

▶ Consult or refer when diagnosis is in question; refer all patients with thalassemia major or intermedia to hematologist, hospitalize for complications. Refer all patients with severe disease to specialty clinics experienced in iron chelation and transfusions.

Follow-up

▶ Depends on severity of disease

Expected Course

▶ Thalassemia minor: Benign

▶ Thalassemia intermedia: Patients have chronic hemolytic anemia but will generally only need transfusions when under stress; live into adulthood.

▶ Children with thalassemia major die in their teens or even younger unless they receive regular transfusions and iron chelation therapy; with compliance, live well into adulthood.

Complications

▶ Limited growth and bony deformities; iron overload (due to frequent transfusions), which can cause cirrhosis, diabetes, cardiac dysfunction (including arrhythmia); failure of sexual maturation; decreased life expectancy

GLUCOSE-6-PHOSPHATE DEHYDROGENASE (G6PD) DEFICIENCY

Description

▶ An anemia of red blood cell destruction (hemolysis), occurring suddenly and episodically when red blood cells are under oxidative stress from acute illness or certain medications

Etiology

▶ Most common form of G6PD deficiency is an X-linked, recessive hereditary enzyme defect.

▶ Lack of enzyme leaves RBCs vulnerable to attack, causing hemolysis

▶ Can result in neonatal hyperbilirubinemia

Incidence and Demographics

▶ Seen in Blacks and people of Mediterranean descent

▶ 7%–15% of Black males affected

▶ Mediterranean variant less common but poses more severe deficiency of G6PD

Risk Factors

▶ Episode of hemolysis may be provoked by infection; oxidant drugs, such as certain antibiotics (e.g., dapsone, nalidixic acid, nitrofurantoin, sulfonamides), antimalarials (e.g., primaquine, quinine), phenazopyridine, doxorubicin, quinidine, and others; ingestion of fava beans; see Box 16–1

Prevention and Screening

▶ Immunizations (influenza, pneumococcal pneumonia, hepatitis B) and measures to avoid infections

▶ Avoidance of known oxidant drugs

▶ Family and genetic counseling as indicated

▶ Avoidance of specific drugs listed in Box 16–1, stress, and fava beans

---

BOX 16-1
SUBSTANCES FOR PEOPLE WITH G6PD DEFICIENCY TO AVOID

Analgesics	**Antimalarials**	**Other**
Aspirin	Primaquine	Vitamin K (OK in the newborn)
Phenacetin	Chloroquine	Probenecid
	Quinacrine	Dimercaprol (BAL)
	Pamaquine	Fava beans
		Mothballs (naphthalene)
		Methylene blue
		Henna

Antibiotics	**Antihelminths**	**Illness**
Sulfonamides	B naphthol	Diabetic ketoacidosis
Chloramphenicol	Stibophen	Hepatitis
Dapsone	Niridazole	Other
Nitrofurans (Macrodantin)		
Nalidixic acid		

Assessment

History

▶ Family history, medication history for oxidative drugs

▶ May be no history of anemia or anemia is mild so patient may only be symptomatic of underlying infection

Physical Exam

▶ Signs of mild anemia, signs of underlying infection

▶ Splenomegaly may be present.

Diagnostic Studies

▶ CBC, reticulocytes, indirect bilirubin, G6PD

▶ In infants, direct and indirect Coombs test should be done to exclude autoimmune hemolytic anemia.

▶ Usual laboratory results: CBC normal between episodes, along with Heinz bodies and low level of G6PD; during episodes of hemolysis, there are increased reticulocytes, increased indirect bilirubin, decreased RBC, decreased Hgb, decreased Hct

Differential Diagnosis

▶ Suspect Mediterranean variant if anemia is severe

▶ Iron deficiency anemia

▶ Combined anemias (e.g., G6PD deficiency and sickle cell anemia)

▶ Acute hemolytic transfusion reactions (Coombs +)

Management

▶ Supportive

▶ Find and eliminate anemia trigger.

Special Considerations

▶ Anemic episodes are self-limiting.

When to Consult, Refer, Hospitalize

▶ Refer severe variants with exacerbations; refer patients with combined anemias.

Follow-up

▶ For exacerbations

Expected Course

▶ There is usually a spontaneous resolution of the anemia as older RBCs with minimal enzyme activity are destroyed and then replaced with new RBCs that have enough (even though reduced) enzyme activity.

Complications

▶ Generally none

▶ Possible severe hemolytic anemia and death with the Mediterranean variant

IMMUNE HEMOLYSIS

Description

▶ Red cell destruction occurs as a result of the binding of antibodies or complement components to the erythrocyte membrane. This may occur as a result of autoimmunization, alloimmunization, or drug reactions.

▶ Warm-reacting antibodies hemolyze optimally at 37° C.

▶ Cold-reacting antibodies hemolyze optimally at 30° C.

Etiology

▶ IgM (cold) and IgG (warm) antibodies induce red cell destruction after binding with antigens on the RBC wall. This binding causes a complementary cascade resulting in defective RBCs, which are prematurely removed and destroyed by hepatic macrophages.

Incidence and Demographics

▶ Seen in all races and in all age groups

▶ Warm agglutinin disease associated with neoplastic or collagen vascular disorder in 40% of the cases

► Cold agglutinin disease seen in patients with lymphoproliferative disorders, infectious diseases (Epstein-Barr virus [EBV], cytomegalovirus [CMV]), and in older adults; usually a diagnosis of exclusion

Risk Factors

► Systemic lupus erythematosus, rheumatoid arthritis

► Adenocarcinoma of the stomach, ovarian teratoma, chronic lymphocytic leukemia

Prevention and Screening

► Screening of prospective parents at risk (ideally before pregnancy), genetic counseling

Assessment

History

► Family or personal history of any of the above states

► Acute episodes may present with dizziness, exertional dyspnea, palpitations, and fatigue.

Physical Exam

► In warm agglutinin disease, chronic effects are mild and may present with jaundice or splenomegaly; acute episodes may present with pallor in addition to above symptoms.

► In cold agglutinin disease secondary to infections, symptoms are short-lived and mild in most cases. In disease associated with neoplastic or idiopathic disorders, exposure to cold may lead to severe acrocyanosis and Raynaud's-type reactions worsened by cold.

Diagnostic Studies

► CBC with attention to RBC morphology; spherocytosis dramatically increased

► In cold agglutinin disease, blood clots at times upon being removed from the vein, distorting the red cell count, MCV, and hematocrit. The serum haptoglobin is decreased and LDH is increased.

Differential Diagnosis

► Thalassemia

► Sickle cell disease

► Paroxysmal nocturnal hemoglobinuria

► Hypersplenism

Management

► Warm agglutinin disease

  » Glucocorticoids

  » Splenectomy

  » Immunosuppressive drugs: Cyclophosphamide, azathioprine

  » Transfusion

▶ Cold agglutinin disease

   » Identify underlying cause.

   » Chlorambucil (Leukeran) 2–4 mg, up to 10 mg daily

   » Advise move to a warmer climate

   » Avoid transfusions; when needed, infuse warmed, well-matched products.

Special Considerations

▶ None

When to Consult, Refer, Hospitalize

▶ Consult with physician or refer to hematologist for acute episodes.

Follow-Up

Expected Course

▶ Warm agglutinin disease is usually chronic, so prognosis affected by the underlying disease.

▶ If cold agglutinin disease is related to an infectious syndrome, complete cure occurs when the infection is cleared.

▶ Otherwise, course is similar to warm agglutinin disease.

Complications

▶ Major cause of death related to a thromboembolic event

OTHER PROBLEMS OF IRON AND RED BLOOD CELLS

HEMOCHROMATOSIS

Description

▶ An autosomal recessive inherited disorder, resulting in an excess of iron stores in the liver, pancreas, heart, kidneys, adrenals, testes, and pituitary gland as hemosiderin

Etiology

▶ Disorder resulting in inefficient erythropoiesis

▶ Most common iron storage and genetic liver disease in the U.S.

Incidence and Demographics

▶ 3/1,000 in the U.S.

▶ Seen in men more than in women

▶ Presentation during middle years

Risk Factors

▶ Alcohol ingestion, iron supplementation, chronic transfusions, ingestion of large amounts of vitamin C

▶ Type 2 diabetes, beta thalassemia

Prevention and Screening

▶ Genetic counseling

▶ Screening of family members of patient with hereditary hemochromatosis

Assessment

History

▶ Often asymptomatic

▶ Weakness, dyspnea on exertion, lassitude, weight loss

▶ Loss of libido, impotence, testicular atrophy, amenorrhea

▶ Slate- or brown-colored skin, alopecia

▶ Abdominal pain

Physical Exam

▶ Hepatosplenomegaly, ascites, cardiomyopathy, peripheral edema, arthropathy

▶ Changes in skin pigmentation: Slate-gray or brown

Diagnostic Studies

▶ Liver biopsy is the diagnostic gold standard.

▶ Laboratory results: Blood glucose elevated, AST increased, serum albumin decreased, FSH and LH decreased, serum ferritin > 300 units/L for men and > 120 units/L for women, transferrin saturation high, urinary iron present

Differential Diagnosis

▶ Cirrhosis   ▶ Excessive iron ingestion   ▶ Repeated transfusions

Management

Nonpharmacologic Treatment

▶ Regular diet; avoid iron-fortified foods and iron supplements, increase tea intake (chelates iron), restrict vitamin C to small amounts between meals

▶ Phlebotomy of 500 mL initially 1–2×/week until mild anemia, then 4–6×/year maintenance

Pharmacologic Treatment

▶ Use iron-chelating agent only if phlebotomy is not feasible or diagnosis is secondary hematochromatosis.

How Long to Treat

▶ Initially until patient is iron-deficient (mild anemia), then lifelong maintenance therapy

Special Considerations

▶ Menstruation delays onset of symptoms in women.

▶ Problem uncommon in people with African or Asian heritage

When to Consult, Refer, Hospitalize

▶ Refer to hematologist to confirm initial diagnosis and consult throughout therapy; hematology office or infusion center for phlebotomy.

Follow-up

Expected Course

▶ Usually normal life expectancy; if more than 18 months needed to achieve mild anemia, life expectancy is decreased

Complications

▶ Cirrhosis, type 1 diabetes, hepatocellular carcinoma, arthritis, cardiomyopathy

POLYCYTHEMIA VERA

Description

▶ Chronic, acquired myeloproliferative disorder showing overproduction of red blood cell mass, resulting in an elevation in hematocrit and red blood cell mass (males Hct > 51%, females Hct > 48%)

Etiology

▶ As a primary disorder, is a hematologic malignancy with excessive erythroid, myeloid, and megakaryocytic elements in the bone marrow

▶ Secondary causes are lung disease, heart disease, kidney disease, and possible other malignancies.

Incidence and Demographics

▶ Prevalence = 1–3/100,000

▶ Most common in newborn or age > 60

Risk Factors

▶ More prevalent in people of Ashkenazi Jewish ancestry

▶ Smoking

▶ Age > 60 years

Prevention and Screening

▶ Cannot prevent onset

▶ No routine screening currently recommended

▶ Often found as a result of blood studies performed for other reasons

▶ Advise patients to seek medical attention for onset of headache; dizziness; blurred vision; tinnitus; vertigo; spontaneous bruising; menorrhagia; peripheral cyanosis; epistaxis; upper GI bleed; pruritus, especially after bathing; rib and sternal bone pain or tenderness; sweating; weight loss; fatigue.

Assessment

History

▶ Might be no symptoms in early stages or only vague symptoms

▶ Headache, dizziness, blurred vision, tinnitus, vertigo

▶ Spontaneous bruising, menorrhagia, peripheral cyanosis, epistaxis, upper GI bleed

▶ Pruritus, especially after bathing

▶ Rib and sternal bone pain or tenderness

▶ Sweating, weight loss, fatigue

Physical Exam

▶ Plethora (reddish flush of skin) on face, hands, feet

▶ Elevated systolic blood pressure, epistaxis, distended retinal veins

▶ Hepatosplenomegaly

▶ Complete exam to look for underlying cause

Diagnostic Studies

▶ CBC with differential, serum B_{12}, chemistries, indirect bilirubin, bone marrow aspiration, CT for underlying malignancy

▶ Laboratory results: Increased Hgb and Hct, thrombocytosis, leukocytosis, increased leukocyte alkaline phosphatase, increased serum vitamin B_{12}, indirect bilirubin elevated

Differential Diagnosis

▶ Secondary polycythemia

▶ Secondary erythrocytosis

▶ Spurious polycythemia

▶ Hemoglobinopathy

Management

Nonpharmacologic Treatment

▶ Phlebotomy to remove 500 cc weekly until hematocrit 45%; patient and family education and support

Pharmacologic Treatment

▶ Medications for hyperacidity, pruritus, uric acid reduction as needed

▶ Hydroxyurea — a myelosuppressive agent — may be used.

How Long to Treat

▶ Lifelong

Special Considerations

▶ Phlebotomy worsens iron deficiency, but iron supplement not recommended

▶ Benign polycythemia caused by high-altitude dwelling

When to Consult, Refer, Hospitalize

▶ Refer to hematologist for management.

Follow-up

Expected Course

▶ Survival with treatment = up to 10 years; without = 6–18 months

Complications

▶ Vascular thrombosis, leukemia, hemorrhage, peptic ulcer, gout

WHITE BLOOD CELL (WBC)–RELATED PROBLEMS

LEUKEMIAS

Description

▶ A collection of disorders that produce a variety of bone marrow and white blood cell abnormalities that may be quickly fatal or may remain asymptomatic for years

▶ Types include:

    ▹ Malignant proliferation of immature lymphocytes (acute lymphocytic leukemia: ALL) or myeloid cells (acute myeloid leukemia: AML; acute nonlymphocytic leukemia: ANLL)

» Proliferation of mature-appearing neoplastic lymphocytes (chronic lymphocytic leukemia: CLL) or immature granulocytes (chronic myeloid leukemia: CML)

» Rarely: Proliferation of mature B cells with prominent projections (hairy cell leukemia)

Etiology

▶ Unknown malignancy that affects the bone marrow and other organs; may be due to exposure to chemicals or ionizing radiation, genetic factors (chromosomal abnormalities), viral agents

▶ Commonly see elevated WBC, abnormal WBCs on blood smear, bone marrow failure, and involvement of other organs

Incidence and Demographics

▶ ALL: Most common childhood malignancy with peak incidence at 4 years of age, most common in Whites and boys, higher incidence in industrialized countries; adult ALL approximately 100 cases/year in U.S.

▶ AML or ANLL: 50% of cases under age 50

▶ CLL: Most common form of adult leukemia in Western countries, occurring during middle age and in older adults

▶ CML: Middle age

▶ Hairy cell leukemia: Rare, disease of old age

Risk Factors

▶ Several immunodeficiency states have an associated risk for lymphoma and leukemia in children (Wiskott-Aldrich, X-linked agammaglobulinemia, severe combined immune deficiency, and ataxia telangiectasia).

▶ Chemical or radiation exposure

▶ Chromosomal abnormalities

▶ Cigarette smoking

▶ Some types increase with age.

Prevention and Screening

▶ Currently there is no standard screening process to detect early stages of leukemia.

▶ There is no way to prevent leukemia, but an individual can make lifestyle changes to lower risk.

▶ Educate patients to report new onset of symptoms early.

▶ Patients with family histories of leukemia should have regular physical examinations.

▶ Patients who have been treated with chemotherapy for other types of cancers should have regular physical examinations.

▶ Avoid exposure to chemicals such as benzene.

▶ Quit smoking or don't start.

Assessment

History

- ▶ General: Fever, malaise, weakness, bruising, bleeding, weight loss
- ▶ ALL: Joint pain, limping, anorexia, infection
- ▶ AML: Sternal tenderness
- ▶ CLL: Might be asymptomatic; dyspnea on exertion
- ▶ CML: Might be asymptomatic; night sweats, blurred vision, anorexia, respiratory distress, sternal tenderness

Physical Exam

- ▶ Lymphadenopathy, confirmation of symptoms
- ▶ ALL: Generalized lymphadenopathy, hepatosplenomegaly, petechiae, purpura
- ▶ AML: Mouth sores, occasional lymphadenopathy
- ▶ CLL: Hepatosplenomegaly, lymphadenopathy, sustained absolute lymphocytosis, bone marrow + lymphocytes
- ▶ CML: Splenomegaly, priapism, Philadelphia chromosome in bone marrow

Diagnostic Studies

- ▶ CBC with differential and platelet, peripheral smear, chemistries, reticulocyte count, bone marrow aspiration
- ▶ Laboratory results: Decreased RBC, neutrophils, platelets, reticulocyte count; elevated LDH and uric acid
- ▶ Consider chest X-ray, ultrasound or CT scan, coagulation profile
- ▶ ALL: Peripheral blood lymphoblasts
- ▶ CLL: Sustained absolute lymphocytosis, bone marrow + lymphocytes
- ▶ CML: Philadelphia chromosome in bone marrow

Differential Diagnosis

- ▶ Aplastic anemia
- ▶ Viral diseases
- ▶ Mononucleosis
- ▶ Pertussis
- ▶ Paroxysmal nocturnal hemoglobinuria
- ▶ Gaucher's disease
- ▶ Myelodysplasia syndromes

Management

Nonpharmacologic Treatment

- ▶ Good diet, compliance with treatment, management of side effects, chronic effects of diagnosis
- ▶ Avoid activities that might cause injury; avoid medications that affect platelets (e.g., aspirin).
- ▶ Bone marrow transplantation

Pharmacologic Treatment

▶ Chemotherapy, infection prevention medications

▶ Hospitalization required for induction of chemotherapy

▶ Interferon treatment for CML

How Long to Treat

▶ Goal is remission

Special Considerations

▶ Children with ALL may benefit from referral to specialty centers involved in clinical trials.

▶ Patients with leukemia are prone to other infections.

When to Consult, Refer, Hospitalize

▶ Refer to hematologist upon suspicion of diagnosis and have followed by hematologist throughout therapy.

Follow-up

Expected Course

▶ ALL: Remission rate is very good.

▶ AML: Remission rate is 60%–80%.

▶ CLL: Depends on stage at diagnosis; median survival is about 9 years.

▶ CML: Usually transforms into the acute phase within 2 years, then poor survival rate

▶ Patients who have undergone stem cell transplantation have a 10-year survival rate of 70%.

Complications

▶ Infections, bleeding, side effects of chemotherapy and radiation, relapses

COAGULATION DISORDERS

IDIOPATHIC THROMBOCYTOPENIA PURPURA (ITP)

Description

▶ An autoimmune disorder characterized by accelerated, spleen-mediated platelet destruction, resulting in a decreased platelet count (< 100,000/mL) that predisposes the patient to a decreased ability for primary clotting. May be acute (with spontaneous resolution within 2 months after an acute infection—usually children) or chronic (persists ≥ 6 months without identifiable cause—usually adults). IgG autoantibody binds to platelets, splenic macrophages bind to antibody-tagged platelets and destroy them.

Etiology

▶ Unknown, perhaps autoimmune response after viral illness

Incidence and Demographics

▶ Predominantly occurs in pediatric population; uncommon in geriatric population

▶ Slight seasonal peaks in winter and spring

▶ Adult female-to-male ratio = 3:1; most common acquired platelet disorder of childhood

Risk Factors

▶ No genetic predispositions described

▶ Acute infection (usually viral, e.g., varicella, EBV, CMV), HIV, cardiopulmonary bypass, hypersplenism, preeclampsia

▶ Exposure to drugs with antiplatelet effects (aspirin, seizure medications, heparin)

▶ History of autoimmune diseases (rheumatoid or collagen vascular symptoms, thyroid disease, hemolytic anemia)

Prevention and Screening

▶ None

Assessment

History

▶ Insidious onset in otherwise well person

▶ Prolonged purpura, bruising tendency, gingival bleeding, menorrhagia, epistaxis, petechiae

▶ History of acute viral illness

Physical Exam

▶ Nonpalpable spleen is essential criterion

▶ Signs of GI bleeding, dysmorphic features

Diagnostic Studies

▶ Often diagnosed on routine CBC with differential and platelets; also get peripheral smear; consider HIV, liver function, CT abdomen, stool guaiac as needed

▶ Laboratory results: Platelets decreased, normal RBC and WBC morphology

Differential Diagnosis

▶ Viral infection

▶ SLE

▶ Bone marrow disorders

▶ AIDS

▶ Drug-induced

▶ Hemolytic-uremic syndrome

▶ Liver disease

▶ Congenital thrombocytopenia (e.g., Fanconi's syndrome)

▶ Sepsis

Management

Nonpharmacologic Treatment

▶ Education and supportive care

▶ Avoid medications that increase bleeding risk.

▶ Decrease activities that might cause bruising and injury.

▶ Monitor patient for platelet count and associated symptoms.

Pharmacologic Treatment

▶ Acute: Prednisone 1–2 mg/kg q.d. for 4 weeks, then taper

▶ Chronic: 60 mg/day for 4–6 weeks, then taper

▶ Severe: IV gamma globulin (IVGG) 0.4 g/kg/day for 3–5 days or high-dose parenteral glucocorticoids

▶ Platelet transfusion *only* during life–threatening hemorrhage

▶ Splenectomy if platelets < 30,000 after 6 weeks of pharmacologic treatment (splenectomy response not good if IVGG response poor)

How Long to Treat

▶ Until remission

Special Considerations

▶ Focus: Bleeding, exclusion of other diagnoses

When to Consult, Refer, Hospitalize

▶ Any febrile child with thrombocytopenia and petechiae (with or without elevated PT and PTT) should be hospitalized and treated for presumed sepsis.

▶ Refer all suspected cases to hematologist; refer to surgeon for splenectomy.

Follow-up

Expected Course

▶ Acute = 80%–85% remission, 15% become chronic; chronic = 20% spontaneous remission

Complications

▶ Cerebral hemorrhage (1% mortality); other blood loss, pneumococcal infection

CASE STUDIES

Case 1. L.O. is a 9-month-old Hispanic male brought to the clinic by his mother for a routine well-child check-up. His mother states all is going well. L.O. lives at home with his mother, father, and maternal grandmother, who cares for him while his parents are at work. He is eating table food and drinking cow's milk.

PMH: UTD on immunizations; no illnesses requiring antibiotics. Current medications: none.

Exam: This is a very plump male infant who is interactive with his mother and the examiner. His vital signs are WNL. His weight is in the 95th percentile for his age, but his height is in the 50th percentile. In your office setting, you perform a Hgb, which is 9 g.

- ▶ What additional history would you like?
- ▶ What type of anemia is most likely in this case?
- ▶ What is the most likely cause of L.O.'s anemia?
- ▶ What corrective actions might you recommend at this time?

Case 2. B.C. is a 48-year-old White female who presents to your clinic complaining of feeling tired all the time. She works full-time and cares for her elderly mother in the home. B.C. reports "getting plenty of sleep and eating well." She finds little time for exercise and "doesn't have the energy to even go for a walk." ROS: Pertinent only for heavy bleeding during her periods, which she states began about 8 months ago. B.C. reports having to stay close to home and using a hand towel to supplement peri-pads.

PMH: Denies any hospitalizations or surgeries. Anemia during pregnancy. LMP: 1 week before clinic visit. Otherwise healthy; does not smoke or drink alcohol.

- ▶ What type of physical exam would you do?
- ▶ At this point, what might you include in your differential diagnosis?
- ▶ What diagnostic studies would you order?

Test results: Hgb 10g; RBC 3.6; MCV 72; TSH 1.56 (normal)

- ▶ What would your recommendations be for B.C. at this point?

Case 3. B.W., an 85-year-old Black male, is brought to clinic by his daughter for evaluation of possible dementia. She is worried that he cannot care for himself, as evidenced by the fact that he forgets his car at church some Sundays and walks home, and by his apparent weight loss. She is concerned that he cannot prepare his own meals anymore.

PMH: Hypertension — controlled; bladder irritability responsive to medication. NKDA; currently taking Vasotec 5 mg q.d., Ditropan 5 mg q.d.

SH: B.W. lives alone in his own home, one block from his church. A neighbor on his block assists him with paying his bills, going to doctor's appointments, and getting medication refills. B.W. reports being able to fix his own meals and denies feeling hungry.

ROS: Denies SOB, CP, anorexia, but admits he has lost some weight. Denies bowel changes. Does have some trouble remembering things but has always been able to find his car because the only place he drives to is church.

▶ What would you include in your differential diagnosis at this time?

Exam: Alert, well-dressed 85-year-old Black male who looks younger than his stated age. His vital signs are WNL. He scores 27 on the MMSE. CN II–XII are intact. He is able to ambulate without assistance. Romberg's intact, no evidence of ataxia. No lymphadenopathy. Lungs are clear without adventitious breath sounds. Heart: regular rate and rhythm without murmur or gallop. Abd: no distention, bowel sounds positive. No palpable masses. No hepatosplenomegaly or CVAT. Genital exam: WNL. Rectal exam: normal size prostate, enlarged without nodules. Stool is brown and heme negative.

▶ What diagnostic studies would you order at this time?

B.W. comes to see you 1 week later and has the following laboratory results: Hgb 9 g; Hct 27.2%; MCV 72; reported as hypochromic; all other parameters are WNL. He has lost two more pounds, despite the fact that his daughter has been cooking for him and encouraging him to eat. His FOBTs are all positive.

▶ What type of anemia does this man most likely have and what would be the next step in your diagnostic work-up of this gentleman?

REFERENCES

Andreoli, T. E. (Ed.). (2010). *Cecil essentials of medicine* (8th ed.). Philadelphia: W. B. Saunders Elsevier.

Baker, R. D., Greer F. R., Committee on Nutrition. (2010). Diagnosis and prevention of iron deficiency anemia in infants and young children (0–3 years of age). *Pediatrics, 126*(5), 1040–1050.

Byrd, L. (2011). Anemia in elders: Diagnosing & treatment strategies. *Geriatric Nursing, 32*(4), 297–298.

Domino, F. (2013). *The 5-minute clinical consult.* Philadelphia: Lippincott Williams & Wilkins.

Dutka, P. (2012). Erythropoiesis-stimulating agents for the management of anemia of chronic disease: Past advancements and current innovations. *Nephrology Nursing Journal, 39*(6), 447–457.

Ferri, F. F. (2013). *Ferri's clinical advisor 201: 5 books in 1.* Philadelphia: Elsevier Mosby.

Friedman, A. J., Chen, Z., Ford, P., Johnson, C. A., Lopez, A. M., Shander, A., Waters, J. H., & van Wyck, D. (2012). Iron deficiency anemia in women across the life span. *Journal of Women's Health, 20*(12), 1282–1289.

G6PD Deficiency Association. (1996). *Drugs that should be avoided — Official list.* Retrieved from www .g6pd.org/en/G6PDDeficiency/SafeUnsafe.aspx

Goolsby, M. J., & Grubbs, L. (2011). *Advanced assessment: Interpreting findings and formulating differential diagnoses* (2nd ed.). Philadelphia: F. A. Davis.

Hardin, S. R. (2010). Anemia of chronic disease, older adults, and Medicare. *Journal of Gerontological Nursing, 36*(10), 3–4.

Headley, C. M., (2012). Anemia management: One protocol does not fit all. *Nephrology Nursing Journal, 39*(1), 63–66.

Hoffman, P. C. (2006). Immune hemolytic anemias. *Hematology: American Society of Hematology Education Program, 13*(8). Retrieved from http://asheducationbook.hematologylibrary.org/cgi/content/full/2006/1/13

Lambing, A., Kachalsky, E., & Muller, M. L. (2012). The dangers of iron overload: Bring in the iron police. *Journal of the American Academy of Nurse Practitioners, 24*(4), 175–183.

Longo, D., Fauci, A., Kaspar, D., Hauser, S., Jameson, J., & Loscalzo, J. (2011). *Harrison's principles of internal medicine, Vol. 1 & 2* (18th ed.). New York: McGraw-Hill.

Marcdante, K J., Kleigman, R. M., Jensen, H. B., & Behrman, R. E. (2011). *Nelson essentials of pediatrics* (6th ed.). Philadelphia: Elsevier Saunders

Metcalf, D. (2012). A promising new treatment for refractory aplastic anemia. *New England Journal of Medicine, 367*(1), 74–75

Papdakis, M. A., McPhee, S. J., & Tierney, L. M. (Eds.). (2013). *Current medical diagnosis and treatment* (52nd ed.). New York: Lange Medical Books/McGraw-Hill..

ENDOCRINE DISORDERS

Shirlee Drayton-Brooks, PhD, FNP-BC

GENERAL APPROACH

Description

- ▶ Defects in aspects of the endocrine regulatory systems that can cause systemic consequences, morbidity, and death
- ▶ Endocrine disorders generally manifest in one of four ways:
  - ▹ Excess hormone (e.g., Cushing's syndrome, excess cortisol secretion)
  - ▹ Deficit hormone (e.g., diabetes mellitus [DM] type1; insulin secretion is low, resistant, or absent)
  - ▹ Abnormal response of end organ to the hormone (e.g., pseudohypoparathroidism)
  - ▹ Gland enlargement (e.g., pituitory adenoma)
- ▶ Endocrine diseases may be associated with a deficiency or hypersecretion of hormones that affect target organs.
- ▶ There are basically three types of hormone:
  - ▹ *Steroids,* such as cortisol (adrenal cortex), estrogen, progesterone (ovaries), and testosterone (testes)
  - ▹ *Amino acids,* such as tyrosine, thyroxine (thyroid), catecholamines (adrenal medulla)
  - ▹ Protein peptides, such as insulin (pancreas).
- ▶ Regulation of hormone secretion is through a negative feedback system.
- ▶ Patients of all ages may need to carry or wear MedicAlert or similar identification for many endocrine disorders.

▶ A total of 25.8 million children and adults in the United State, comprising 8.3% of the population, have diabetes, while 79 million people have prediabetes.

▶ The FNP must consider normal physiologic changes occurring with growth, development, and aging when managing various endocrine diagnoses across the life span.

▶ The FNP must consider lifestyle management and certain risk factors, such as obesity, when caring for individuals with endocrine diseases such as DM type 2.

RED FLAGS

▶ *Type 1 diabetes* may present with acute ketoacidosis: nausea, fatigue, abdominal pain, thirst, hunger, polyuria progressing to vomiting, confusion, lethargy, hypotension, fruity breath odor

▶ *Type 2 diabetes* may present with hyperglycemic, hyperosmolar, nonketotic syndrome (HHNKS), characterized by confusion and lethargy, blood glucose > 600 mg/dL, minimal ketosis, serum osmolality > 340, and profound dehydration.

▶ Prediabetes generally starts years before diagnosis, with macrovascular and microvascular changes.

▶ *Hypoglycemia* may present as initial headache, hunger, difficulty problem-solving, sweating, shakiness, tremor, anxiety, irritability, behavior change; without treatment, progresses to coma and seizures

▶ *Thyroid nodules* are common, but < 10% of solitary nodules are malignant.

▶ *Acute adrenal insufficiency* or Addisonian crisis may present as severe abdominal pain, nausea and vomiting, hypotension, hypoglycemia, and shock; precipitated by surgery, infection, exacerbation of comorbid illness, and sudden withdrawal of long-term glucocorticoid replacement.

▶ *Pituitary adenoma* may present as headache with visual changes, amenorrhea, or galactorrhea; obtain prolactin level and MRI of brain or CT with attention to sella turcica.

Risk Factors

▶ For malignancy, include family history of thyroid cancer or multiple endocrine metaplastic type 2 carcinoma; male gender; extremes in age (< 15 and > 70); exposure to radiation of head, neck, or chest; single nodule

DISORDERS OF THE PANCREAS

DIABETES MELLITUS TYPE 1

Description

▶ A syndrome produced by disorders in metabolism of carbohydrate, protein, and fat due to absolute lack of insulin resulting in hyperglycemia. Without insulin therapy, ketoacidosis occurs rapidly. Formerly called insulin-dependent diabetes mellitus (IDDM), juvenile-onset. Some genetically predisposed individuals develop autoimmune beta-cell destruction in response to some environmental triggers.

Etiology

▶ Destruction of beta cells in pancreatic islets and absolute deficiency or failure to produce insulin, related to autoimmune response or environmental trigger (e.g., virus)

▶ Human leukocyte antigens HLA, HLA-DR3, or HLA-DR4 associated with type 1

▶ May be triggered in susceptible individuals by viruses, toxic chemical agents, or cytotoxins

▶ Genetic susceptibility influenced by environmental factors

▶ Hyperglycemia from inability of glucose to enter cell for use as energy

▶ Ketoacidosis from use of free fatty acids for energy

Incidence and Demographics

▶ Type 1 accounts for 10%–12% of all diabetes cases in United States.

▶ Usually occurs in children and adolescents at puberty between ages 8 and 14

▶ Highest prevalence in Scandinavia where 20% of people with diabetes have type 1; Japan and China < 1%

▶ Can develop in adulthood but rarely occurs after 30 years of age; very rare to develop in older adults

▶ Idiopathic etiology most common in people of Asian or African descent

Risk Factors

▶ First-degree relative with type 1 diabetes mellitus; other autoimmune disorders

Prevention and Screening

▶ No prevention and no routine screening in childhood

Assessment

History

▶ Acute onset of polyuria, polydipsia, polyphagia, weight loss, blurred vision, fatigue, abdominal pain, nausea and vomiting, vaginal itching or infections, unhealed wounds, skin infections or rashes, dehydration, hypoglycemic or ketotic episodes

▶ Nightmares, night sweats, or headache may indicate nocturnal hypoglycemia in both children and adults.

▶ Parent report of frequent diaper changes, bed-wetting, listlessness or fatigue, frequent sick days from school or daycare, changes in school performance or behavior

▶ Pediatric patients: Birth weight and history of complications at birth, health status at birth

▶ Family history of diabetes

Physical Exam

▶ Exam may be normal or patient may be ill-looking with fruity odor to breath

▶ Weight loss, thin (children and adults) or failure to thrive (infants), signs of dehydration, orthostatic hypotension

► Presence of skin infections, oral or vaginal candidiasis (more common in type 2)

► Diabetic ketoacidosis: Dehydration, labored breathing, confusion or disorientation, lethargy

► Signs of complications

 » Delayed sexual maturation (adolescents)

 » Late disease: Ophthalmic changes—microaneurysm with soft and hard exudates; deep retinal hemorrhages, neovascularization, cataracts, glaucoma; peripheral vascular insufficiency; diminished deep tendon reflex

 » Possible cardiovascular changes occurring in late disease: Postural hypotension, resting tachycardia, "silent" myocardial infarctions

 » Possible peripheral vascular changes occurring in late disease: Cool extremities due to decreased circulation, decreased pulses, edema, delayed capillary refill

 » Possible neurologic changes occurring in late disease: Diminished pain sensation, proprioception, vibration, light touch, absent lower extremity reflexes, dysfunction in extraocular movements, weakness, ataxic gait, paresthesias; may have change in level of consciousness

Diagnostic Studies

► Diagnosis of type 1 diabetes

 » HbA1C ≥ 6.5%

 » Fasting plasma glucose (FPG) ≥ 126 mg/dL (7.0 mmol/L)

 » 2-h plasma glucose ≥ 200 mg/dL (11.1 mmol/L) during an OGTT

 » A random plasma glucose ≥ 200 mg/dL (11.1 mmol/L)

 » When no symptoms of hyperglycemia (polyuria, polydipsia, polyphagia, etc.) are present, the diagnosis of diabetes must be confirmed on another day by repeat measurement, repeating the same test for confirmation. If results of two different tests (A1C and FPG) are available and are both indicative of diabetes, additional testing is not needed.

► A random plasma glucose ≥ 200 mg/dL (11.1 mmol/L), FPG > 110 mg/dL, is diagnostic of prediabetes.

► Oral glucose tolerance test (OGTT) no longer recommended for routine clinical use except in screening for gestational diabetes

► May consider serum C peptide or insulin level (decreased)

► Glucose and ketones in urine

► Baseline diagnostic studies: BUN, serum creatinine, urinalysis, urine microalbumin, and fasting lipid profile; glycosylated hemoglobin (HbA1C; 5.5% to < 7% = good control)

► ECG and chest X-ray for coronary and pulmonary pathology in adults

► Elevated BUN and creatinine if dehydrated; hypertriglyceridemia: Triglyceride levels > 150 mg/dL

► Thyroid-stimulating hormone (TSH) level

Differential Diagnosis

▶ Diabetes mellitus type 2

▶ Diabetes insipidus

▶ Pancreatitis or pancreatic disease

▶ Pheochromocytoma

▶ Cushing's syndrome

▶ Acromegaly

▶ Liver disease

▶ Salicylate poisoning

▶ Glucosuria w/o hyperglycemia in renal tubular disease or benign renal glucosuria

▶ Secondary effects of oral contraceptives, corticosteroids, thiazides, phenytoin, nicotinic acid

▶ Severe stress from trauma, burns, or infection

▶ Urinary tract infection (UTI)

Management

Nonpharmacologic Treatment

▶ Patient education: Basic pathophysiology, cause, general management and long-term complications of type 1 diabetes, administration of insulin, medications

▶ Short- and long-term goals of treatment: Whole blood glucose average 80–120 mg/dL preprandially and 100–140 mg/dL bedtime; HbA1C goal < 7%

▶ Lifestyle modifications: Diet, exercise, smoking cessation (if appropriate), alcohol avoidance

▶ Medical nutrition therapy prescribed by a registered dietician, following American Diabetes Association (ADA) guidelines; constant reinforcement by all providers

▶ General guidelines for adults: 10%–20% calories from protein, < 10% from saturated fats, < 10% from polyunsaturated fats, and 50%–70% from carbohydrates and monounsaturated fats; cholesterol 300 mg/day, fiber to 25–35 g/1,000 calories

▶ General guidelines for children: Consistent timing and amount of meals (3 meals and 3 snacks). However, for those on fast-acting insulin (such as NovoLog) and insulin glargine, or using fast-acting insulin in an insulin pump, exact timing and amount of meals is not as critical. A well-balanced, healthy diet is recommended, with dosing adjusted to number of carbohydrates consumed at any meal and adjustments made for high or low blood sugar. Diet should include 15% of calories from protein, 30% of calories from fats, and 55% of calories from carbohydrates.

▶ Daily exercise regimen for adults and physical activity for children

▶ Use a multidisciplinary approach to help work with the patient and the family, including the patient, parents (if appropriate), primary care provider, endocrinologist, nurse educator, and dietician.

   » Teach patient and parent recognition and management of episodes of hypoglycemia due to inadequate oral intake, increased exercise without adequate increase in caloric intake, or excess insulin

   » Self or parental glucose monitoring education: t.i.d., before meals and bedtime; check for urine ketones if blood glucose is > 300 mg/dL; during illness, stress, pregnancy, or symptoms of ketosis such as nausea, vomiting, or abdominal pain; keep self-monitoring blood glucose (SMBG) log

▶ Establish a foot care plan.

▶ Establish a dental care plan.

▶ Annual eye examination

▶ Teach patient or parent how to modify therapy if ill. "Sick day guidelines" require continuing usual dose of insulin, frequent SMBG, and adjustment of insulin if necessary; checking urine for ketones if SMBG > 300 mg/dL, increased intake of fluids

▶ Referral to local support groups and American Diabetes Association

▶ Recommend wearing a MedicAlert or similar identification bracelet or necklace.

▶ Inform school, work, and friends of condition.

▶ Pneumococcal vaccine and annual influenza vaccines

Pharmacologic Treatment

▶ Insulin therapy (see Tables 17–1, 17–2, and 17–3) and other treatments

▶ Individual presenting with ketones must be started on insulin.

▶ Glycemic goals should be individualized, based on a patient's duration of diabetes, age, life expectancy, comorbid conditions, known cardiovascular disease (CVD) or advanced microvascular complications, unawareness of hypoglycemia, and other considerations.

▶ Goal of therapy is to maintain blood sugar:

  » Preprandial 70–130 mg/dL

  » Peak postprandial < 180 mg/dL; postprandial glucose measurements should be made 1–2 h after beginning of meal

▶ Children should be managed by an endocrinologist.

  » Preschoolers: FPG range 90–140 mg/dL, postprandially 90–200 mg/dL

  » School-age: FPG range 80–120 mg/dL, postprandially 80–180 mg/dL

▶ Insulin doses in general can be divided into 2–4 injections per day or continuous subcutaneous insulin infusion (insulin pump) once stabilized; typical regimen for children and adults is 2 injections per day; adolescents may require 3 injections per day.

▶ Adjust insulin doses according to glucose monitoring.

▶ A "honeymoon period" or remission phase after diagnosis may last from several months to 2 years.

Insulin Therapy

Insulin therapy has become more effective with advancements such as insulin analogs and combination therapy. Bolus insulin with advance infusion technology also has led to increase glycemic control and less risk of hypogylcemia. Insulin treatment is usually prandial, basal, combination basal/prandial, and premixed biphasic (see Tables 17–1, 17–2, and 17–3). Basal/prandial insulin management is general 50% basal and 50% prandial, with the prandial divided into 3 doses, one at each mealtime with consideration for the largest meal. For instance, if the total daily dose of insulin (TDDI) is 60 units, then 30 units would be basal insulin and 5 units prandial could be given for breakfast, 10 units prandial for lunch, and 15 prandial for dinner, assuming dinner is the meal with the highest caloric intake.

Insulin injections must be given subcutaneously with sites of injected rotated to avoid lipohypertropy. Although insulin with needles to be drawn up from vials is still commonly used, the insulin pen provides an easy and efficient means for patients to deliver precise, accurate insulin doses.

TABLE 17–1
PRANDIAL INSULINS, GIVEN AT MEALTIMES

	REGULAR/ HUMAN SHORT-ACTING	ANALOG LISPRO RAPID-ACTING	ANALOG ASPART RAPID-ACTING	ANALOG GLUTISINE RAPID-ACTING
Onset	0.5–1 hr	0.3–0.5 hr	0.25 hr	0.25 hr
Peak	2–3 hr	0.5–2.5 hr	0.5–1.0 hr	1.0–1.5 hr
Duration	3–6 hr	3–6.5 hr	3.5 hr	3.5 hr
Administration	30–45 min	15 min before or immediately after	5–10 min	15–20 min

TABLE 17–2
BASAL INSULINS

	GLARGINE	DETEMIR BID
Duration	Up to 24 hrs	Up to 24 hrs

TABLE 17–3
PREMIXED OR BIPHASIC INSULINS

HUMAN BIPHASIC	ANALOG BIPHASIC	ANALOG BIPHASIC	ANALOG BIPHASIC
Human insulin (70/30) NPH/Regular	Humalog 75-25 (75-25 insulin Lispro suspension and 25 insulin Lispro)	Humalog mix 50-50 (insulin Lispro)	70% insulin aspart protamine suspension and 30% insulin aspart 70/30

Newer insulin therapies include exenatide b.i.d. with glargine insulin and liragludide with detemir insulin.

Special Considerations

▶ Puberty: Initially, increased caloric need, followed by decrease to 35 calories/kg of ideal body weight as growth is completed; pubertal growth spurt will require insulin adjustment (1.25–1.5 units/kg/day)

▶ Co-management with pediatrician or pediatric endocrinologist

When to Consult, Refer, Hospitalize

▶ Hospitalization is recommended for all newly diagnosed pediatric patients.

- ▶ Hospitalize adults and children with diabetic ketoacidosis (DKA) and severe infections.
- ▶ Co-manage pediatric type 1 DM patients with a pediatrician or pediatric endocrinologist.
- ▶ Refer unstable adult or geriatric patients; consider co-management of all type 1 DM patients.
- ▶ Refer all families to diabetes educator and registered dietician (RD).
- ▶ Ophthalmologist: Initial screening and annual exam for diabetic retinopathy and visual problems; all patients > 9 years who have diabetes for 3–5 years, and all patients > 30 years
- ▶ Dentist: Routine check-ups and for dental complaints for all ages
- ▶ Podiatrist: Routine foot care in older adults and foot problems as indicated
- ▶ Consider psychological counseling if needed, to address issues of altered body image and individual and family stressors related to disease and management

Follow-up

- ▶ Continue ongoing follow-up and consultation with endocrinologist and diabeted educator.
- ▶ Routine diabetes visits: Daily for initiation of insulin or change in regimen, at least quarterly for patients not meeting their goals, and semiannually for other patients
- ▶ 24-hour urine collection or spot urine collection for microalbuminuria beginning at puberty and at 5 years' duration
- ▶ HbA1cC every 3–6 months
  - » Glycosylated hemoglobin (HbA1C): Target goal = 6%; normal range 4%–6%; each % correlates to 30 mg/dL FPG elevation; provides index of glycemic control for life of red blood cells, 8–12 weeks
- ▶ Serum fructosamine: Glycosylated protein (primarily albumin); normal value 1.5–2.4 mmol/L; provides index of glycemic control for preceding 2–3 weeks; low albumin levels will lower fructosamine levels; useful when hemolytic states affect HbA1C measures
- ▶ Annual physical exam or routine well-child exam with primary care provider
- ▶ Thyroid function tests initially, then every 2–3 years for adults; annually for children

Expected Course

- ▶ Chronic, lifelong disease with no cure

Complications

- ▶ Hypoglycemia signs and symptoms: Shakiness, weakness, sweating, headache, tachycardia, nervousness, dizziness, hunger, irritability, convulsions, coma
- ▶ Somogyi effect: Early morning rebound hyperglycemia due to nocturnal hypoglycemia; around 3:00 a.m. serum glucose falls and patient is hypoglycemic; counterregulatory hormones compensate by mobilizing glucose stores; patient rebounds and becomes hyperglycemic by early morning; treated with reducing or eliminating p.m. or h.s. doses to eliminate nocturnal hypoglycemia
- ▶ Dawn phenomenon: Hyperglycemia due to hepatic gluconeogenesis in early morning. Peripheral tissue insulin receptors become desensitized to insulin nocturnally, believed to be due to insulin receptor desensitizing property of growth hormone. Around 3:00 a.m., blood sugar measures either normal or high normal and gets progressively higher

throughout the night; is elevated at 7 a.m. Treatment is to increase p.m. long-acting insulin or add an h.s. dose.

▶ Lipodystrophy (destruction of subcutaneous fat at injection sites): Seen less with use of synthetic human insulin, rather than beef or pork insulin

▶ Retinopathy

▶ Nephropathy and renal failure

▶ Cardiovascular disease with lipid abnormalities; premature atherosclerosis

▶ Cerebrovascular disease

▶ Diabetic ketoacidosis

▶ Insulin resistance with long-term, high-dose therapy

▶ Peripheral neuropathy

▶ Autonomic nervous system problems, incontinence, and erectile dysfunction

▶ Infections

▶ Foot and skin ulcerations

▶ Insulin allergy

DIABETES MELLITUS TYPE 2

Description

▶ Metabolic disease causing hyperglycemia, characterized by a relative insufficiency of insulin due to resistance to the action of insulin in target tissues, decrease in insulin receptors, impairment of insulin secretion, or combination of these

▶ Formerly non–insulin-dependent diabetes mellitus (NIDDM), adult or maturity onset, type 2, nonketotic diabetes (because there is some endogenous insulin activity, diabetic ketoacidosis usually does not develop)

Etiology

▶ Genetically and clinically a heterogeneous disorder with familial pattern

▶ Influenced by environmental factors, lack of physical activity, diet high in refined carbohydrate and fat with low fiber

▶ Two major types

   » Obese type 2 diabetes: Most common

      ▷ Initial peripheral insulin receptor insensitivity, possibly due to cellular distention secondary to increased fat accumulation

      ▷ Beta cell compensates by increasing insulin release; hyperglycemia does not occur.

      ▷ Eventually, beta cells may "burn out," insulin release falls, and hyperglycemia occurs as result of insulin receptor insensitivity.

   » Non-obese

      ▷ Initial problem may be blunted response of beta cell to glucose

▷ Glucose does not trigger adequate insulin release.

▷ Insulin resistance is not clinically significant.

▷ More common in certain Asian populations

► No human leukocyte antigen or islet cell antibodies

► Syndrome of hyperinsulinemia and insulin resistance, resulting in hyperglycemia, hypertension, and hyperlipidemia to varying degrees in all patients

Incidence and Demographics

► Occurs predominantly in obese adults > 30 years but occasionally in adolescents with a genetic predisposition or obesity

► Incidence higher in females than males

► Accounts for nearly 90% of all diabetes mellitus cases in U.S.

Risk Factors

► Obesity and inactivity, > 20% above ideal body weight, or body mass index (BMI) > 30 kg/m²

► Family history of diabetes, mostly type 2

► Gestational diabetes increases risk for developing type 2 diabetes within 5–10 years postparturition

► Delivery of macrosomic infant, weight > 9 lbs

► Previously impaired glucose tolerance

► Age > 45

► Black, Asian American, Hispanic, Native American, or Pacific Islander

► Metabolic syndrome (syndrome X or insulin resistance syndrome): Cluster of disorders, including hypertension, insulin resistance, truncal obesity, abnormal lipid levels, hyperinsulinism

► High-density lipoprotein (HDL) cholesterol ≤ 35 mg/dL, triglycerides > 250 mg/dL, or both

Prevention and Screening

► Adults > 45 years screened every 3 years; more often with FPG near 126 mg/dL

► Screening of pregnant women for gestational diabetes at 24–28 weeks' gestation

► Secondary prevention of complications essential

Assessment

History

► More insidious onset; may not have classical signs of type 1 diabetes at early onset

► Obesity, blurred vision, chronic skin infections, polyuria, polydipsia, polyphagia, weight loss, fatigue, slow-healing wounds, recurrent infections (especially *Candida* and urinary tract infections), spontaneous abortion

► History related to type 2 diabetes: More prominent macrovascular changes than microvascular, such as vascular insufficiency, cardiovascular or cerebrovascular disease, and atherosclerosis

► History of hyperosmolar hyperglycemic nonketotic syndrome (HHNKS): Precipitating factors such as treatment with calcium channel blockers, propranolol, corticosteroids, thiazides, phenytoin

Physical Exam

► Usually discovered on routine exam with elevated glucose level

► Central obesity, hypertensive

► With more advanced stage

   ▸ Orthostatic blood pressure changes

   ▸ Weight loss

   ▸ Skin infections present

   ▸ Visual and funduscopic changes: Microaneurysms with soft (cotton wool) and hard exudates, deep retinal hemorrhages, neovascularization, cataracts, glaucoma

   ▸ Oral *Candida* infections

   ▸ Peripheral vascular: Decreased circulation, cool extremities, decreased pulses, edema, capillary refill > 3 seconds

   ▸ Neurologic: Decreased sensation of pain, proprioception, vibration, light touch, absent lower extremity reflexes, dysfunction in extraocular movements, weakness, ataxic gait

Diagnostic Studies

► Diagnosis of Type 2 diabetes

   ▸ HbA1C ≥ 6.5%

   ▸ Fasting plasma glucose (FPG) ≥ 126 mg/dL (7.0 mmol/L)

   ▸ 2-h plasma glucose ≥ 200 mg/dL (11.1 mmol/L) during an OGTT

   ▸ A random plasma glucose ≥ 200 mg/dL (11.1 mmol/L)

   ▸ When no symptoms of hyperglycemia (polyuria, weight loss, polydipsia, etc.) are present, the diagnosis of diabetes must be confirmed on another day by repeat measurement, repeating the same test for confirmation. If results of two different tests (A1C and FPG) are available and are both indicative of diabetes, additional testing is not needed.

► A random plasma glucose ≥ 200 mg/dL (11.1 mmol/L) or FPG > 110 mg/dL is diagnostic of prediabetes.

► Oral glucose tolerance test (OGTT) no longer recommended for routine clinical use except in screening for gestational diabetes

► FPG > 100 mg/dL and < 126 mg/dL represents impaired fasting glucose (IFG)

► Urinalysis for protein, glucose, and ketones; microalbuminuria screening at initial diagnosis (ketonuria may occur but ketone accumulation in serum is rare)

► BUN, urine, and serum creatinine

► Fasting serum cholesterol and lipid profile

▶ Adult recommendations:

» Glycemic control: Glycosylated hemoglobin A1C (HbA1C) < 7.0%, preprandial capillary plasma glucose 90–130 mg/dL, peak postprandial capillary plasma glucose < 180 mg/dL

» Blood pressure 130/80 mm Hg

» Lipids: Low-density lipoproteins (LDL) < 100 mg/dL, trigylcerides < 150 mg/dL, high-density lipoproteins (HDL) > 40 mg/dL for men; goal HDL > 50 mg/dL for women

▶ ECG and chest X-ray if clinically indicated for coronary and pulmonary pathology

▶ TSH

▶ Glycated serum protein: Index of glycemic control over past 1–2 weeks

▶ C-peptide levels normal or above normal with type 2

Differential Diagnosis

▶ Diabetes mellitus type 1

▶ Diabetes insipidus

▶ Pancreatitis or pancreatic disease

▶ Pheochromocytoma

▶ Cushing's syndrome

▶ Liver disease

▶ Glucosuria w/o hyperglycemia in renal tubular disease or benign renal glucosuria

▶ Secondary effects of oral contraceptives, corticosteroids, thiazides, phenytoin, nicotinic acid

▶ Severe stress from trauma, burns, or infection

Management

▶ Common treatment plan with goal of FPG 80–100 mg/dL and HbA1C < 7.0%

» Diet and exercise

» Oral monotherapy

» Add a 2nd drug class

» Add a 3rd drug class or insulin

Nonpharmacologic Treatment

▶ Patient education: Basic pathophysiology, cause, general management, and long-term complications of type 2 diabetes; oral glucose-lowering medications dosage, administration, and side effects

▶ Mainstay of treatment is correction of insulin resistance through diet, exercise, and weight loss; patients with FPG < 250 mg/dL may be treated initially with medical nutritional therapy

» Lifestyle modifications: Diet, exercise, smoking cessation (if appropriate), alcohol avoidance

» Medical nutrition therapy prescribed by a registered dietician

» Nutrition counseling following American Diabetes Association (ADA) guidelines; weight reduction of 5–10 lbs increases insulin sensitivity

- » General guidelines for adults and children: 10%–20% calories from protein, < 10% from saturated fats, < 10% from polyunsaturated fats, and 50%–70% from carbohydrates and monounsaturated fats

- » Moderate weight loss (10–20 lbs) and hypocaloric diets based on average daily intake can improve blood glucose levels.

- » Daily exercise regimen for adults and physical activity for children reduces insulin resistance by increasing number of insulin receptors, increases glucose uptake for 48–72 hours, and contributes to lipid control and weight loss.

▶ SMBG should be encouraged as appropriate and when medications are initiated or altered: Before each meal, at bedtime, and 2–4 in a.m. for 3 days, then before breakfast and dinner for 7 days. Once glucose is controlled, monitor daily at random times; maintain SMBG log.

▶ Teach patient or parent how to modify therapy if ill. "Sick day guidelines" for adults require continuing usual dose medication, frequent SMBG, increase intake of fluids; for pediatric patients, consult with pediatrician or pediatric endocrinologist.

▶ Counsel regarding contraception and discuss importance of glucose control before and during pregnancy.

▶ Perform stress test if > 35 years with DM

▶ Referral to local support groups and American Diabetes Association.

▶ MedicAlert or similar identification bracelet or necklace

▶ Foot care plan

▶ Annual influenza and pneumococcal vaccinations

▶ Avoid HHNKS with hydration

Pharmacologic Treatment

▶ Step approach

▶ If FPG > 250 mg/dL and < 400 mg/dL without symptoms of acidosis, dehydration, or ketosis, in addition to nutrition therapy and exercise, begin monotherapy with oral antidiabetic agent (30%–40% patients may not respond)

▶ Antidiabetic agents listed in Table 17–4: Select based on blood glucose level, age, and weight of the patient, taking into consideration precautions and contraindications specific to the classification of agent selected

▶ For obese patients: Begin metformin with a low dose, increase dosage every 1–2 weeks on basis of glycemic control; treatment should continue for 4 weeks before changing to another agent; then add insulin-release stimulator if control inadequate; then add thiazelolidinedione if first 2 agents do not provide adequate control. If no control, then stop oral insulin-release stimulator and add or switch to insulin.

▶ For nonobese patients: Use insulin-release stimulator as initial agent; metformin if inadequate control with the first agent, thiazelolidinedione if the first 2 agents do not provide adequate control, then add insulin if needed, but do not discontinue the oral insulin-release stimulator.

▶ Alpha-glucosidase inhibitors may also be added to the regimen to achieve better control in some patients.

▶ If FPG > 400 mg/dL or patient has signs of ketoacidosis, insulin therapy is required.

TABLE 17-4
COMMONLY USED ORAL ANTIDIABETIC AGENTS

GENERIC AND CLASS	BRAND NAME	ACTION	DOSAGE RANGE	USUAL MAXIMUM DOSAGE	COMMENTS AND MAJOR SIDE EFFECTS
Sulfonylureas: Pancreatic islet beta cell insulin-release stimulator					
Glipizide 2nd generation	Glucotrol	Intermediate-acting	5–15 mg daily 5–40 mg/day divided	15 mg/day or 40 mg divided	Hypoglycemia
	Glucotrol XL	Long-acting	5–10 mg daily	20 mg/day	Good in controlling postprandial hyperglycemia
Glyburide 2nd generation	DiaBeta Micronase	Intermediate-acting	1.25–20 mg, single or divided	20 mg/day	Hypoglycemia
Glyburide, micronized 2nd generation	Glynase Pres Tab	Intermediate-acting	0.75–12 mg single or divided	12 mg/day divided	Hypoglycemia
Meglitinides: Pancreatic islet beta cell insulin-release stimulator					
Repaglinide	Prandin	Short-acting	0.5–4 mg within 30 min of meals 2–4×/day	16 mg/day	Take with meals, quick onset; hypoglycemia; many drug interactions
Nateglinide	Starlix	Short-acting	60–120 mg t.i.d. within 30 min before meals	120 mg t.i.d.	Quick onset, which may be useful in adolescents with irregular eating schedules; do not take if a meal is skipped. Use with caution in severe renal disease. May be used as an adjunct with metformin.
Biguanides: Decrease hepatic glucose production; increase action on muscle glucose uptake					
Metformin	Glucophage	Intermediate-acting	500 mg–2.55 g divided into 2 or 3 doses	2.55 g/day	Contraindicated in renal dysfunction, chronic heart failure requiring treatment; use cautiously in many conditions that may predispose to lactic acidosis

CONTINUED

TABLE 17–4 CONTINUED

GENERIC AND CLASS	BRAND NAME	ACTION	DOSAGE RANGE	USUAL MAXIMUM DOSAGE	COMMENTS AND MAJOR SIDE EFFECTS
Thiazolidinediones: Increase insulin action on muscle and fat glucose uptake					
Pioglitazone	Actos	Long-acting	15 or 30 mg daily	45 mg/day	Precautions with hepatic dysfunction, cardiac disease, anovulatory conditions
Rosiglitazone	Avandia	Long-acting	4–8 mg single or divided into 2 doses	8 mg/day	Precautions with hepatic dysfunction, cardiac disease, anovulatory conditions
Alpha-Glucosidase Inhibitors: **Delay carbohydrate digestion and decrease postprandial glucose**					
Acarbose	Precose	Short-acting	50–100 mg t.i.d.	< 60 kg: 150 mg/day divided > 60 kg: 300 mg/day divided	Take before meals. Contraindicated in inflammatory bowel disease and other intestinal conditions; use glucose rather than sucrose for hypoglycemia
Miglitol	Glyset	Short-acting	50 mg t.i.d.	300 mg/day divided into 3 doses	Take before meals. Contraindicated in inflammatory bowel disease and other intestinal conditions; use glucose rather than sucrose for hypoglycemia

▶ If insulin is required, follow regimen of type 1 regarding insulin and SMBG.

▶ Treat to the target; start with 10 units insulin q.h.s. and adjust weekly based on mean FBG on preceding 2 days:

   ▹ > 180, increase 8 units

   ▹ 140–180, increase 6 units

   ▹ 120–140, increase 4 units

   ▹ 100–120, increase 2 units

▶ Alternative is the body weight approach: 0.1–0.24 u/kg/day. If FPG < 70, reduce 4 u or 10% of TDD (total daily dose). If FPG > 130, increase 2–4 u every 3 days/ (ADA)

▶ Another approach is to increase the dose 2 u every 3 days until FPG is in the range of 70 to 100 mg/dL or increase 1 u daily until FPG, < 110 mg/dL.

▶ Goal of therapy: HbA1C control is looser than in type 1 DM; tight control is associated with fewer long-term microvascular complications but may increase the risk of severe hypoglycemia and weight gain.

▶ In metabolic syndrome (syndrome X or insulin resistance syndrome), it is theorized that the insulin receptors' insensitivity leads to hyperinsulinemia; this leads to increased hepatic, very low-density lipoprotein (VLDL) production, which leads to increased sodium retention. Hyperinsulinemia also leads to endothelial proliferation, accelerating atherosclerosis with associated hypertension. These patients require treatment for hyperglycemia, hypertension, dyslipidemia, and weight loss.

▶ New therapies include DPP-4 inhibitors, incretins (sitagliptin [Januvia], saxagliptin [Onglyza], and linagliptin [Tradjenta]). DPP-4 inhibitors block dipeptidyl peptidase IV (DPP-4), an enzyme that breaks down gut peptides, especially GLP-1. DPP-4 inhibitors work indirectly to raise GLP-1.

Special Considerations

▶ Pregnancy

  » Routine screening at 24–28 weeks' gestation in all pregnant women with OGTT: Oral 50 g glucose (regardless of fasting) solution with a 1-hour blood glucose assay

  » High-risk women (previous gestational diabetes, other risk factors) should be screened at the first prenatal visit.

    ▷ Positive screening (> 140 mg/dL) necessitates a standard glucose tolerance test before diagnosis

  » Criteria for diagnosis of gestational diabetes following 75-g OGTT glucose load: Fasting ≥ 92 mg/dL, 1 h ≥ 180 mg/dL, 2 h ≥ 153 mg/dL (8.5 mmol/L)

    ▷ IFG refers to higher than normal serum glucose levels but not diagnostic of diabetes mellitus

  » Gestational diabetes is treated through a multidisciplinary approach, including nutrition therapy and insulin, if necessary.

    ▷ Pregnant patients with gestational diabetes requiring insulin management should be managed by an endocrinologist and perinatologist.

    ▷ Refer all patients with gestational diabetes who require insulin therapy.

  » Screen women with GDM for persistent diabetes at 6–12 weeks postpartum, using the OGTT and nonpregnancy diagnostic criteria.

  » Women with a history of GDM should have lifelong screening for the development of diabetes or prediabetes at least every 3 years.

▶ Older adults

  » Frail or mentally disabled older adults are likely to have hypoglycemic events resulting from forgetting to take medication as prescribed; incidence of falls may increase.

When to Consult, Refer, Hospitalize

▶ Endocrinologist referral for uncontrolled hyperglycemia

▶ Pediatric endocrinologist for pediatric DM type 2 patients until stabilized

▶ Hospitalize for severe infections or HHNKS, characterized by blood glucose > 600 mg/dL, minimal ketosis, serum osmolality > 340, and profound dehydration.

▶ Diabetes educator for further teaching for all patients and for pregnancy and lactation

▶ Registered dietitian for further nutritional teaching

▶ Ophthalmologist: Initial screening and annual exam for diabetic retinopathy and visual problems; all patients > 9 years who have diabetes for 3–5 years, and all patients > 30 years

▶ Podiatrist for routine foot care in older adults and any patients with foot problems as indicated

Follow-up

▶ When first diagnosed or when adjusting medications, see weekly, then biweekly, monthly; well controlled patients, see every 6 months

▶ Annual urine protein, FPG, lipid profile, creatinine, ECG, full physical exam with funduscopic and neurologic exams, complete foot inspection

▶ If treated with medication, obtain HbA1C every 3–6 months; goal < 7%

▶ Thyroid function tests as indicated

Expected Course

▶ Chronic, lifelong disease that requires long-term control to minimize complications

Complications

▶ Hyperglycemic hyperosmolar nonketotic coma, Charcot foot is a weaking of bones in the foot,a nd develops secondary to neuropathy; also see type 1 DM complications

HYPOGLYCEMIA

Description

▶ Plasma glucose concentration < 50 mg/dL (value may vary by lab); may be asymptomatic; plasma glucose level of < 30 mg/dL usually symptomatic

▶ Can be classified as reactive (within 5 hours of eating) or fasting (occurs > 5 hours after a meal)

  ▹ Reactive hypoglycemia rare; more likely is pseudo hypoglycemia (symptoms without the drop in blood glucose; unclear cause)

Etiology

▶ Most commonly caused by excess exogenous insulin in people with diabetes, but may result from use of some oral antihyperglycemic agents; precipitated by change in quantity and timing of activity and food

▶ At onset, parasympathetic nervous system is activated, causing hunger, which is followed by activation of the sympathetic nervous system (nervousness, sweating, tachycardia); known as "Whipple's Triad," which consists of low plasma glucose, parasympathetic and sympathetic symptoms, and relief with ingestion of carbohydrates

▶ Other causes: Benign functional disturbance of insulin secretion, pancreatic beta-cell tumor (insulinoma); autoimmune process (very rare); ethanol ingestion; glucocorticoid and growth hormone deficiencies; malnutrition; gastrointestinal surgery; chronic disease states (hepatic, renal, chronic heart failure [CHF])

▶ In neonates, due to erythroblastosis fetalis, insulinomas, β-cell nesidioblastosis, functional β-cell hyperplasia, Beckwith's syndrome, panhypopituitarism, infants of mothers with DM and gestational DM, very ill or immature, intrauterine malnutrition, metabolic defects

Incidence and Demographics

▶ Most prevalent in patients with diabetes on insulin and sulfonylureas

▶ Occurs in 1–3 per 1,000 live births, including approximately 5%–15% of infants with intrauterine growth retardation (IUGR)

Risk Factors

▶ Type 1 DM, type 2 DM on insulin or sulfonylureas

▶ Enzyme defects

▶ Liver disease, insulinoma

▶ Medication use, such as disopyramide (Norpace), pentamidine, quinine

▶ Pregnancy, 3rd trimester

▶ Pituitary or adrenal insufficiency

▶ Alcohol abuse

▶ Neonatal: Prematurity, hypoxia, hypothermia, IUGR, maternal DM, maternal glucose infusion during labor, small-for-gestational age (SGA)

Assessment

History

▶ Symptom history, especially whether it occurs postprandially or when fasting; may follow excessive exercise

▶ Initial symptoms of headache, hunger, difficulty problem-solving; may be sweating, shakiness, tremor, anxiety, irritability, behavior change

▶ Progresses to coma and seizures without treatment

▶ Insulinoma: Morning headaches, morning confusion, nocturnal or early morning seizures

▶ Infants and children: SGA (highest risk), IUGR, prematurity

  ▹ Hypothermia, hypoxia, or drug withdrawal at birth

  ▹ Maternal DM, gestational DM history, or glucose infusion at birth

  ▹ History of apnea of prematurity

Physical Exam

▶ Altered mental status; tachycardia; hypotension; pale, cool, and clammy skin; coma; positive Babinski

▶ In neonates, onset may be a few hours to 1 week after birth with jitteriness; convulsions; episodic cyanosis, apnea, or tachycardia; lethargy and poor feeding; high-pitched cry; diaphoresis; pallor; hypothermia

Diagnostic Studies

▶ Adults: Serum glucose level < 50 mg/dL indicates hypoglycemia (varies by laboratory)

▶ Consider drug testing for ethyl alcohol or sulfonylurea, liver function, BUN, creatinine, cortisol tests to identify associated factors in patients with diabetes

▶ In patients without diabetes, also get C-peptide levels, insulin, insulin antibodies, oral glucose tolerance test

▶ If cause not identified, additional testing after 72-hour fast may be done by specialist.

▶ Neonates and children: Serum glucose level < 35 mg/dL at 1–3 hours of age; < 40 mg/dL at 3–24 hours of age; < 45 mg/dL after 24 hours of age

Differential Diagnosis

▶ Pseudo hypoglycemia

▶ Anxiety and panic

▶ Pheochromocytoma

▶ Factitious hypoglycemia

▶ Other causes of coma

▶ See conditions listed under Etiology

Management

Nonpharmacologic Treatment

▶ Avoid fasting, alcohol use; snack before exercise.

▶ Caffeine restriction (mimics symptoms)

▶ Avoid simple carbohydrates or beverages with high sugar content.

▶ Diet: High-protein with complex carbohydrates, frequent small meals approximately 6×/day

▶ Avoid causative agents.

▶ Insulinomas and nesidioblastosis: surgery

▶ In neonates: Oral or gavage feeding of high-risk, normoglycemic neonates and monitor for hypoglycemia

Pharmacologic Treatment

▶ If able to take oral substances, consume 2 glucose tablets or 5 Life Savers candies (equivalent to 10–15 g glucose) at onset of symptoms, followed by complex carbohydrates after the acute reaction is controlled

▶ If unconscious or unable to swallow, home or office management could include 1 mg glucagon IM or SC (adult and adolescent); 0.5–1 mg glucagon (5–10 years); 0.25–0.5 mg (< 5 years): roll patient on side in case of vomiting; transport to an acute care facility for further monitoring and treatment.

▶ If oral or gavage feedings are not tolerated in a normoglycemic, high-risk neonate, refer to neonatal specialist for further care.

Special Considerations

▶ Some drugs, such as beta-adrenergic antagonists, mask symptoms of hypoglycemia.

▶ Men can fast for 72 hours and maintain plasma glucose level above 50 mg/dL, while women exhibit progressive decrease in plasma glucose during prolonged fasting.

▶ Geriatric patients may have blunted autonomic response, and present with confusion and impaired central nervous system (CNS) function.

When to Consult, Refer, Hospitalize

▶ Refer for suspected insulinoma and nesidioblastosis to adult or pediatric surgeon as appropriate.

▶ Consult with physician or refer to endocrinologist for any unknown or uncontrollable cause.

▶ Activate the emergency medical system for all unconscious patients.

Follow-up

▶ Educate patient and family about prevention, symptoms, and treatment of hypoglycemia.

▶ Monitor insulin and sulfonylurea dosage carefully, based on patient's diet and activity.

▶ Monitor children with hypoglycemia for attainment of developmental milestones because intellect can be affected, especially in low birth weight infants and infants of mothers with diabetes.

Expected Course

▶ Variable and dependent on etiology, but favorable prognosis with appropriate treatment

Complications

▶ Brain damage and tissue death from prolonged low glucose level

THYROID DISORDERS

HYPERTHYROIDISM (THYROTOXICOSIS)

Description

▶ Clinical condition caused by increased level of thyroid hormones T4 (thyroxine) and T3 (triiodothyronine)

▶ Manifestations include excessive metabolic activities.

Etiology

▶ Excessive and uncontrolled secretion of thyroid hormone from a variety of causes:

　» Autoimmune Graves' disease (diffuse toxic goiter); most common cause

　» Hyperfunctioning single nodular and multinodular goiter (toxic nodular goiter, Plummer's disease)

　» Solitary hyperfunctioning adenoma; transient subacute thyroiditis; postpartum

　» Drug-induced, such as iodide and iodide-containing drugs (amiodarone) and contrast media

　» Exogenous ingestion of thyroid hormone (factitia)

» Rare causes: Toxic thyroid carcinoma, hCG-secreting tumors (choriocarcinoma, hydatiform mole), TSH-secreting pituitary tumors, testicular embryonal carcinoma

Incidence and Demographics

▶ Graves' disease accounts for > 85% of cases of hyperthyroidism; autoantibodies against diffuse fractions of the gland catalyze accelerated hormone production and release.

▶ Affects women > men, 8:1

▶ Typical age at onset in adulthood: Mid-20s through 30s, but can occur in older adults

▶ Typical age at onset in childhood: 12–14 years, can occur at any age; less likely in neonates

Risk Factors

▶ Family history of thyroid disorders and autoimmune disorders

▶ Thyroid replacement hormone ingestion

▶ Other history of autoimmune disorder

▶ Mother with Graves' disease (neonates)

Prevention and Screening

▶ Monitor TSH and T4 for patients taking thyroid replacement hormones.

Assessment

History

▶ Weight loss, increased appetite, nightmares, hypersensitivity to heat, fatigue, weakness, palpitations

▶ Mental: Insomnia, irritability, nervousness, anxiety, psychosis; in older adults, severe depression

▶ GI: Increased frequency of bowel movements, diarrhea, pernicious vomiting

▶ Medication history, past medical history, and family history of autoimmune diseases

Physical Exam

▶ Adrenergic: Nervousness, sweating, tachycardia, palpitations, tremor, lid lag, excitability

▶ Skin: Onycholysis, myxedema, hyperpigmentation, flushes, diaphoresis, thin or fine hair, spider angiomas

▶ Eyes (only Graves' disease): Periorbital edema, exophthalmos, chemosis, ophthalmoplegia, papilledema, blurred vision, photophobia, diplopia

▶ Neck: Goiter smooth or nodular, thyroid bruit or thrill

▶ Cardiac: Arrhythmia, such as atrial fibrillation, sinus tachycardia, systolic flow murmurs, heart failure, widened pulse pressure

▶ Respiratory: Dyspnea on exertion, tachypnea

▶ Muscle: Proximal myopathy, periodic paralysis, progressive wasting of muscles

▶ Lymph nodes: Lymphadenopathy, splenomegaly

▶ Bone: Osteoporosis, hypercalcemia

▶ Reproductive: Abortion, infertility, abnormal menses, testicular atrophy, gynecomastia

▶ Neurologic: Hyperactive reflexes, tremors

▶ Thyroid storm (rare in children): Hyperpyrexia, tachyarrhythmia, encephalopathy, shock brought on by infection, trauma, noncompliance with antithyroid drugs, or other precipitating event

Diagnostic Studies

▶ TSH decreased or undetectable; free T4 (unbound thyroxine) usually elevated; if normal, order T3 (5% hyperthyroid patients have normal T4); T3 elevated; hypercalcemia; elevated alkaline phosphatase; low hemoglobin and hematocrit; elevated serum antinuclear antibody; elevated TSH receptor antibody

▶ Urine pregnancy test in females if abnormal menses present

▶ CT scan for unilateral eye findings to rule out tumor; ECG in older adult patient

▶ High radioactive iodine uptake scan for Graves' disease, goiter; low radioactive iodine uptake scan for thyroiditis

▶ Thyroid uptake scan or ultrasound for palpable nodules to rule out cold nodule (possibly cancer)

▶ Biopsy

Differential Diagnosis

▶ Psychological disorders (e.g., anxiety, panic, psychosis)

▶ Pheochromocytoma

▶ Infection

▶ Thyrotoxic phase of Hashimoto's thyroiditis

▶ Hormone ingestion

▶ Plummer's disease

▶ Acromegaly

▶ Malignancy

▶ Chronic heart failure

▶ New onset or worsening angina

▶ Orbital tumors (cause exophthalmos)

▶ Myasthenia gravis (ophthalmoplegic changes)

Management

Nonpharmacologic Treatment

▶ Treatment may not be necessary in mild cases.

▶ Surgery is a last option due to complications of hypoparathyroidism and vocal cord paralysis.

▶ Educate parents about thyroid disease if appropriate.

Pharmacologic Treatment

▶ Radioactive iodine (I^{131}) treatment choice for Graves' disease, symptomatic multinodular goiter, and single hyperfunctioning adenoma; treatment of choice in older adults

  » 1–2 doses orally; euthyroid in 2–6 months

» Contraindicated in pregnancy and children

» Hypothyroidism can occur.

► Adjunctive therapy to control symptoms

» Propranolol (Inderal) 10–60 mg q6h to abate catecholamine symptoms; children 1 mg/kg/day

» Atenolol 50–100 mg q.d.; not recommended in children

► Antithyroid medication is often first-line therapy for children

» Propylthiouracil (PTU) 100–150 mg q8h initially, then 50–100 mg b.i.d. maintenance dose

▷ Neonates and children: 5–7 mg/kg/day in divided doses

▷ 6 –12 weeks to reach euthyroid state

▷ Relapses with PTU rarely occur except postpartum

» Methimazole (Tapazole) 20–30 mg q12h initially, then 5–10 mg q.d. or b.i.d. maintenance

▷ Children: 0.4 mg/kg/day in divided doses, then 0.2 mg/kg maintenance dose

▷ 4–6 weeks to reach euthyroid state

» Usually remain on drug for 1–2 years, then gradually withdrawn

» Agranulocytosis: Rare side effect of drugs; order WBC before initiating antithyroid drugs

► Other medications as needed

» Diltiazem (Cardizem) for patients unable to take beta-blockers

» Gradually discontinue as euthyroid develops

» Multivitamin, calcium replacement, and vitamin D rebuild bone density.

» Ophthalmopathy: Eye lubricants for mild cases

Special Considerations

► Older adults may develop arrhythmia (usually atrial fibrillation), CHF, and angina.

► Pregnancy: Thyroid autoantibodies, including TSH receptor antibody, may be ordered.

► Nonthyroidal illnesses, such as active hepatitis, cirrhosis, nephrotic syndrome, infections, malnutrition, and severe acute illness, can affect thyroid functioning serum tests.

► PTU at lowest doses during pregnancy, does not cross placenta

► Spontaneous remission in 25% of children within 2 years, and in 50% of children within 4–5 years; relapse can occur in 30%–40% of cases

When to Consult, Refer, Hospitalize

► Refer to endocrinologist for management of all patients; may co-manage after initial therapy.

► Hospitalize for thyroid storm.

► Pituitary tumor: Immediate referral to neurosurgeon

► Surgical referral for thyroidectomy

► Ophthalmologist for evaluation of eye pathology

Follow-up

▶ Monitor free T4 and TSH every 4–8 weeks until patient becomes euthyroid or hypothyroid, then thyroid replacement therapy

▶ Maintenance visits every 3 months, then 6 months, then annually

▶ After radioactive iodine therapy, order TSH every 6 weeks, 12 weeks, 6 months, then annually

▶ Baseline CBC, LFT every 3–6 months, ECG

Expected Course

▶ Usually requires long-term maintenance for replacement therapy, or follow-up for recurrence after remission

Complications

▶ Thyroid storm

▶ Hypothyroidism following surgery or radiation

▶ Severe depression post-treatment

▶ Visual disturbance from ophthalmopathy

▶ Hypoparathyroidism and vocal cord paralysis postsurgery

HYPOTHYROIDISM

Description

▶ Decreased secretion of thyroid hormone due to dysfunction in thyroid gland or pituitary gland, occurring after the neonatal period

▶ Congenital hypothyroidism is present at birth

Etiology

▶ Primary: Inability of thyroid gland to produce TSH

  ▹ Autoimmune thyroiditis (Hashimoto's) is the most common.

  ▹ Transient hypothyroidism in acute or subacute thyroiditis (viral etiology): Transient postpartum thyroiditis

  ▹ Ablation of gland due to surgery, radiation, thioamide drugs, radioactive iodine

  ▹ Congenital: Ectopic thyroid gland; aplasia of the thyroid gland; ineffective synthesis or utilization of thyroid hormones; transient hypothyroidism related to maternal antithyroid medications or fetal or neonatal exposure to high levels of thyroid hormone; congenital hypopituitarism

  ▹ Iodine deficiency

▶ Secondary: Lesions in pituitary gland (less common)

  ▹ Pituitary adenoma

▹ Certain drugs, such as lithium and para-aminosalicylic acid; previously treated hyperthyroidism, especially postpartum; coexisting autoimmune disorders (lupus, pernicious anemia, rheumatoid arthritis

▶ Tertiary: Thyrotropin-releasing hormone (TRH) deficiency from hypothalamus

Incidence and Demographics

▶ Predominant age > 40; more frequent in women

▶ Hashimoto's thyroiditis can occur < age 3 years but usually > age 6 years, with an increasing incidence in adolescence

▶ Congenital hypothyroidism occurs in 1 in 3,700 live births in North America; more frequent in East Asian and Hispanic descent

Risk Factors

▶ Previous hyperthyroidism treatment

▶ Autoimmune diseases; presence of thyroid antibodies

▶ Family history of thyroid or autoimmune disorders

▶ Pituitary disease; hypothalamic disease

▶ Postpartum women, maternal TSH-binding antibodies

▶ Lithium treatment

▶ Diabetes mellitus type 1 (10% will develop hypothyroidism)

▶ Infertility problems, repeated spontaneous abortions

▶ Fetal or newborn exposure to antithyroid drugs or excessive amounts of iodine

▶ Children with Down, Turner, Klinefelter, or Noonan syndrome

Prevention and Screening

▶ No official screening guidelines; however, periodic TSH screening for patients treated for hyperthyroidism or those who are symptomatic; some clinicians screen adult women > 45 or 50

▶ Mandatory newborn screening at 2–6 days (5%–10% false-negative rate); thyroid dysfunction must be confirmed with a venous sample

▶ Retest children with Down syndrome at age 3 months and periodically thereafter.

▶ Screen those with autoimmune diseases.

Assessment

History

▶ Adults: Anorexia, dry skin, coarse dry hair, alopecia, receding hairline, constipation, cold intolerance, lethargy, increase in weight, irregular or heavy menses, memory loss, depression, muscle aches, paresthesias, medication history (especially lithium)

▶ Neonates: Persistent jaundice, constipation, poor feeding, lethargy or somnolence, prolonged gestation, increased birth weight

▶ Children: Family history, poor growth, learning disabilities or poor school performance, fatigue, constipation, weight gain, cold intolerance

Physical Exam

▶ Weight gain, short stature in pediatric patients, failure to grow, subnormal temperature, decreased level of consciousness

▶ Face: Dull, blank expression, swollen; eyes: periorbital edema; ears: decreased auditory acuity

▶ Skin: Dry skin; coarse, dry hair; brittle nails; hair loss; temporal thinning of eye brows

▶ Mouth: Swollen tongue, slow speech, hoarseness; thyroid: enlarged gland or atrophy, tender, nodules

▶ Cardiac: Bradycardia, decrease heart tones, mild hypotension or diastolic hypertension, cardiomegaly

▶ Respiratory: Dyspnea, pleural effusion

▶ Breasts: Galactorrhea

▶ Electrolytes: Hyponatremia

▶ Abdominal: Hypoactive bowel sounds, ascites

▶ Extremities: Swollen hands and feet, leg edema

▶ Neurologic: Dementia, paranoid ideation, slow or delayed reflexes, cerebellar ataxia, carpal tunnel syndrome

▶ Hematologic: Anemia; hyperlipidemia, hypercholesterolemia

▶ Neonates: Occasional large birth weight, jaundice, large fontanels, respiratory distress, hoarse cry, large abdomen, umbilical hernia (possibly), hypothermia, cool or mottled extremities, bradycardia with murmurs and cardiomegaly, anemia

Diagnostic Studies

▶ TSH assay (use third-generation assay): Elevated in primary hypothyroidism; TSH will be low in cases due to pituitary insufficiency

▶ Order free T4 when TSH elevated; low free T4 confirms diagnosis of hypothyroidism.

▶ Subclinical hypothyroidism: Normal T4 and elevated TSH

▶ If secondary to pituitary or hypothalamic failure: Normal TSH, low or mildly elevated T4

▶ Further tests when secondary hypothyroidism suspected, such as serum prolactin level, neuroradiologic studies, pituitary-adrenal and pituitary-gonadal function

▶ CBC, serum electrolytes, BUN, creatinine, glucose, calcium, phosphate, albumin levels, pregnancy test, urine protein, lipid studies as indicated

▶ Free thyroxine index (FTI) in most cases provides indirect estimate of T4

▶ Children: Bone age if short stature is suspected

▶ Neonates: Thyroid scan

Differential Diagnosis

- Depression
- Obesity
- Dementia
- Ischemic heart disease
- Chronic heart failure (CHF)
- Kidney failure
- Cirrhosis
- Nephrotic syndrome

- Chronic renal disease
- Coexisting secondary cause
- Congenital hypothyroidism
- Transient hypothyroidism
- Hypopituitarism
- Sick euthyroid
- Iodine ingestion
- Thyroid hormone resistance

Management

Nonpharmacologic Treatment

- Education, high-fiber diet for constipation, diet and exercise for weight loss if obese
- Avoid drug interactions: Cholestyramine (Questran); ferrous sulfate; aluminum hydroxide antacids; sucralfate; foods such as cabbage, turnips, kale, and soybeans that increase the loss of thyroid hormone, because they may interfere with levothyroxine absorption, should be spaced 4 hours from these medications
- Take medication in the morning on an empty stomach to increase absorption.
- For congenital hypothyroidism, monitor growth and development and be alert for signs of behavior changes.

Pharmacologic Treatment

- Primary hypothyroidism: Correct hormone deficiency with thyroxine replacement.
    - Levothyroxine (Synthroid; T4) first-line therapy for primary hypothyroidism
    - Adults: Starting dose 50–100 mcg p.o. q.d., increase 25 mcg every 1–3 weeks based on clinical condition and laboratory results. Average dose 125 mcg q.d. with maximum dose of 300 mcg.
    - Older adults with coronary artery disease: Start levothyroxine at 25–50 mcg p.o. q.d. with gradual increase every 4–6 weeks as tolerated, maximum dose of 75–150 mcg.
- Children: Congenital hypothyroidism is a true endocrine emergency; goal is to begin therapy by 14 days of life.
    - Levothyroxine at 2–5 mcg/kg/day; recheck T4 and TSH at 1 month and titrate to maintain normal levels.
- Subclinical hypothyroidism
    - Treat pharmacologically if TSH > 10 mU/mL with presence of thyroid autoantibodies.
    - Just monitor older adults, due to risk of coronary artery disease (CAD) with treatment.
- Transient, subacute hypothyroidism
    - Self-limited with symptoms resolving after 2–3 months
    - No therapy for minimal symptoms

▶ Congenital hypothyroidism

» Initially, levothyroxine 10–15 mcg/kg/day p.o.; recheck thyroid function tests within 2–3 weeks (goal: raise T4 and decrease TSH; TSH may not decrease to normal levels for several months, despite normal T4)

» Management is usually with a pediatric endocrinologist.

» May consider stopping levothyroxine at age 2–3 years in children with congenital hypothyroidism to reevaluate, if medication was started before a thyroid scan or if child had a normal gland on initial scan

» Hashimoto's thyroiditis may be self-limited in older children; reevaluate periodically throughout life.

Special Considerations

▶ Adults: Concomitant use of CNS depressants, digoxin, insulin may decrease efficacy of thyroid replacement dosage; older adults are at risk for angina as thyroid levels increase.

▶ Pregnancy: If hypothyroidism is present during pregnancy, monitor TSH every trimester.

▶ Children: T4 may be normally low and TSH high in premature infants; soy-based formula may interfere with absorption of levothyroxine; untreated hypothyroidism in children leads to facial edema, hirsute forehead, growth delays, and mental retardation or intellectual development disorder.

When to Consult, Refer, Hospitalize

▶ Refer developing myxedema coma, hypothermia, decreased mentation, respiratory acidosis, hypotension, hyponatremia, hypoglycemia, hypoventilation, significant cardiac disease, secondary hypothyroidism, or radically abnormal thyroid function tests to an endocrinologist.

▶ Consult or refer for co-management of congenital hypothyroidism.

▶ Refer pregnant and pediatric patients to an endocrinologist for ongoing management.

▶ Hospitalization is not usually required.

Follow-up

▶ Adults: Measure TSH 4–6 weeks after initial dosage, then every 2 months until within normal limits, then every 6–12 months (TSH levels may remain elevated for several months despite effective treatment); if drug dosage changed, recheck TSH levels in 2–3 months.

▶ Annual lipid levels

Expected Course

▶ Improvement within 1 month of starting medication; symptoms resolve within 3–6 months

▶ Treatment usually lifelong; maintain medication at lowest dosage to maintain euthyroid state

▶ Excellent prognosis with appropriate treatment

Complications

▶ Chronic heart failure

▶ Depression, psychoses

▶ Miscarriages during pregnancy

▶ Thyrotoxicity, myxedema coma (rare)

▶ Bone demineralization due to overtreatment

▶ Mental retardation or intellectual developmental disorder in children

THYROID NODULE

Description

▶ Localized enlargements within thyroid gland; may function independently of hypothalamic-pituitary feedback

▶ Evaluation of thyroid nodule is important to detect thyroid cancer.

Etiology

▶ Unknown

▶ Autonomously functioning nodules (hot nodule on thyroid scan) are usually benign and may cause symptoms of hyperthyroidism.

▶ Nonfunctioning nodule (cold nodule) may be malignant carcinoma.

Incidence and Demographics

▶ Solitary nodules in 4%–7% of U.S. population

  » More common with age, women, exposure to ionizing radiation, living in areas with iodine deficiency

▶ < 10% of solitary nodules are malignant.

▶ 10,000–20,000 new cases of thyroid cancer per year

▶ Papillary carcinoma 75% of thyroid cancers; follicular carcinoma (aggressive) < 10% of thyroid cancers

▶ Papillary nodules twice as common in women than men; slow-growing

▶ Cysts comprise 15%–25% of thyroid nodules.

▶ Uncommon in children; if they occur, usually asymptomatic and 25%–75% malignant

Risk Factors

▶ For thyroid nodule

  » Female, increasing age, residing in area of endemic iodine deficiency

▶ For thyroid cancer

  » Family history of thyroid cancer or multiple endocrine metaplastic type II carcinoma

  » Male gender, extremes in age (< 15 and > 70)

  » Exposure of head, neck or chest to radiation

  » Single nodule

Assessment

History

▶ Hoarseness, cough, dysphagia, obstruction, neck tenderness, neck swelling or enlargement

▶ History of hypo- or hyperthyroidism; external radiation to head, neck, chest; or nuclear fallout

▶ Family history of thyroid disease

▶ Medication history

▶ Pregnancy status

▶ Benign or malignant nodules often asymptomatic but may have symptoms of hypo- or hyperthyroidism

Physical Exam

▶ Malignant: Hoarseness; enlarged cervical lymph nodes; dyspnea; tumor palpable as fixed, painless, hard, irregular-shaped mass; does not move with swallowing

▶ Benign: Multiple nodules palpable (nodular Hashimoto's thyroiditis or multinodular goiter)

Diagnostic Studies

▶ Fine-needle biopsy aspiration initial test with palpable nodules > 1.5 cm

▶ Serum TSH; if low, order free T4

▶ Multinodular goiter is usually euthyroid

▶ Radionuclide scans to determine cytologic results; hot nodules are benign in 98% of cases; 5%–10% of cold nodules are malignant (meaning decreased amount of radionuclide uptake).

▶ Ultrasound to determine if cystic

▶ Serum calcitonin with family history of medullary thyroid carcinoma

▶ Evaluate anithyroperoxidase antibodies and antithyroglobulin antibodies to rule out thyroiditis

Differential Diagnosis

▶ Malignant nodules vs. benign nodules   ▶ Thyroiditis

▶ Cysts

Management

Nonpharmacologic Treatment

▶ Adequate iodine intake

▶ Surgery for malignant or disfiguring tumors

▶ Carefully follow patients with benign nodules (see Follow-up)

▶ Instruct patients to follow up for size changes, lymphadenopathy, dysphasia, hoarseness, or new or worsening symptoms of hypo- or hyperthyroidism.

Pharmacologic Treatment

▶ Treat abnormal thyroid hormone levels following guidelines for hypo- and hyperthyroidism.

Special Considerations

▶ Pregnancy and lactation: Avoid radionuclide scan.

When to Consult, Refer, Hospitalize

▶ Refer all patients with thyroid nodules to endocrinologist for evaluation to rule out malignancy.

Follow-up

▶ Reevaluate euthyroid patients with benign nodules annually to check size and TSH.

▶ Benign nodules with abnormal thyroid function require frequent monitoring according to hypothyroidism and hyperthyroidism guidelines.

▶ Patients with malignancy must be followed up by an endocrinologist and possibly oncologist.

Expected Course

▶ Good survival rate with malignant nodules unless due to follicular carcinoma

Complications

▶ Tumor recurrence

▶ Hypo- or hyperthyroidism

ADRENAL DISORDERS

CUSHING'S SYNDROME

Description

▶ Syndrome of clinical abnormalities resulting from exogenous glucocorticoid excess (mainly cortisol)

▶ Due to endogenous hypercorticosolism related to adrenal or pituitary dysfunction

Etiology

▶ Excess glucocorticoid production caused by adrenocorticotrophic hormone (ACTH)–secreting pituitary tumor (⅔ of cases), ectopic production by a nonpituitary tumor (small cell carcinoma of lung), or ACTH-independent adrenal tumor

▶ Prolonged use of glucocorticoids

▶ Serum concentration of glucocorticoids is regulated by the negative-feedback loop of the hypothalamic-pituitary-adrenal (HPA) system. Corticotropin-releasing hormone (CRH)

stimulates the production and release of ACTH by the anterior pituitary, which stimulates the adrenal cortex to produce cortisol. Cortisol levels increase in response to increased ACTH levels and will decrease in response to decreasing ACTH levels.

Incidence and Demographics

▶ Cushing's syndrome and primary adrenal tumors more common in women

▶ Pituitary tumors 5 times more frequent in women than men

▶ Age of onset 20–40 years

▶ Rare in childhood and infancy

Risk Factors

▶ Adrenal tumor

▶ Pituitary tumor

▶ Long-term or frequent high-dose corticosteroid use

Prevention and Screening

▶ Limit corticosteroid use

▶ Screen for unprescribed steroid use.

Assessment

History

▶ Acne, back pain, headache, emotional lability, depression, mental changes, muscle weakness, fatigue, poor wound healing, thin skin, menstrual disorders or amenorrhea, hyperglycemia, susceptibility to infections, weight gain, easy bruising, decreased libido, insomnia

▶ Therapeutic or factitious use of corticosteroids

Physical Exam

▶ High blood pressure

▶ Truncal obesity with thin extremities, dorsal fat pad ("buffalo hump"), moon face

▶ Skin: Thin, atrophic, acne, hirsutism, ecchymosis, hyperpigmentation; purple striae around breasts, abdomen, thighs

▶ Eyes: Increased intraocular pressure

▶ Musculoskeletal: Weakness, atrophy of muscles, thinning bones

Diagnostic Studies

▶ Glycosuria and elevated urine cortisol (24-hour urine for free cortisol)

▶ Plasma cortisol level elevated evenings (> 5–7.5 mcg/dL)

▶ Serum glucose elevated, hypokalemia without hypernatremia

▶ Screening tests: Refer to endocrinologist.

▸ Dexamethasone overnight suppression test: Suppression cortisol level < 5 mcg/dL normal result. If abnormal, more reliable suppression test performed by giving dexamethasone 0.5 mg p.o. q6h for 2 days

▶ CT scans, chest and abdomen, for adrenal tumors and MRI for pituitary tumors

Differential Diagnosis

▶ Alcoholism

▶ Obesity

▶ Depression

▶ Familial cortisol resistance

▶ Hirsutism

▶ Anorexia nervosa

▶ Drugs such as phenytoin, phenobarbital, primidone accelerate dexamethasone metabolism, causing "false-positive" dexamethasone suppression test

Management

Nonpharmacologic Treatment

▶ High-protein diet

▶ Reduce pituitary ACTH by transsphenoidal resection or radiation.

▶ Reduce adrenal cortisol secretion by bilateral adrenalectomy.

▶ Surgically remove ectopic ACTH-secreting tumors.

Pharmacologic Treatment

▶ Refer to endocrinologist for ongoing management.

▶ Replacement glucocorticoid therapy up to 1 year post adrenal surgery, lifelong if bilateral adrenalectomy

▶ Patient taken off glucocorticoid therapy may need to restart if they become ill.

Special Considerations

▶ Pregnancy can exacerbate symptoms.

When to Consult, Refer, Hospitalize

▶ Refer all cases to endocrinologist and coordinate their primary care.

▶ Refer to surgeon and oncologist for adrenal or pituitary tumor.

Follow-up

▶ For recurrence of symptoms, measure urine-free cortisol.

Expected Course

▶ Posttreatment for pituitary adenoma: Normal ACTH suppressed and requires 6–36 months to recover to normal function; hydrocortisone replacement therapy necessary

▶ Normal HPA function within 3–24 months after surgery if one adrenal gland left

▶ 10%–20% failure rate with transsphenoidal surgery; patients with complete remission will have 15%–20% recurrence rate over next 10 years

Complications

▶ Hypertension, CAD

▶ Osteoporosis, compression fractures of spine, aseptic necrosis of femur head

▶ Diabetes mellitus

▶ Overwhelming infection

▶ Nephrolithiasis

▶ Psychosis

▶ If untreated, morbidity and death

ADRENAL INSUFFICIENCY AND ADDISON'S DISEASE

Description

▶ Primary adrenal insufficiency is a loss of all adrenal hormones, including mineralocorticoids, glucocorticoids, and adrenal androgens. It is an insidious, chronic disease of adrenal destruction, also known as Addison's disease or primary adrenal failure.

▶ Secondary adrenal insufficiency is a lack of glucocorticoids due to pituitary dysfunction.

▶ Tertiary adrenal insufficiency is lack of glucocorticoids caused by hypothalamic failure.

Etiology

▶ Autoimmune destruction of the adrenal gland accounts for 80% of Addison's disease, followed by tuberculosis as second leading cause.

▶ Rarer causes include AIDS and other infections, genetic disorder, carcinoma, amyloid disease, hemochromatosis, antineoplastic chemotherapy, and bilateral adrenal hemorrhage, or it may be idiopathic.

▶ Secondary and tertiary adrenal insufficiency result from suppression of HPA axis through glucocorticoid replacement or adrenalectomy; pituitary tumor, trauma, surgery, or infarction; or hypothalamic disease.

Incidence and Demographics

▶ Usually affects those age 30–50, but may occur at any age; females > males

▶ Prevalence approximately 4:100,000

Risk Factors

▶ Autoimmune disease

▶ Family history of adrenal insufficiency

▶ Prolonged steroid use followed by infection, trauma, surgery

▶ Medications: Ketoconazole, Dilantin, rifampin, opiates

Assessment

History

▶ Progressive weakness, fatigue, weight loss, lightheadedness, anorexia, possible nausea and vomiting, diarrhea, cold intolerance, abdominal pain (like peptic ulcer disease), salt craving, emotional changes

Physical Exam

▶ Postural hypotension

▶ 90% systolic blood pressure < 110 mm Hg and rarely > 130 mm Hg

▶ Skin: Hyperpigmentation (especially hand creases, knuckles, elbows, buccal mucosa) in Whites, multiple freckles, change in body hair distribution with scant axillary and pubic hair, areas of vitiligo

▶ Breasts: Dark nipples and areola

▶ Cardiac: Small heart

▶ Lymph: Hyperplasia, lymphadenopathy

▶ Acute adrenal insufficiency or Addisonian crisis may present with profound fatigue, dehydration, severe abdominal pain, nausea and vomiting, hypotension, hypoglycemia, and shock with vascular collapse and renal shut-down, and is precipitated by surgery, infection, exacerbation of comorbid illness, or sudden withdrawal of long-term glucocorticoid replacement.

Diagnostic Studies

▶ Diagnostic: Low plasma cortisol < 5 mcg/dL at 8 a.m.

▶ Sodium, chloride, glucose, and bicarbonate levels low with high potassium level

▶ BUN, plasma renin, ACTH, calcium all elevated

▶ CBC, decreased hemoglobin, neutrophils, and eosinophils

▶ Serum anti-adrenal antibodies in 50% cases of autoimmune Addison's disease

▶ ECG: Nonspecific changes

▶ EEG: Generalized slowing

▶ Abdominal CT scan: Small adrenals

▶ Chest X-ray: Small heart size and adrenal calcification

Differential Diagnosis

▶ Hyperparathyroidism

▶ Depression

▶ Mild thyrotoxicosis in elderly

▶ Gastrointestinal malignancy

▶ Chronic infection

▶ Heavy metal poisoning

▶ Hemochromatosis, anemia

▶ Salt-wasting nephritis

▶ Myopathies

▶ ACTH-secreting tumors

Management

Nonpharmacologic Treatment

▶ Monitor fluid and electrolytes.

▶ Ensure adequate dietary intake of sodium.

▶ Treat all infections immediately and vigorously and raise cortisol dose.

Pharmacologic Treatment

▶ Chronic phase: Management initiated by endocrinologist; replace deficient hormones

▶ Cortisol 10–20 mg p.o. every morning; 5–10 mg p.o. at 4–6 p.m. (total of 15–25 mg of hydrocortisone daily in two divided doses with ⅔ morning and ⅓ afternoon) *or* prednisone 3 mg p.o. every morning, 2 mg p.o. every evening

  » Dose will be increased in case of stress, trauma, surgery, stressful diagnostic procedures, postural hypotension, hyperkalemia, or weight loss.

▶ Fludrocortisone acetate 0.05–0.3 mg p.o. q.d. or q.o.d. for cases of primary adrenal insufficiency if insufficient sodium retention with cortisol alone

  » If edema, hypokalemia, or hypertensive crisis occurs, lower dose.

  » Salt additives for excess heat or humidity

▶ Acute adrenal insufficiency: Hospitalize for IV hydrocortisone, mineralocorticoid, and normal saline.

When to Consult, Refer, Hospitalize

▶ Refer all suspected cases to endocrinologist for management.

▶ Hospitalize for acute crisis, dehydration, severe stress.

Follow-up

▶ Periodic evaluations of blood pressure, weight, electrolytes and other labs, muscle strength, appetite, cardiac status

▶ MedicAlert or similar identification bracelet or necklace

Expected Course

▶ Excellent prognosis with lifelong steroid replacement therapy

Complications

▶ Acute adrenal crisis

▶ Complications of steroid therapy: Osteoporosis, psychosis, hyperglycemia, Cushing's syndrome

PITUITARY DISORDERS

PITUITARY ADENOMA

Description

▶ Pituitary adenoma or tumor can manifest by disturbance of function (hyper- or hyposecretion of trophic hormones), anatomic invasion into surrounding structures (enlargement of tumors), or a combination.

▶ Microadenoma is < 10 mm and macroadenoma is > 10 mm in size.

Etiology

▶ Largely unknown

▶ Occasionally part of multiple endocrine neoplasia type 1 (MEN1) syndrome, autosomal dominant chromosomal mutation

▶ If adenoma is secretory, usually only one hormone is secreted (frequently growth hormone, ACTH, or prolactin), causing characteristic symptoms. Secretion of prolactin (common) causes syndrome of hyperprolactinemia.

Incidence and Demographics

▶ More frequent in women

▶ Growth hormone secretion with gigantism almost always occurs in males.

▶ Fairly common and may be asymptomatic; often found on autopsy

Assessment

History

▶ Headaches, visual field loss due to pituitary enlargement; rare: loss of consciousness, seizures, mental state changes, brainstem dysfunction

▶ Amenorrhea, infertility, galactorrhea, impotence due to hyperprolactinemia

▶ Symptoms of Cushing's syndrome with ACTH secretion (acne, weight gain, depression)

▶ Symptoms of acromegaly with growth hormone secretion (enlargement of head and face, feet and hands)

Physical Exam

▶ Body habitus for signs of gigantism, acromegaly, Cushing's syndrome

▶ Eyes: Ocular motor dysfunctions, pupillary dysfunction, limited visual fields

▶ Breast exam: Bilateral galactorrhea (milky discharge)

Diagnostic Studies

▶ Serum prolactin, growth hormone, adrenal steroids may be elevated

  » Prolactin should be considered for complaint of headache with visual changes, amenorrhea, or galactorrhea.

▶ MRI of brain preferred over CT scan for pituitary imaging; angiography, visual field testing

　　» Imaging indicated for men or women with serum prolactin > 200 ng/mL.

Differential Diagnosis

▶ Pituitary inflammation

▶ Other causes of headache

▶ Other causes of amenorrhea and galactorrhea

▶ Aneurysm

▶ Cushing's syndrome

Management

Nonpharmacologic Treatment

▶ Transsphenoidal surgery or stereotactic radiosurgery to remove pituitary adenoma

▶ Radiation to pituitary

Pharmacologic Treatment

▶ Dopamine agonist bromocriptine (Parlodel) for hyperprolactinemia; may shrink tumors by 50% in 40% of patients within 3 months; treatment many be long-term. Withdrawal from drug may result in recurrent hyperprolactinemia.

▶ Octreotide (Sandostatin), a somatotropin for treatment of acromegaly

▶ Postoperative substitution, including adrenal steroids, thyroxin, and testosterone or estrogen may be given.

Special Considerations

▶ Stop bromocriptine treatment with pregnancy and lactation.

When to Consult, Refer, Hospitalize

▶ Refer all suspected cases to endocrinologist; neurologist if surgery indicated.

Follow-up

▶ MRI scans at 6 months, 12 months, and annually for patients treated with bromocriptine

▶ Growth of tumor indicates need for surgery or radiation therapy.

Expected Course

▶ Possible recurrence within 5–10 years

Complications

▶ Hypopituitarism

▶ Pituitary hemorrhage, infarct

▶ Diabetes insipidus

▶ Surgical complications including infertility and cessation of menstruation

SHORT STATURE

Description

▶ Genetic: Height below the 3rd percentile (or 2.5 standard deviations below the norm) with no known etiology with appropriate growth in relation to parents' heights; normal growth rate and bone age

▶ Constitutional delay in growth also a normal variant of short stature: Well child who is short, takes longer to get to his or her eventual height (which is usually average height), with a biologically slower maturation and delay in puberty; delayed bone age by about 2 years; often progresses to delayed puberty; parents' heights are normal; predicted final height is comparable to target height.

▶ Turner's syndrome: Short stature in females due to absence or abnormality of an X chromosome

Etiology

▶ Genetic: Usually normal variant; possible genetic tendency toward growth hormone (GH) deficiency or GH receptor defect; possible inherited pathologic condition, e.g., hypochondroplasia

▶ Constitutional delay in growth: Often no known cause; possible causes include decreased GH secretion, abnormal GH structure, GH receptor defect

▶ Turner's syndrome: Absence or defect of an X chromosome, usually 45,X (monosomy) or 46,XX (mosaicism)

Incidence and Demographics

▶ Genetic: 3% of all normal children are below the 3rd–5th percentile in height; equal incidence in boys and girls

▶ Constitutional delay in growth: Increased incidence in boys

▶ Turner's syndrome: Occurs in 1 in 2,000 live female births (no males)

Risk Factors

▶ Genetic: Parents who are below the 3rd–5th percentile in height or with a pathologic cause for short height (e.g., hypochondroplasia)

▶ Constitutional delay in growth: Usually a positive family history of growth delay

▶ Turner's syndrome: No known risk factors

Prevention and Screening

▶ No known prevention

▶ Assess parents' heights.

▶ Fetal ultrasound may detect abnormality associated with Turner's syndrome (no known prevention).

▶ Amniocentesis or chorionic villus sampling may detect Turner's syndrome, but also has the potential to overdiagnose an X-chromosome abnormality.

Assessment

History

▶ Genetic: Normal birth size; no intrauterine growth retardation; short parents below the 3rd–5th percentile with or without known pathologic reason

▶ Constitutional delay in growth: Normal birth weight and size; gradual decrease in rate of growth in first 2 years of life, then maintains growth curve approximately 2 standard deviations (SDs) below normal

▶ Turner's syndrome: No family history, slightly small birth size, puffy hands and feet in neonatal period; short stature with a marked deviation of a decreased height on the normal growth curve

Physical Exam

▶ Genetic: Gradual decrease in growth rate within the first 2 years of life; normal growth rate after age 2 years; normal onset of puberty

▶ Constitutional delay: Aside from short stature, healthy; reduced growth rate until about age 2 years secondary to delayed bone age; in early adolescence, rate of growth decreases secondary to delayed puberty but then resumes after onset of puberty with some catch-up growth noted (see Table 17–5)

▶ Turner's syndrome: Short stature, small jaw, short or webbed neck (20%–30% cases), high arched palate; absence of or delayed puberty with ovarian failure; skeletal abnormalities; possible cardiovascular and renal abnormalities; recurrent otitis media, hearing loss, Hashimoto's thyroiditis, usually normal intelligence

▶ Height should be assessed on a carefully calibrated scale with a built-in level for children and on measuring boards for infants.

Diagnostic Studies

▶ X-rays for bone age: Normal in genetic, delayed in constitutional delay

▶ Check for decreased serum GH and GH receptor defect.

▶ Diagnostic tests for Turner syndrome should be directed by a pediatric endocrinologist and may include chromosomal karyotype, FSH and LH, thyroid function tests, glucose tolerance test, echocardiogram, and renal and pelvic ultrasound.

Differential Diagnoses

▶ Constitutional short stature
▶ Familial short stature
▶ Malnutrition
▶ Chronic renal failure
▶ GI malabsorption
▶ Skeletal defects
▶ Pulmonary disease
▶ Cardiac disease
▶ Failure to thrive
▶ Metabolic diseases
▶ DM type 1
▶ Anemia
▶ Hypothyroidism
▶ GH deficiency
▶ Turner's syndrome
▶ IUGR
▶ Chromosomal abnormalities

TABLE 17–5
COMPARISON OF NORMAL VARIANTS

	FAMILIAL SHORT STATURE	CONSTITUTIONAL DELAY
Parents	Short (or family history)	Average height
Birth History and Early Years	Normal; often born at 25th–75th percentile followed by a deceleration period until age 2, at which point they are in 3rd–5th percentile	Same growth shift as genetic short stature
Growth Velocity	Steady after age 2 to adulthood; parallels growth curve	Steady until puberty and because pubertal growth spurt is delayed, begins to fall further in growth chart
Puberty Changes	Normal age	Males: Failure to achieve Tanner genital 2 by age 13.8 years, or Tanner pubic 2 by 15.6 years. Females: Failure to achieve Tanner breast 2 by age 13.3 years
Bone Age	Normal	Delayed (usually 2–4 years)
Ultimate Height	Short	Average (can be tall) Males > 163 cm (64 inches) Females > 150 cm (59 inches)
Diagnostic Studies	All normal	All normal except delayed bone age; a more extensive work-up likely will be done because of the delayed puberty
Treatment	Reassurance	None

Management

Nonpharmacologic Treatment

▶ Genetic: No treatment is necessary because this is usually a normal variant; occasional uses of subcutaneous injections of GH have not proven to significantly increase final height

▶ Reassurance that child is healthy aside from short stature

Pharmacologic Treatment

▶ Constitutional delay: Treatment with injections of GH occasionally renders a brief increase in growth, but is unclear whether final height is truly affected; appropriate time to discontinue therapy is controversial.

▶ Adolescents with constitutional delay may be treated with low doses of androgen.

▶ Turner's syndrome: Use hormone replacement at puberty, GH therapy, and anabolic steroid therapy managed by a pediatric endocrinologist.

Special Considerations

▶ Educate families that growth hormone treatment will not make their child tall but will restore the normal growth pattern.

When to Consult, Refer, or Hospitalize

▶ Consult with pediatrician or pediatric endocrinologist for evaluation and diagnosis; no further referral needed for genetic short stature.

▶ Constitutional delay and Turner's syndrome: Refer to pediatric endocrinologist for management.

Follow-up

▶ Continue to assess growth and development in routine physical exams.

▶ Follow up with pediatric endocrinologist and other pediatric specialists as appropriate for clinical manifestations.

▶ Periodic monitoring of thyroid function in all ages and lipid levels in adults is indicated at 6-month intervals for patients treated with GH who have constitutional delay.

▶ Carefully monitor bone maturation and serum glucose levels in patients with Turner's syndrome.

PUBERTAL DISORDERS

Normal onset of puberty is 8–13 years in girls and 9–14 years in boys; see Table 3–10 for classification of sexual maturity (Tanner staging).

PRECOCIOUS PUBERTY

Description

▶ Early onset of pubertal changes (secondary sexual development)

　▫ Girls < 6–8 years of age

　▫ Boys < 9 years of age

▶ Normal development sequence is thelarche followed closely by pubarche and menarche 2–3 years later.

▶ Normal variants of early onset puberty

　▫ Premature thelarche: Benign breast development (typically Tanner 2), usually in toddlers (see next section)

　▫ Premature adrenarche: Small amounts of pubic hair < age 8 in girls and < age 9 in boys (possibly axillary hair and body odor); no growth spurt, breast development, testicular enlargement (needs to be differentiated from true and pseudo precocious puberty)

Etiology

▶ True precocious puberty or central precocious puberty (CPP) results from premature activation of the hypothalamic-pituitary-gonadal axis; referred to as gonadotropin-releasing hormone–dependent. Hypothalamic-pituitary (CNS) stimulation of gonads produces estrogen and testosterone, which induces the pubertal changes. May be:

- » Idiopathic: No identifiable cause (system turns on spontaneously at an earlier than expected age); 75% of precocious puberty in females is idiopathic; approximately 33% in males
- » Neurogenic: Damage to areas of the CNS that affect the hypothalamic pituitary axis and may include CNS tumors, infections, trauma, radiation, cerebral malformations, hydrocephalus, seizure disorders, neurofibromatosis, and tuberous sclerosis

► Pseudo (or peripheral) precocious puberty

- » Cause is from a source outside the central hypothalamic-pituitary system, such as the ovaries or adrenals; hypothalamic-pituitary system is not activated and does not mature
- » Results in the same secretion of pubertal amounts of estrogen and testosterone
- » Can occur from ovarian or testicular tumors, liver tumors (hepatomas), congenital adrenal hyperplasia, exposure to exogenous sex steroids from food (e.g., soybeans), drugs (e.g., oral contraceptives or estrogen-containing creams), or familial trait (e.g., familial testotoxicosis)

Incidence and Demographics

► More common in girls than in boys

► Usually idiopathic in girls

► In boys, approximately 50% related to a tumor, congenital adrenal hyperplasia, or familial testotoxicosis

Risk Factors

► CNS insult

► Family history

Prevention and Screening

► No known prevention

Assessment

History

► Pubertal changes: Age of onset, progression and specific symptoms (e.g., breast budding, hair, menses)

► Symptoms of possible underlying etiology such as headaches, weight loss, fatigue, and constipation (hypothyroid)

► History of CNS insult (meningitis, radiation)

► Exogenous sources of hormones

► Family history of early-onset puberty

Physical Exam

- ▶ Assess all pubertal changes: Breast development, testicular size, pubic hair staging, presence of adult body odor, acne, any growth spurt (plot on growth chart)
- ▶ Obtain blood pressure: Increased blood pressure may be consistent with increased intracranial pressure or congenital adrenal hyperplasia.
- ▶ Thorough neurologic exam, including funduscopic exam (papilledema), visual acuity, and visual fields
- ▶ Palpate scrotum and testicles for any masses; abdomen for possible hepatomegaly or enlarged ovary or uterus
- ▶ Assess skin for café-au-lait spots, myxedema
- ▶ Palpate thyroid

Diagnostic Studies

- ▶ Results of tests will vary depending on the etiology.
- ▶ Levels of FSH and LH are usually in the prepubertal ranges with true precocious puberty; therefore, to document the premature activation of the hypothalamic-pituitary axis, a gonadotropin-stimulating test must be obtained. If premature activation has occurred, an increase in LH in response to a GnRH stimulation (i.e., serum concentration > 10 IU/L 30–40 minutes after administering GnRH SQ) will occur. A positive response indicates the presence of true precocious puberty (not the cause but the presence). If LH/FSH is high, follow with prolactin.
- ▶ In both true and pseudo precocious puberty, levels of testosterone or estradiol will be elevated. Levels are normal for normal variants such as premature adrenarche.
- ▶ Adrenal androgens, particularly dehydroepiandrosterone sulfate (DHEAS), are obtained to rule out congenital adrenal hyperplasia. Levels would be elevated.
- ▶ Thyroid function studies (free T4 and TSH) if hypothyroidism suspected
- ▶ Bone age should be obtained on all patients to assist with determining etiology (e.g., advanced with true precocious puberty, normal with normal variants), height potential, and whether treatment is warranted; may need to be repeated in the follow-up of patients.
- ▶ Pelvic and testicular ultrasounds may be obtained to rule out tumors.
- ▶ Cranial CT scan or MRI of the hypothalamic-pituitary region can determine tumors or structural abnormalities.
- ▶ CT scan of the adrenals if adrenal tumor suspected

Differential Diagnosis

- ▶ Premature thelarche
- ▶ Premature adrenarche
- ▶ Ovarian tumors
- ▶ Ovarian cysts
- ▶ Adrenal tumors
- ▶ McCune-Albright syndrome
- ▶ Exogenous sex steroids
- ▶ Congenital adrenal hyperplasia
- ▶ Familial testotoxicosis (Leydig cell tumors)
- ▶ Cerebral lesions

Management

Nonpharmacologic Treatment

▶ Treatment directed at underlying cause

▶ Reassurance if pubescent or postpubescent if evaluation negative and lack of pathology

▶ Referral to surgeon if fibrous tissue present causing breast enlargement, or breast mass present

▶ Weight reduction

Pharmacologic Treatment

▶ Anti-estrogens (tamoxifen, clomiphene), dehydrotestosteroney

▶ Eliminate or decrease any medication that may have a side effect of gynecomastia.

▶ Treat specific hormone disorders.

Special Considerations

▶ None

When to Consult, Refer, Hospitalize

▶ Refer to adult endocrinologist if diameter > 4 cm or abnormalities persist > 2 years, physical abnormalities in addition to gynecomastia, males > 18 years, or history or work-up compatible with pathologic origin.

▶ Urologist if cryptorchidism, testicular neoplasm

▶ Surgeon for removal of mass if indicated

Follow-up

▶ Pubescent males every 3–6 months

▶ Watch for signs of abnormal progression of puberty, chronic illness, or emotional or psychological disorders.

▶ Perform or repeat diagnostic work-up if clinical picture changes.

Expected Course

▶ Pubescent males should normalize within a 2-year period.

▶ Usually good prognosis

Complications

▶ Self-image problems

▶ Increased risk of breast cancer in patients with Klinefelter's syndrome

OBESITY

Description

▶ Condition involving accumulation of excess adipose tissue > 20% over ideal body weight or body mass index (BMI) > 30

Etiology

▶ May be secondary to disease processes or a primary result of overeating and inadequate exercise

▶ Genetic predisposition; 60% risk of obesity if one parent obese, 90% risk if both

▶ Multifactorial, including environmental and psychological factors

▶ Abdominal fat (visceral fat) is associated with metabolic disorders (diabetes mellitus, Cushing's syndrome) and cardiovascular disease.

▶ Hip and thigh fat (subcutaneous fat) more common in women and pose less medical risk than abdominal fat

▶ Waist measurements > 35 inches in women and > 40 inches in men pose significant health risk for cardiovascular disease; risk of death increases with BMI > 30.

▶ Secondary causes such as adrenal problems, hypothyroid, polycystic ovary disease cause < 1% of cases

▶ Many medications cause increased appetite and weight gain, including steroids, antidepressants, hormones, mood stabilizers, and antipsychotics.

Incidence and Demographics

▶ Most prevalent chronic medical disorder in world

▶ Incidence and prevalence increasing in all genders and ages

▶ One-third of U.S. population obese

▶ Prevalence rates higher in Hispanic and Black women, Asian and Pacific Islanders, Native Americans, Native Hawaiians, and Alaskan Natives

▶ Childhood obesity has more than doubled in children and tripled in adolescents in the past 30 years.

　▹ Data from 2010 show children 6–11 years in the U.S. who were obese increased from 7% in 1980 to almost 18% in 2010. Adolescents age 12–19 years who were obese increased from 5% to 18% over the same period.

▶ New onset in elderly is rare, requires investigation

Risk Factors

▶ Overeating or other poor dietary habits

▶ Sedentary lifestyle

▶ Genetic predisposition

Prevention and Screening

▶ Balanced dietary intake throughout life span

▶ Exercise regularly

Assessment

History

▶ Obtain weight history of life span.

▶ Collect comprehensive diet history including food categories, amount of servings, number of meals per day, fluid intake, snacks.

▶ Exercise history

▶ Motivation to lose weight and prior attempts to lose weight

▶ Smoking and alcohol intake

▶ Occupational history

▶ Past medical history of diabetes mellitus, thyroid disease, cardiovascular disease, cerebral vascular disease, hypertension, orthopedic problems

▶ Medication use, with particular attention to laxatives, diuretics, hormones, nutritional supplements, OTC medications

▶ Family history of obesity, overeating, metabolic disorders, cardiovascular disease, cerebral vascular disease, hypertension, diabetes mellitus

Physical Exam

▶ Height and weight: Calculate BMI by using tables or formula (see Diagnostic Studies).

▶ Obtain waist and hip measurement; waist > 35 inches in females and > 40 inches in males is dangerous.

▶ Children: Weight exceeds 120% of that expected for their height (95th percentile on weight-for-height plot)

▶ Complete physical exam to assess for conditions associated with obesity

  ▸ Skin: Assess for changes of Cushing's syndrome or intertrigo caused by obese skin folds, striae, dermatitis, poor wound healing

  ▸ Respiratory: Compromise due to restrictive lung disease, hypoventilation

  ▸ Cardiovascular: Hypertension, coronary artery disease

  ▸ Peripheral vascular: Venous insufficiency

  ▸ Musculoskeletal: Arthritis

Diagnostic Studies

▶ Adults: Calculate BMI = weight in kg ÷ height in meters squared.

  ▸ Pounds ÷ 2.2 = kg; inches × 0.0254 = meters

  ▸ Also can be calculated by [weight in pounds ÷ height in inches ÷ height in inches] × 703

    ▹ BMI between 18.5 and 25 is healthy, normal weight.

    ▹ BMI 30–34.9 = Class I obesity; 35–39.9 = Class II obesity; > 40 = Class III obesity

- Asian populations have lower BMI thresholds.
  - ▷ 18.5–23.9 healthy weight range, 24–26.9 overweight , > 27 obese
► Waist–hip ratio: Estimate fat distribution using waist–hip ratio by measuring waist at navel and measure hips over buttocks, then divide waist measurement by hip measurement to get ratio.
  - Men: Low risk < 0.85, moderate risk 0.85–0.95, high risk > 0.95
  - Women: Low risk < 0.75, moderate risk 0.75–0.85, high risk > 0.85
  - Upper body obesity has more significant health consequences than lower body obesity; therefore, large abdominal circumference or increased waist-to-hip ratio suggests increased risk of diabetes or vascular disease.
► Calculate ideal body weight.
  - Men: Height (cm) = 64.19 − (0.04 × age) + (2.02 × knee height)
  - Women: Height (cm) = 84.88 − (0.24 × age) + (1.83 × knee height)
  - A rough estimate of ideal body weight can be obtained by starting with 100 lbs (women) or 106 lbs (men) and adding 5 lbs (women) or 6 lbs (men) for each inch over 5 feet.
► Instruments to quantify body adipose tissue: Hydrostatic densitometry (gold standard), skin-fold thickness measurement (simplest, most common), dual energy X-ray absorptiometry (DEXA) scan (most reliable and accurate, especially in older adults)
► Lipid profile, fasting blood glucose, metabolic and chemistry panel, thyroid function, consider urine-free cortisol measures for work-up of secondary cause of obesity, or complication of obesity
► Children: Calculate BMI (interpretation depends on the child's age) and plot the BMI-for-age according to sex-specific charts through puberty.
  - BMI = [weight in pounds ÷ height in inches ÷ height in inches] × 703
  - Fractions and ounces must be entered as decimal values.
    - ▷ BMI-for-age < 5th percentile = underweight
    - ▷ BMI-for-age ≥ 85th percentile = at risk of overweight
    - ▷ BMI-for-age ≥ 95th percentile = overweight

Differential Diagnosis

► Endocrine disorders presenting with obesity include hypothalamic disease, thyroid disease, pituitary dysfunction, Cushing syndrome, and polycystic ovary disease.

Management

Nonpharmacologic Treatment

► U.S. Preventive Services Task Force suggests that a combination of diet, exercise, and behavioral modifications is essential to obtain and maintain weight reduction.
► Children: Develop an alliance with the family; treat parents also; use positive reinforcement; emphasize the importance of family involvement in physical activity program.

- ▶ Long-term lifestyle changes
- ▶ Comprehensive multidisciplinary approach to weight reduction includes dietary control, exercise, eating behavior modifications, and psychosocial modification.
- ▶ To lose 1 pound, 3,500 more calories must be expended than consumed (500 calories/day to lose 1 pound per week).
- ▶ Moderate calorie deficit or low-calorie diet for obese men and women attempting to lose weight
  - ▹ 800–1,200 cals/day for adult women; 800–1,500 cals/day for adult men
- ▶ Follow U.S. Department of Agriculture (USDA) My Plate guidelines; avoid controversial fad diets; high-fiber, low-fat diets have proven most successful.
- ▶ Exercise: For energy expenditure, exercise 5–7 times a week for minimum of 30 minutes of moderate-intensity activity (walking, jogging, cycling, ice or roller skating, swimming).
- ▶ May require cardiac stress test before initiating exercise plan
- ▶ Eating behavior modification: Emphasize planning and record-keeping.
- ▶ Psychosocial modification: Support for losing weight essential, whether form of close friend, peer, therapist, or formal organization of people (such as Overeaters Anonymous, TOPS, Weight Watchers)
- ▶ Surgical approach with morbid obesity includes gastric operations, such as vertical-banded (Mason) gastroplasty and gastric bypass.
- ▶ Pediatric obesity is best managed by increasing the child's activity level and improving nutrition; avoid medication or hypocaloric approaches.

Pharmacologic Treatment

- ▶ Recommended for BMI > 30 in conjunction with diet modification and exercise regimen or BMI > 27–29 with at least one major comorbidity
- ▶ Appetite suppressant: Sibutramine (Meridia) 5, 10, or 15 mg dosage q.d.; initial dosage usually 10 mg q.d.
  - ▹ Monitor blood pressure and CNS side effects.
- ▶ Fat blocker: Orlistat (Xenical) 120 mg t.i.d. with meals (no systemic absorption); discuss GI side effects; consider fat-soluble vitamin supplementation
- ▶ Over-the-counter products are not recommended.

How Long to Treat

- ▶ Sibutramine is approved for 1 year; orlistat is approved for 1–2 years if no nutritional deficits result.

Special Considerations

- ▶ Encourage patient to set goal of 10% weight loss for improved health and repeat as necessary.

When to Consult, Refer, Hospitalize

▶ May consider registered dietician when designing a low-calorie diet after determination of caloric requirements based on daily energy intake, expenditure, and average weight loss goal of 1 pound per week after the first month

▶ Counselor for behavior modification.

▶ Refer adults and children with morbid obesity to specialists.

Follow-up

▶ Frequently, at least initially, to evaluate progress

▶ Monthly to monitor blood pressure if taking sibutramine

▶ Regular monitoring and reinforcement of progress until goal weight reached

Expected Course

▶ Slow progress with expected loss from ½ lb to 2–3 lbs per week maximum

▶ Continue to monitor for obesity complications.

▶ Many regain if do not maintain the lifestyle modifications

Complications

▶ Cardiovascular disease: Hypertension, coronary artery disease, varicose veins, CVA

▶ Metabolic disorders: Hyperinsulinemia, diabetes mellitus type 2, hyperlipidemia

▶ Pulmonary: Sleep apnea syndrome, chronic respiratory infections, hypoventilation

▶ Cholelithiasis; nephrotic syndrome

▶ Depression, loss of self-esteem; psychosocial disability

▶ Degenerative joint disease, chronic orthopedic problems

▶ Structural disorders; skin disorders

▶ Cancers: Colon, rectum, prostate, uterine, biliary tract, breast, ovary

▶ Surgery increases perioperative morbidity and mortality.

CASE STUDIES

CASE 1. A 52-year-old Hispanic female arrives at your clinic. She states she has been fatigued for 3 months, has gained weight since her last visit (6 months ago), and is urinating more frequently, but that she is consuming more water and relates the urination to increased intake of fluids.

PMH: Hypertension and obesity; medications benazepril (Lotensin) 10 mg q.d. and Prempro 0.625 mg/2.5 q.d.

▶ What additional history would you ask for?

Exam: Vital signs: BP 130/88, HR 72, RR 12, temperature 97.9° F, weight 196 lbs, height 5'4", BMI 33.7; general appearance is alert without distress. HEENT exam is normal, lungs clear, and heart rate and rhythm regular without murmurs; abdomen is obese with waist circumference 39 inches; no masses or tenderness. Extremity pulses are normal; skin is warm and dry, sensation intact without lesions. Neuro exam is within normal limits.

▶ What diagnostic tests would you order?

▶ If your suspicions were correct, what actions would be required?

▶ What is your treatment plan and follow-up?

CASE 2. A mother arrives at your clinic with her 7-year-old daughter, stating that she is developing breasts early and has hair under her arms.

PMH: Normal growth and development at well-child visits; current on immunizations.

▶ What additional history would you ask for?

Exam: Vital signs within normal limits, height 95th percentile on the growth curve, Tanner stage III; the rest of the exam is normal.

▶ What diagnostic tests would you order?

▶ What is your next course of action?

CASE 3. Black parents bring their 11-year-old son to the community clinic, stating he has lost 15 pounds in 3 weeks and is urinating frequently. He is also "drinking a lot."

PMH: Recent recovery from chickenpox (4 weeks); otherwise normal growth and development; immunizations up to date.

▶ What additional history would you ask for?

Exam: Alert and oriented but appears ill, thin; fruity odor to breath, vital signs stable; mucous membranes slightly dry

▶ What are your differential diagnoses?

▶ What diagnostic tests would you order?

  ▸ The lab results return with a glucose of 420 mg/dL (fasting) and urine dip positive for ketones and glucose. What is your next course of action?

REFERENCES

American Association of Clinical Endocrinologists. (2010). *Medical guidelines for clinical practice for the diagnosis and management of thyroid nodules.* Retrieved from www.aace.com/publications/guidelines

American Association of Clinical Endocrinologists. (2011a). *Hyperthyroidism and other causes of thyrotoxicosis: Management guidelines of the American thyroid.* Retrieved from www.aace.com/publications/guidelines

American Association of Clinical Endocrinologists. (2011b). *Medical guidelines for developing a diabetes mellitus comprehensive care plan.* Retrieved from www.aace.com/publications/guidelines

American Association of Clinical Endocrinologists. (2012). *Medical guidelines for clinical practice: Clinical practice guidelines for hypothyroidism in adults.* Retrieved from www.aace.com/publications/guidelines

American Diabetes Association Guidelines. (2013). Diagnosis and classification of diabetes mellitus. *Diabetes Care, 36*(Suppl. 1), S67–S74.

Centers for Disease Control and Prevention. (2012a). *Childhood obesity facts.* Retrieved from www.cdc.gov/healthyyouth/obesity/facts.htm

Centers for Disease Control and Prevention. (2012b). *Diabetes fact sheet.* Retrieved from www.cdc.gov/diabetes/pubs/factsheets.htm

Centers for Disease Control and Prevention. (2012c). *Overweight and obesity.* Retrieved from www.cdc.gov/obesity/

Cook, D. M., Yuen, C. J., Biller, B. M., Kemp, S. F., & Vance, M. L. (2009). American association of clinical endocrinologists medical guidelines for clinical practice for growth hormone use in growth hormone-deficient adults and transition patients—2009 update. *Endocrine Practice, 15*(Suppl 2). Retrieved from www.aace.com/files/growth-hormone-guidelines.pdf

Dambro, M. R. (2013). *Griffith's five-minute clinical consult.* Philadelphia: Lippincott Williams & Wilkins.

Edmunds, M. W., & Mayhew, M. S. (2009). *Pharmacology for primary care providers* (3rd ed.). St. Louis, MO: Mosby.

Goroll, A. H., & Mulley, A. G. (2009). *Primary care medicine* (6th ed.). Philadelphia: Lippincott Williams & Wilkins.

Hay, W., Hayward, A. R., Levin, M. J., & Sondheimer, J. M. (2012). *Current pediatric diagnosis and treatment* (20th ed.). New York: Lange Medica Book/McGraw Hill.

Joslin Diabetes Center. (2013). *Asian American Diabetes Initiative: BMI calculator.* Retrieved from http://aadi.joslin.org/content/bmi-calculator

Kleigman, R. M., Marcdante, K. J., Jensen, H. B., & Behrman, R. E. (2011). *Nelson essentials of pediatrics* (6th ed.). Philadelphia: Elsevier Saunders.

National Center for Chronic Disease Prevention and Health Promotion. (2012). *Body mass index-for-age: BMI is used differently with children than it is with adults.* Retrieved from www.cdc.gov/healthyweight/assessing/bmi/adult_bmi/

National Guideline Clearinghouse. (2012). Standards of medical care in diabetes III. Detection and diagnosis of gestational diabetes mellitus (GDM). *Diabetes Care 35*(Suppl 1), S15–16. Retrieved from http://guideline.gov/content.aspx?id=35246

Papadakis, M. A., McPhee, S. J., & Tierney, L. M. (2013). *Current medical diagnosis & treatment* (52nd ed.). Norwalk, CT: Appleton & Lange.

Schwartz, M. W. (2012). *The five-minute pediatric consult* (6th ed.). Philadelphia: Lippincott Williams & Wilkins.

PSYCHIATRIC AND MENTAL HEALTH DISORDERS

Dawn Aubel, MS, MPH, FNP-BC

Note: The 2013 ANCC test content outline for this exam does not incorporate the fifth edition of the *Diagnostic and Statistical Manual of Mental Disorders*; the exam includes information from the fourth edition. Therefore, this review manual includes information from DSM-IV.

GENERAL APPROACH

Description

- ▶ Mental illnesses are common, serious brain disorders that affect thinking, motivation, emotions, and social interactions. An estimated 1 in 4 adults suffers from a diagnosable mental disorder in a given year.

- ▶ Untreated mental illness contributes adversely to other physiological illnesses.

- ▶ Obtain a complete history, including past medical, family, social history, medications, and review of systems.

- ▶ Obtain a mental status exam, using specific screening tools as appropriate.

- ▶ Distinguish between a mental disorder and a medical condition or substance abuse.

- ▶ The U.S. standard psychiatric diagnostic system (*Diagnostic and Statistical Manual of Mental Disorders*, Fourth Edition, DSM-IV) uses a categorical approach in which each disorder has its own set of criteria.

- ▶ Concomitant disorders are common.

- ▶ Most mild mental disorders can be treated effectively in a primary care setting.

▶ With the presence of a developmental delay in a child, the clinician should consider a psychiatric disorder.

▶ Approximately 20%–25% of children visiting pediatric outpatient settings have psychiatric disorders, either diagnosed or undiagnosed.

RED FLAGS

▶ People with mental illness often self-medicate with alcohol or other substances.

▶ Consult, refer, or hospitalize when presenting symptoms are severe, chronic, or unresponsive.

▶ Suicidal ideation and attempt are always psychiatric emergencies.

▶ Patients who represent clear and present danger to themselves or others should never be left alone and should be hospitalized immediately even when it is contrary to their wishes.

ANXIETY DISORDERS

Description

▶ Anxiety is an acute or chronic fearful emotion with associated physical symptoms.

Subtypes

▶ Panic disorder

  ▹ Episodes of recurrent and intense fear or feeling of impending doom that occur without apparent warning

  ▹ Physical symptoms including palpitations, shortness of breath, tachycardia, sweating, abdominal distress, dizziness, tightness in chest; fear of dying, "losing one's mind," "going crazy"; a sense of unreality

  ▹ May be accompanied by agoraphobia, in which patients rigidly avoid situations that they perceive as dangerous or threatening, often due to the environment's vastness or crowdedness. They prefer to be accompanied by a friend or family member in tunnels, elevators, crowded streets, subways, airplanes, etc. Some patients may refuse to leave their homes.

▶ Obsessive–compulsive disorder (OCD)

  ▹ Recurrent, repetitive, and intrusive thoughts, behaviors, or both that are extremely difficult or impossible to control, unreasonable, or excessive, and that interfere significantly with a person's ability to function

▶ Posttraumatic stress disorder (PTSD)

  ▹ Exposure to an extreme traumatic stressor such as rape, sexual or physical abuse, natural disasters, war, or other perceived or actual threat to a person's physical being or self-concept

  ▹ Results in persistent symptoms, including nightmares, flashbacks, numbing of emotion, dissociative episodes, or inability to recall specific events

- Acute form identified as lasting less than 3 months; chronic form lasting 3 months or longer

▶ Acute stress disorder (ASD)

- Exposure to a traumatic event that involved actual or threatened death or serious injury

- Response to event is intense fear, helplessness, or horror

- Results in same symptoms as PTSD, but occur within 4 weeks of the event

- Lasts for minimum of 2 days and maximum of 4 weeks

▶ Phobias

- Social phobia

  ▷ Severe, persistent fear of social or performance situations provoking an immediate and intense anxiety response; extreme, irrational fear leads to avoidance of people or social situations

- Specific phobia

  ▷ Extreme, irrational fear of specific objects, such as elevators, snakes, or insects, that leads to avoidant behavior of that particular object

▶ Generalized anxiety disorder (GAD)

- Excessive worry, feelings of apprehension, panic, or dread accompanied by symptoms of physiological arousal (palpitations, muscle tension and restlessness, fatigue, sweating, difficulty concentrating); anxiety may seem groundless, or appear disproportionate to issue

- Symptoms present at least 6 months, occurring more days than not, with person reporting little or no control, along with significant distress and impairment in social, occupational, and interpersonal areas

Etiology

▶ Psychodynamic theory

- Severe conflict between the id and superego

- Irrational guilt and shame

▶ Behavioral theory

- Conditioned behavioral response to earlier interpersonal or social experiences

▶ Biologic theory

- Genetic predisposition

- Overstimulated autonomic nervous system, stress response

- Abnormalities of neurotransmitter receptors in the central nervous system (CNS), specifically GABA receptors

▶ Existential theory

- Response to an awareness of a vast void in existence and meaning

Incidence and Demographics

▶ Anxiety disorders are one of the most common mental illnesses in the United States.

▶ Anxiety disorders account for 15% of the population seen in general practice settings.

▶ Panic disorders occur more frequently in women than men.

▶ Anxiety is a common concomitant disorder in patients with a history of early traumatic experiences such as abuse, separation, or loss of a parent.

▶ Anxiety disorders frequently co-occur with depressive disorders or substance abuse.

▶ Separation anxiety and overanxious disorders are syndromes unique to pediatric patients.

▶ Phobias affect children and adults, with a lifetime prevalence of 10%.

▶ Adult onset of obsessive-compulsive disorder affects men and women equally; childhood onset is more common in boys.

▶ Generally, onset of anxiety is before the early-adult years. If a first episode occurs after this age, consider other non-psychological source.

Risk Factors

▶ Family history; genetic predisposition

▶ Exposure to traumatic events; history of depression or substance abuse

Prevention and Screening

▶ Public and patient education and awareness

▶ Reduced exposure to real or potential trauma

▶ Strong social support systems and strategies to develop personal resilience

Assessment

History

▶ **General**

   ▷ Determine onset, frequency, and duration of symptoms.

   ▷ Determine degree of distress and symptom interference with daily function.

   ▷ Elicit predisposing factors or stressors, such as divorce, financial difficulties, job loss, or victimization.

   ▷ Obtain complete medical history, including medications, over-the-counter drugs (OTCs), and supplements taken.

   ▷ Obtain history and current patterns of use of caffeine, alcohol, nicotine, and other substances.

   ▷ Ask about:

      ▷ Feelings of loss of control, panic, impending doom or dread, depersonalization, difficulty concentrating

      ▷ Excessive worry, irrational fear, concern over "losing one's mind" or death, memory changes

  ▷ Difficulty concentrating, making decisions, irritable, agitated mood, motor restlessness

  ▷ Sleep disturbances (insomnia, frequent awakenings), fatigue, irritation, agitated mood

  ▷ Nausea, diarrhea, vomiting, frequent urination

  ▷ Feeling of lump in the throat, difficulty swallowing, dry mouth

▶ **Obsessive–Compulsive Disorder (OCD)**

  ▸ Either recurrent and persistent unwanted thoughts that are difficult or impossible to control, or

  ▸ Repetitive, uncontrollable behaviors such as excessive handwashing or counting

  ▸ Present most days for > 2 weeks

▶ **Posttraumatic Stress Disorder (PTSD)**

  ▸ Recurring dreams or nightmares of a previously experienced traumatic event, or intrusive recollections of the event

  ▸ Hyper-arousal

  ▸ Avoidance of stimuli associated with the event

  ▸ Intense psychological distress at exposure to reminders of the original event

▶ **Phobias**

  ▸ Excessive, persistent fear and avoidance of specific objects or situations

  ▸ In children: Avoidance of school; impaired social, family, and academic functioning

  ▸ In adults: Avoidance of work, social activities

▶ **General Anxiety and Panic Attacks**

  ▸ Palpitations, tachycardia, tightness in chest or chest pain

  ▸ Difficulty breathing, tachypnea, hyperventilation

  ▸ Light-headedness, dizziness, diaphoresis

  ▸ Tingling, numbness in extremities

  ▸ Fear of losing control or going crazy

  ▸ Fear of dying

Physical Exam

▶ Perform general exam to rule out serious central nervous system, cardiopulmonary, or endocrine disorder.

▶ Focus on vital signs, cardiac, pulmonary, and neurologic exam.

Diagnostic Studies

▶ Diagnostic labs such as ECG, TSH, CBC, chemistry panel to rule out medical conditions

▶ Minnesota Multiphasic Inventory (MMPI-II), Hamilton Anxiety Scale, Adult Manifest Anxiety Scale (AMAS), Children's Manifest Anxiety Scale (RCMAS) may be done.

Differential Diagnosis

- ▶ Any medical condition with central nervous system involvement
- ▶ Substance abuse, including acute withdrawal or intoxication
- ▶ Metabolic disorders
- ▶ Seizure disorders
- ▶ Mood disorders
- ▶ Caffeine, nicotine
- ▶ Delirium, especially in older adults

Cardiac Disorders

- ▶ Arrhythmias
- ▶ Myocardial infarction (MI)
- ▶ Cardiovascular disease
- ▶ Chronic heart failure (CHF)

Endocrine Disorders

- ▶ Cushing's syndrome
- ▶ Hyperthyroidism
- ▶ Hypoglycemia

Pulmonary Disorders

- ▶ Chronic obstructive pulmonary disease (COPD)
- ▶ Asthma
- ▶ Pulmonary embolism
- ▶ Pneumothorax

Medications That May Produce Anxiety as a Side Effect

- ▶ Anticholinergics
- ▶ Antihistamines
- ▶ Corticosteroids
- ▶ Antihypertensives
- ▶ Antipsychotics
- ▶ Antidepressants
- ▶ Bronchodilators
- ▶ Amphetamines
- ▶ Anesthetics

Management

- ▶ Mild cases of anxiety disorders and GAD are responsive to treatment in primary care settings.
- ▶ Refer primary anxiety disorders that meet DSM-IV criteria to a mental health provider.
- ▶ Provide patient education to ensure compliance and effective treatment.

Nonpharmacologic Treatment

- ▶ Cognitive–behavioral therapy; supportive psychotherapy, insight-oriented psychotherapy, group therapy (especially for PTSD)
- ▶ Stress management education, courses, workshops; behavioral conditioning, biofeedback
- ▶ Community self-help and support groups
- ▶ Education of patient and family about the disorder and treatment

Pharmacologic Treatment

- ▶ Benzodiazepines are effective in the short-term management of some anxiety disorders (see Table 18–1).
  - ▻ Significant potential for dependence and abuse; limit use to 1 month
  - ▻ Rapid onset of action with quick symptom relief

- Alprazolam (Xanax) and clonazepam (Klonopin) frequently used to treat panic disorders
- Patients with substance abuse histories at risk for abuse so avoid these medications

TABLE 18-1
BENZODIAZEPINE THERAPY FOR ADULT ANXIETY DISORDERS

BENZODIAZEPINES	INITIAL DOSE	THERAPEUTIC DOSE
Alprazolam (Xanax)	0.25–0.5 mg t.i.d.	0.5–4 mg/day
Clonazepam (Klonopin)	0.25–1 mg b.i.d.	1–4 mg/day
Lorazepam (Ativan)	1–1.5 mg b.i.d.	2–6 mg/day
Diazepam (Valium)	2–10 mg b.i.d.	4–40 mg/day

▶ Other anti-anxiety medications

- Buspirone (Buspar): 7.5 mg b.i.d. up to 20–30 mg a day

  ▷ Slower onset of action—may take up to 4 weeks for anti-anxiety effects

  ▷ Maximum therapeutic effect may not be reached for 4–8 weeks.

- Antidepressants are commonly the first-line drug of choice for anxiety disorders (see Table 18–2).

  ▷ Potential for substance abuse and dependence is significantly less than with benzodiazepines

  ▷ Main therapeutic effect may take 2–4 weeks

  ▷ Educating patient on time required to reach main effect of drug is essential for compliance

TABLE 18-2
SSRI/SNRI THERAPY IN ANXIETY DISORDERS

SSRI/SNRI MEDICATIONS	INITIAL DOSE	THERAPEUTIC DOSE
Fluoxetine (Prozac)	20 mg q.d.	20–60 mg/day
Paroxetine (Paxil)	20 mg q.d.	20–50 mg/day
Sertraline (Zoloft)	25 mg q.d.	25–200 mg/day
Fluvoxamine (Luvox)	50 mg q.h.s.	100–300 mg/day
Venlafaxine (Effexor)	12.5–25 mg b.i.d.	150–375 mg/day
Escitalopram (Lexapro)	10 mg q.d.	20 mg/day

How Long to Treat

▶ Length varies according to individual response and symptom management.

▶ Mild and situational anxiety usually resolves within 2 months.

▶ Long-term use of antidepressants can be required.

▶ Chronic, disabling anxiety requires a psychiatric consultation and referral.

Special Considerations

▶ It is common for anxiety disorders to occur concomitantly with other disorders, such as depression, eating disorders, and substance abuse, or with ADHD, depression, OCD, and Tourette's syndrome in children.

▶ Anxiety disorders are commonly seen with medical disorders. Always rule out underlying medical causes and ensure appropriate treatment of any concomitant disorders.

▶ Patients with anxiety disorders need reassurance that their disorders can be effectively treated.

▶ Establishing a trusting, safe, therapeutic relationship with the primary practitioner is essential for compliance and effective treatment.

When to Consult, Refer, Hospitalize

▶ Severe panic attacks, intense PTSD, and disabling OCD always require a psychiatric consult or referral and usually require a combination of pharmacotherapy and cognitive-behavioral therapy.

▶ There have been few studies documenting the results of treatment of anxiety in children and adolescents and few anti-anxiety agents are approved in children. Referral to a psychiatrist is indicated for anxiety in children.

Follow-up

▶ Patients should be seen weekly during the acute phase of treatment.

▶ Medications need to be monitored for effectiveness, appropriate dose, and potential abuse.

Complications

▶ Drug abuse or dependence, dysfunctional social or occupational performance

▶ Treatment resistance or undertreatment, side effects from medications

MOOD DISORDERS

Description

▶ Include symptoms of depressed mood and include depressive disorder, dysthymic disorder, and bipolar disorder

GRIEF OR BEREAVEMENT

Description

▶ A normal emotional and physiological reaction to loss; situational and time-limited

▶ May cause varying degrees of symptoms, such as feeling of profound sadness, crying spells, insomnia, loss of appetite, survivor guilt

Incidence and Demographics

▶ All people, for uncomplicated grief

Risk Factors

▶ Risk of developing more complicated mood disorders: Poor coping skills, lack of support, history of previous mood disorder, alcohol or substance abuse

Management

Nonpharmacologic Treatment

▶ Encourage the expression of grief and mourning over loss.

▶ Offer reassurance that grief is a normal, nonpathologic reaction to loss and is self-limited.

▶ Encourage participation in support groups.

Pharmacologic Treatment

▶ Mild anti-anxiety agents at the lowest effective dose may be used to treat symptoms, but do not treat symptoms of major depression.

When to Consult, Refer, Hospitalize

▶ Grief that lasts longer than 2 months should be evaluated for mood disorders and referred to a mental health specialist.

▶ Suicidal ideation is a psychiatric emergency — the patient should be referred immediately for psychiatric evaluation.

Follow-up

▶ The duration of normal grief reaction varies among different individuals and may vary among cultures, but usually begins to show marked improvement within 8 weeks.

▶ The diagnosis of major depressive disorder is not given unless symptoms are still present after 2 months and represent a significant change in function and impairment.

▶ Older adults and patients without adequate social or familial support are at high risk for developing major depression and suicidal ideation.

▶ Children may harbor feelings of guilt and responsibility, and may require referral to psychiatrist or mental health specialist.

DEPRESSIVE DISORDERS

Description

▶ Major depression is a complex mood disorder lasting at least 2 weeks, with sad, "blue" mood that may or may not be accompanied by the loss of interest or pleasure in nearly all activities, every day.

▶ In children, the mood may be irritable rather than sad.

▶ Depression is associated with abnormalities in neurotransmission, neurophysiology, and neuroendocrine function.

▶ Clinical manifestations of childhood depression vary according to the child's developmental age.

Subtypes

▶ Adjustment disorder with depressed mood

▶ Depressive disorders

▶ Major depressive disorder: Single or recurrent episodes of depression associated with other symptoms lasting at least 2 weeks but without mood elevation, elation, or mania

▶ Dysthymic disorder: Chronic, sustained depressed mood ongoing for a minimum of 2 years, more days than not, symptoms less severe than depressive disorder

▶ Premenstrual dysphoric disorder

▶ Mood disorders due to illness and drugs

▶ Bipolar disorder (mania, cyclothymic disorder): Recurrent episodes of depression with episodes of mania characterized by lack of impulse control, excessive energy, grandiose or delusional thinking, elated mood, inappropriate behaviors, hyperactivity, pressured speech, decreased need for sleep

▶ Atypical depression: Characterized by hypersomnia, fatigue, rejection sensitivity, overeating

▶ Melancholic depression: Characterized by insomnia, early morning or frequent awakenings, anxiety, loss of appetite, difficulty concentrating, fatigue

▶ Postpartum: Symptom onset within 2 weeks to 6 months postpartum

Etiology

▶ Genetic predisposition

▶ Biological dysregulation of the hypopituitary axis (stress response). The core symptoms of depression — such as sleep, appetite, and mood disturbances — are related to the functions of the hypothalamus and the pituitary glands and associated hormones such as cortisol, leptin, and corticotropin-releasing hormone (CRH).

▶ Abnormalities in neurotransmitters in the brain are associated with serotonin, acetylcholine, dopamine, norepinephrine, epinephrine, and GABA; possible structural changes in the brain.

▶ Additional environmental factors and learned behaviors may influence neurotransmitter function or exert independent influence.

Incidence and Demographics

▶ Depression is the most common mental illness seen in primary care practices.

▶ Depressive disorders often co-occur with anxiety disorders and substance abuse.

▶ The lifetime prevalence for the U.S. population is 7% for women and 3% for men.

▶ Patients with depression have 2–3 times the normal death rate at any age (independent of suicide) and are more likely to incur long-term medical consequences, such as premature osteoporosis, coronary artery disease, dysfunction of inflammatory mediators and the immune system, and increased insulin resistance.

▶ Bipolar disorder has a mean age of 30 and ranges from age 5 to 50.

▶ Mean age for onset of major depressive disorder is age 32.

▶ Dysthymic disorder occurs up to 7× more often in women than in men.

▶ Suicide rates are highest in older adults.

Risk Factors

▶ Recent stressful life events are the most powerful predictors of onset of a depressive disorder.

▶ Prior episodes of depression

▶ People without close interpersonal relationships

▶ Losing a parent before age 11

▶ Family history, especially having first-degree relative who is diagnosed

▶ Alcohol and substance abuse

▶ Postpartum period

▶ Significant psychosocial stressors such as divorce, finances, job loss, trauma, or abuse

▶ Chronic medical illness

▶ Risk factors for suicide

  » Personal or family history of one or more mental or substance abuse disorders

  » Severe psychosocial stressors: Divorce, unemployment, legal problems, perception of poor health

  » Anxiety

  » Depression in childhood or adolescence

  » Previous suicide attempt(s)

  » Family or domestic violence, including physical or sexual abuse

  » Firearms in the home

  » Specific plan

  » Family history of suicide

Prevention and Screening

▶ Patient education and public awareness of signs, symptoms, and treatment modalities available

▶ Early recognition, intervention, and initiation of treatment

Assessment

History

▶ Establish frequency, type, and duration of symptoms.

▶ Degree of disruption or impairment in daily activities

▶ Past medical history, including thyroid disease

▶ Prior personal psychiatric history

▶ Social history including alcohol and substance use

▶ Family psychiatric and psychosocial history

▶ Identify acute and chronic stressors.

▶ Ask about suicidal thoughts, impulses, and history of prior attempts or current plans. Inquire about homicidal ideations.

▶ According to the DSM-IV-TR, sad, blue, or depressed mood, absence of pleasure (or any combination of these) plus 4 or more of listed symptoms must be present for a minimum of 2 weeks and represent a change from previous function to diagnose major depression. Classic symptoms of major depression (DSM-IV-TR):

  » Depressed mood most of the day, nearly every day; in children, can be irritable mood

  » Significant weight loss when not dieting, or weight gain, or increase or decrease in appetite

  » Markedly diminished interest or pleasure in all or almost all activities

  » Psychomotor agitation or retardation

  » Difficulty concentrating or making decisions

  » Change in sleep patterns (insomnia or hypersomnia)

  » Low self-esteem; feelings of worthlessness or excessive, inappropriate guilt

  » Recurrent thoughts of death, suicidal ideation with or without a specific plan, prior suicide attempt

  » Decreased energy and fatigue; increased somatic complaints such as headache

  » Feelings of hopelessness

▶ Use a scale such as the Patient Health Questionnaire–9 item (PHQ-9), which has good test-retest reliability, internal consistency, and sensitivity to change in depression over time. It has been extensively studied as a screening measure for major depression in primary care settings.

▶ Adjustment disorder

  » A less severe form of depression in which symptoms occur within 3 months of identifiable stressor, mild sadness, inability to concentrate, excess worry, somatic complaints

▶ Bipolar disorder

  » Extreme swings in mood, hyperactivity, flight of ideas, decreased need for sleep, grandiosity, impaired judgment, depression, aggressive behavior, sexual acting out, delusions, or ideation

► Depression in children

- ⯈ Sadness, crying, withdrawal, fatigue, anger, irritability or agitation, somatic complaints, separation anxiety, difficulty concentrating, feelings of guilt or worthlessness, weight change, change in sleep patterns, increased social isolation, substance abuse, or suicidal ideation

► Dysthymic disorder

- ⯈ Depressed mood most of the day, present almost continuously; complaint that has always been depressed

Physical Exam

► Complete physical exam with a mental status exam to rule out any underlying medical conditions

► Observation of personal appearance, grooming, hygiene, affect

Diagnostic Studies

► Primarily a clinical diagnosis; tests (CBC, TSH, sedimentation rate, chemistry profile, B_{12} and folate, RPR, CT scan) used to rule out suspected underlying medical causes

► ECG before initiation of tricyclic antidepressants (TCA)

► Cortisol levels, EEG may be done by specialist

► Psychometric tests include Minnesota Multi Personality Index (MMPI-2)

► Self-report scales commonly used are Beck Depression Inventory, Hamilton Rating Scale for Depression, Zung Self-Rating Depression Scale, and Geriatric Depression Scale

Differential Diagnosis

► Electrolyte imbalances

► Chronic fatigue syndrome

► COPD

► Bereavement or grief reaction over recent loss

► Bipolar disorders

► Psychotic disorders, schizophrenia

► Alcohol and substance abuse

► Mononucleosis

Endocrine Disorders

► Hypothyroidism

► Hyperthyroidism

► Cushing syndrome

► Addison's disease

► Diabetes

Cardiac Disorders

► Arrhythmia

► CHF

► MI

► Hypertension

Neurologic Disorders

► Neoplasms

► Stroke

► Severe trauma

► Head injury

► Multiple sclerosis

► Seizure disorders

► Parkinson's disease

► Dementia

► Chronic pain

Medications That Can Induce Depression

- ▶ Opioids
- ▶ Steroids
- ▶ Estrogen
- ▶ Antihypertensive agents
- ▶ Digoxin
- ▶ Anti-Parkinson drugs
- ▶ NSAIDs

- ▶ Beta-blockers
- ▶ Sedatives and hypnotics
- ▶ Antibacterials, antifungals
- ▶ Antineoplastic drugs
- ▶ Psychotropic drugs
- ▶ Analgesics
- ▶ Antiinflammatories

Management

- ▶ Mild depression or hypomania may be safely managed by a primary practitioner with frequent evaluation.
- ▶ Frequent follow-up is necessary to educate patient regarding the illness and to adequately treat.
- ▶ Tricyclic antidepressants and SSRIs may precipitate a manic episode in patients prone to manic depressive or bipolar illness.
- ▶ Patient education concerning the nature of the illness, course of treatment, and expected outcome is essential.
- ▶ A complete diagnostic evaluation is essential, with evaluation of suicide risk.

Nonpharmacologic Treatment

- ▶ Psychotherapy, alone or in combination with antidepressant medication, is an option for patients with mild to moderate major depression.
- ▶ Cognitive-behavioral therapy and dialectical behavior therapy with a focus on cognitive distortions and behaviors that exacerbate depressive illness
- ▶ Psychoanalysis or psychotherapy with a focus on interpersonal skills
- ▶ Suicidal ideation or behavior is a psychiatric emergency and should always be evaluated further and treated by a mental health practitioner immediately.
- ▶ Electroconvulsive therapy is indicated for severely depressed or suicidal patients who don't respond to pharmacologic agents; main side effect is temporary memory impairment that may last up to 2 weeks
- ▶ Provide community resources, hotlines, and a list of local support groups.

Pharmacologic Teatment

- ▶ SSRIs (Table 18–3) are the first-line drug of choice, due to their effectiveness and safety record in adults.
  - ▹ Fluoxetine (Prozac) is the SSRI with a pediatric indication. Use of other SSRIs in children is off-label. Treatment of children should be initiated and managed by a mental health specialist.
  - ▹ Information from an increasing number of studies indicates an increase in suicidal and homicidal behavior with SSRI use in some children. An FDA advisory panel has recently recommended warnings on all antidepressants, indicating that suicide risk

may be increased in children taking these products, therefore they should be seen once a week when initiating treatment or when changing dosages until stable.

- ▹ Other cautions include abrupt withdrawal of SSRIs may cause unpleasant somatic complaints (fatigue and irritability), so SSRIs should be tapered; during treatment, children may experience "behavior activation" (the underactive child may become agitated and impulsive).

TABLE 18-3
COMMON SSRI THERAPY FOR TREATMENT OF ADULT DEPRESSION

MEDICATION	INITIAL DOSE	TARGET DOSE
Fluoxetine (Prozac)	20 mg q.d. in a.m.	20-80 mg q.d.
Sertraline (Zoloft)	50 mg q.d.	50-200 mg q.d.
Paroxetine (Paxil)	20 mg q.d. in a.m.	20-50 mg q.d.
Citalopram (Celexa)	20 mg q.d.	40-60 mg q.d.
Escitalopram (Lexapro)	10 mg q.d.	10-20 mg q.d.
Duloxetine (Cymbalta)	40 mg q.d.	40-60 mg q.d. in divided dose

- ▶ Tricyclic antidepressants (see Table 18-4) are also effective, but are associated with greater incidence of side effects.
  - ▹ Tricyclics block cholinergic muscarinic receptors, resulting in possible constipation, dry mouth, urinary retention, blurred vision, and sinus tachycardia; other side effects include sedation, postural hypotension, weight gain, potentiation of CNS medications, and dizziness.
  - ▹ Tricyclics are contraindicated in patients with cardiac conduction disorders, narrow angle glaucoma, and prostatic hypertrophy.
  - ▹ Tricyclics cause weight gain; monitor weight and BMI.

TABLE 18-4
COMMON TRICYCLIC ANTIDEPRESSANTS

MEDICATION	INITIAL DOSE	TARGET DOSE
Amitriptyline (Elavil)	25 mg q.h.s.	50-150 mg divided
Desipramine (Norpramin)	25 mg q.d.	75-300 mg q.d.
Imipramine (Tofranil)	25 mg q.h.s.	75-300 mg q.h.s.
Nortriptyline (Pamelor)	10-25 mg q.h.s.	75-150 mg q.d. or divided

- ▶ Monoamine oxidase inhibitors (MAOIs), such as phenelzine (Nardil) and tranylcypromine (Parnate), are used in the treatment of refractory or treatment-resistant depression. Potentially serious and lethal side effects, such as hypertensive crisis, may occur. These drugs should be ordered by psychiatrist.

▶ Other antidepressants and antidepressants used in adults and children are listed in Table 18–5. Dose should be increased weekly until therapeutic dose is reached.

TABLE 18-5
OTHER ANTIDEPRESSANTS COMMONLY USED IN TREATING ADULTS AND CHILDREN

MEDICATION	INITIAL DOSE	TARGET DOSE
Bupropion (Wellbutrin)	75 mg b.i.d; avoid bedtime dosing	300–400 mg/day divided 3–4× daily
Mirtazapine (Remeron)	15 mg q.h.s.	15–45 mg q.h.s.
Nefazodone (Serzone)	200 mg/day divided 2×/day	300–600 mg/day divided 2× daily
Venlafaxine (Effexor)	25–50 mg q.d. with food in 2–3 doses	75–375 mg q.d. divided

How Long to Treat

▶ Duration and course of treatment is individualized, depends upon severity of illness and response to treatment.

▶ If the patient is nonresponsive to medication, increase to maximum dose slowly. If no response, change within class (one SSRI to another) or to another antidepressant (Wellbutrin, Effexor, Remeron); next to second-line tricyclics; and, finally, refer out for MAOIs.

▶ Depression is a chronic illness with frequent episodes of recurrence.

▶ Antidepressants are most effective when taken for at least 1 year after remission of symptoms.

▶ If patient has had 2 or more episodes, consider remaining on antidepressants.

Special Considerations

▶ Patients treated for major depression in a general practice setting have more pain, physical illness, and social and interpersonal impairment than other patient populations.

▶ Sustained release (SR) or extended release (XR) versions are more easily tolerated.

▶ Tricyclic medications have a high potential for lethality in overdose.

▶ Depression in older adults may be difficult to diagnose, due to the greater incidence of dementia and number and types of medications taken for other medical conditions.

▶ Older adult patients require smaller starting doses, but may require same therapeutic dosage as younger adults and frequently require closer medical management.

When to Consult, Refer, Hospitalize

▶ All patients who present with suicidal ideation, prior attempt, or plan should immediately be referred to an emergency room or psychiatrist for further evaluation and treatment.

▶ All patients should be referred to the appropriate mental health practitioner for therapy.

▶ Consult for all women who are pregnant or plan on becoming pregnant before initiating medication.

▶ Patients who are severely impaired by their symptomology or present with comorbid disorders, such as obsessive–compulsive disorder, substance abuse, eating disorders, or no social support, should be referred to a psychiatrist or other mental health specialist.

▶ Patients who represent a clear and present danger to themselves or others should be hospitalized immediately.

▶ Children should be referred to a child and adolescent psychiatrist.

▶ *Antidepressant medication in children should be managed by a mental health professional.*

Follow-up

▶ Patients should initially be seen weekly to titrate dosage and monitor symptom management and compliance.

▶ Medication compliance is a serious issue, with patients often discontinuing treatment before medication has time to work and symptoms subside.

▶ Educate patients concerning risks, benefits, and possible side effects of medications.

Expected Course

▶ Most patients respond to antidepressants within 2–3 weeks of treatment, but should be educated that drug therapy may take months to reach full effect.

▶ Risk factors for recurrence are several prior episodes and early discontinuance of medication.

▶ To ensure the most effective response, antidepressants need to be taken at least 1 year after remission of symptoms because depression is a chronic disease with frequent episodes of recurrence.

Complications

▶ Social isolation, impairment of vocation and interpersonal relationships, suicide

SUBSTANCE USE DISORDERS

TOBACCO DEPENDENCE

Description

▶ Tobacco is smoked, chewed, and snuffed. Electronic cigarettes use a liquid nicotine cartridge, rather than tobacco. Nicotine is the main source of dependence.

Incidence and Demographics

▶ Prevalence of smoking in the U.S. was 19.3% in 2010

▶ Greater incidence of smoking in men than women

▶ An estimated 4,000 youths under age 18 begin smoking each day.

▶ Almost every adult who smokes started by the age of 18.

Risks of Tobacco Use

▶ More than 400,000 Americans die each year of tobacco-related illnesses.

▶ Deaths from use include cardiovascular disease, cancer, and COPD

▶ Direct and indirect health costs each year are estimated at more than $100 billion.

▶ > 40% of U.S. children are exposed to environmental tobacco smoke in their own homes.

▶ 23% of high school students currently use some form of tobacco, most commonly cigarettes.

Prevention and Screening

▶ Discuss the effects of tobacco use at all healthcare visits with children, adolescents, and adults.

▶ Screen patients for exposure to second-hand smoke.

▶ Inquire at adolescent health visits whether a teen's friends are smokers. If a teen's friends smoke, the teen is more likely to smoke.

▶ Take a complete smoking history at all healthcare visits and encourage attempts to quit.

Assessment

▶ Use 5A's algorithm: **Ask** about their smoking status; **Advise** smokers to quit; **Assess** their readiness to quit; **Assist** them with smoking cessation effort; **Arrange** for follow-up visits or contact.

Management

Smoking Cessation

▶ Combination of education, support, behavioral strategies, pharmacotherapy (with nicotine replacement, bupropion, or varenicline) is more effective than any method alone.

▶ Encourage patient to quit and offer therapy at every visit.

▶ Brief tobacco dependence treatment is effective. Clinicians should offer at least brief treatments to every patient who uses tobacco.

▶ Individual, group, and telephone counseling are effective, and their effectiveness increases with treatment intensity. Two components of counseling are especially effective; clinicians should use practical counseling (problem-solving skills training) and social support delivered as part of treatment.

▶ Numerous effective medications are available for tobacco dependence; clinicians should encourage their use by all patients attempting to quit smoking — except when medically contraindicated or with specific populations for which there is insufficient evidence of effectiveness (i.e., pregnant women, smokeless tobacco users, light smokers, and adolescents).

▶ Seven first-line medications (5 nicotine and 2 nonnicotine) reliably increase long-term smoking abstinence rates:

  ▹ Patient must stop smoking before nicotine preparation is used.

  ▹ Nicotine gum (Nicorette): 2–4 mg p.o. every 1–2 hours. Taper use after 6 weeks. Max 24 pieces/24 hours.

- » Nicotine inhaler (Nicotrol): 4 mg per cartridge. Taper use. Maximum 16 cartridges/ 24 hours.

- » Nicotine lozenge (Nicorette): 2–4 mg p.o. every 1–2 hours. Taper use after 6 weeks.

- » Nicotine nasal spray (Nicotrol NS): 10 mg/mL (0.5 mg/spray). 1 spray each nostril every 1–5 hours for 8 weeks. Then taper. Maximum 80 sprays (40 mg) per 24 hours.

- » Nicotine transdermal patch: Dose based on cigarette consumption; 7 mg, 14 mg, 21 mg patches. Tapered dosing.

- » Bupropion SR (Wellbutrin SR): 150 mg b.i.d. for 7–12 weeks

- » Varenicline (Chantix): Start drug 1 week before planned quit date. Increase dose first week, then 1 mg p.o. b.i.d. for 11 weeks. May continue additional 12 weeks if initial treatment is unsuccessful.

▶ Consider combination therapies.

▶ Nicotine replacement product adverse reactions include local irritation of skin or mucous membranes, withdrawal symptoms, GI upset, tachycardia, and spontaneous abortion. Avoid use immediate post-MI, accelerated hypertension, severe angina, chronic nasal disorders (spray), hepatic and renal dysfunction, hyperthyroidism, and other disorders.

▶ Counseling and medication are effective when used by themselves for treating tobacco dependence. The combination of counseling and medication, however, is more effective than either alone. Thus, clinicians should encourage all patients making a quit attempt to use both counseling and medication.

▶ Telephone quit-line counseling is effective with diverse populations and has broad reach, so clinicians should promote quit-line use.

Follow-up

▶ Pregnant women should be encouraged to stop smoking without pharmacologic support.

▶ Relapse is common and frequently occurs within the first 1–2 weeks during withdrawal.

▶ Provide weekly visits during attempts to quit.

▶ Long-term success is greater with multiple attempts.

ALCOHOL DEPENDENCE

Description

▶ Alcohol dependence is defined as a maladaptive pattern of use associated with 3 or more of the following: tolerance; withdrawal; taking in more than intended; persistent desire to cut down or control use; time spent obtaining, using, or recovering from the substance; social, occupational, or recreational tasks sacrificed; and uses despite physical and psychological problems.

Etiology

▶ Alcohol is absorbed rapidly from the gastrointestinal tract and acts as a CNS depressant.

▶ Excessive quantity will cause stupor, coma, and death (from respiratory depression or toxicity to neurons).

▶ Physical and psychological dependence vary; there may be genetic predisposition to alcoholism, as well as social and cultural conditioning to its use.

Incidence and Demographics

▶ Alcohol dependence and abuse are prevalent worldwide.

▶ The first episode of alcohol intoxication is likely to occur in adolescence.

▶ Alcohol is the most frequently used depressant in the world.

▶ Increased risk of alcohol dependence is associated with male sex, being single, lower income, and White or Native American ethnicity.

▶ Middle-age adults are at the highest risk of abuse; abuse and dependence are prevalent across the age spectrum, but decline with age.

▶ It is estimated that more than 50% of violent crimes committed occur under the influence of alcohol.

Risk Factors

▶ Family history; 40% of Japanese have aldehyde dehydrogenase deficiency, which increases susceptibility to alcoholism; Native Americans

▶ Abuse of other substances; presence of a psychiatric disorder

▶ Cultural conditioning, college students

▶ Domestic violence or abuse

Prevention and Screening

▶ Screen using a brief, simple questionnaire, such as the Single-Item Screening or AUDIT-C.

  » How often do you have a drink containing alcohol?

  » How many drinks containing alcohol do you have on a typical day that you are drinking?

  » How often do you have 6 or more drinks on one occasion?

▶ Use CAGE questionnaire (see Table 18–6) if someone screens positive on the simple questionnaire.

▶ Early public education as to the nature, course, and consequences of alcohol

▶ Primary intervention programs in the community and schools

▶ Increased social and public awareness through educational mass media campaigns

▶ Community groups such as Mothers Against Drunk Drivers (MADD)

TABLE 18-6
CAGE QUESTIONNAIRE

MEMORY CLUE	QUESTION TO ASK
C	Have you ever felt you ought to **Cut** down on your drinking?
A	Have people **Annoyed** you by criticizing your drinking?
G	Have you ever felt bad or **Guilty** about your drinking?
E	Have you ever had a drink the first thing in the morning (**Eye**-opener) to steady your nerves or get rid of a hangover?

Scoring and interpretation: Person receives one point for each positive answer. One "yes" answer indicates hazardous drinking. Two or more "yes" answers indicate alcohol abuse or dependence.

Adapted from "Screening for Alcohol Abuse Using the CAGE Questionnaire," by B. Bush, S. Shaw, P. Cleary, T. L. Delbanco, & M. D. Anderson, 1987, *American Journal of Medicine, 82,* 231–235.

Assessment

History

▶ Inquire about patterns of use; however, denial is a common coping mechanism.

▶ History of prior substance abuse treatment

▶ Psychiatric history and mental status exam

▶ Current use of prescribed and OTC medications

Physical Exam

▶ Clinical manifestations of alcoholism and alcohol abuse include:

　» Withdrawal symptoms such as tremors, confusion, hallucinations, disorientation, seizures

　» Neurologic: Memory impairment, forgetfulness, loss of time or blackouts, hyperreflexia, ataxia, confabulation

　» Cardiovascular: Cardiomyopathy, hypertension, and arrhythmias

　» Compromised immune system, frequent infections

　» Gastrointestinal: Peptic ulcer; diarrhea; nausea; gastric distention; ascites; enlarged liver; hepatitis; cirrhosis; pancreatitis; malnutrition; thiamin, folic acid, and vitamin B deficiency

　» Musculoskeletal: Muscle wasting, frequent fractures

　» Generally unkempt appearance, poor personal hygiene

　» Integumentary: Cushing appearance, flushed face, spider nevi, ecchymosis

　» HEENT: Nystagmus, angiomas, smell of alcohol on breath, blurred vision

　» Impotence, sexual dysfunction

　» Generalized edema

　» Higher incidence of STDs, HIV infections

► Acute intoxication: Ataxia, drowsiness, disinhibition, delayed responses, nystagmus, psychomotor dysfunction

► Overdosing: Coma, respiratory depression, seizures, stupor

► Chronic indicators of alcoholism: Flushed face, frequent accidents, positive response to CAGE questionnaire, scleral injection, unexplained work or school absences

Diagnostic Studies

► Blood alcohol levels; CBC: decreased WBC, platelets, hematocrit; increased MCV

► Chemistry profile for liver function studies (AST, ALT, GGT, LDH, alkaline phosphatase, total bilirubin), cholesterol, triglycerides, uric acid, amylase all increased (AST > ALT by factor of 2)

► Consider HIV, thyroid function tests, glucose, electrolytes to clarify the diagnosis

► Prothrombin time, PTT if liver disease suspected

► Urinalysis, ECG, chest X-ray to fully evaluate health

Differential Diagnosis

► Major depressive mood disorders

► Anxiety disorders

► Bipolar disorder

► Personality disorders

► Polysubstance abuse disorder

► Endocrine disorders such as Cushing's syndrome

► Neurologic disorders, seizure disorders

► Cardiovascular disease

Management

Nonpharmacologic Treatment

► Substance abuse counseling; treatment program such as Alcoholics Anonymous, employee assistance programs

► Cognitive–behavioral therapy, psychoanalysis

Pharmacologic Treatment

► Detoxification for symptoms of withdrawal; commonly used agents include the benzodiazepines lorazepam (Ativan), chlordiazepoxide (Librium), oxazepam (Serax); use of atenolol (Tenormin) to reduce need for benzodiazepines; clonidine, carbamazepine when benzodiazepines are not a good choice.

► Maintenance therapy includes disulfiram (Antabuse), naltrexone (ReVia), thiamine, folic acid, and B complex.

► Pharmacologic and medical management of underlying medical disorders as appropriate

How Long to Treat

► Physical withdrawal can be treated in 1 week; however, psychological dependence is long-term.

► Treatment for maintenance can be 2 to 6 months of medication with an additional 6 months of follow-up.

Special Considerations

▶ Alcohol abuse during pregnancy can lead to severe birth defects or fetal alcohol syndrome.

▶ Alcoholism and alcohol abuse have long-term medical, social, and legal consequences.

▶ Severe intoxication is a medical emergency and may lead to coma, respiratory depression, aspiration, and death.

When to Consult, Refer, Hospitalize

▶ Refer patients diagnosed or suspected of alcoholism to a substance abuse specialist.

▶ Hospitalize for acute intoxication and withdrawal.

▶ Refer social issues to a mental health specialist for long-term management.

▶ Refer all legal issues to the appropriate legal authority.

Follow-up

Expected Course

▶ Treatment and outcome are variable for each individual, with recovery as a lifelong commitment.

Complications

▶ Peak at 65–74 years of age, depending on length of exposure, frequency, and quantity of consumption

▶ See Assessment for list of medical complications; fetal alcohol syndrome

SUBSTANCE ABUSE AND DEPENDENCE

Description

▶ A maladaptive pattern of substance use manifested by recurrent and significant adverse medical, psychosocial, and legal consequences related to the repeated use of the substance

▶ Drug dependence manifests as substance-seeking behaviors, physical dependence, tolerance, and withdrawal.

Etiology

▶ Acquired brain disease; not well-understood

▶ Neurons in the locus caeruleus are thought to adapt to chronic opiate exposure and fire at a higher than normal rate when withdrawal occurs, and are responsible for producing the physical symptoms of withdrawal.

▶ Contributing factors to individual vulnerability:

  ▹ Genetic predisposition

  ▹ Neurotransmitter abnormalities

  ▹ Environmental stressors

» Psychodynamic factors, such as unstable childhood, impaired developmental stages, personality disorders

» Sociocultural factors, such as increased availability and prevalence, cultural acceptance and peer pressure, impaired family and peer relations, stress, lack of valued alternatives

Incidence and Demographics

▶ Abuse and dependence are more common in men than in women.

▶ The average onset age of substance use is 12–14 years of age.

▶ There is a link between substance use and suicide in adolescents.

▶ Usage crosses all cultural and socioeconomic barriers.

▶ Marijuana is the most commonly used substance, excluding alcohol and tobacco.

▶ Strong links occur among alcohol, substances, and nicotine abuse.

▶ The highest prevalence of abuse occurs during ages 18–25.

▶ 70% of all admissions to treatment programs are men, 30% are women.

▶ 76% of men and 65% of women with a diagnosis of substance abuse have psychiatric disorders.

Risk Factors

▶ Genetic vulnerability

▶ Personal or family history

▶ Social, cultural, peer acceptance, and frequent use

▶ Psychiatric diagnosis, history of previous addiction

▶ Chronic pain

Prevention and Screening

▶ National and local public education and awareness through mass media educational campaigns

▶ Early prevention and education programs in school systems

▶ All patients interviewed for possible substance abuse disorder

▶ Cognitive-behavioral therapy to enhance coping skills

Assessment

History

▶ Personal, family history of abuse

▶ Patterns of use, substances of choice

▶ History of accidents, traumas, overdoses; legal difficulties

▶ Effects in Table 18–7

TABLE 18-7
EFFECTS OF DRUG ABUSE

NAME OF DRUG	EFFECT	METHOD OF USE	CHARACTER-ISTICS	EFFECTS ON USER
Tobacco	No alterations in mood or effect	Smoked, chewed	Addicting	Frequent respiratory symptoms, infections. Lowered HDL cholesterol, increased heart disease. Smokeless tobacco increases incidence of oral cancer, periodontal disease.
Alcohol	Initial euphoria, impaired judgment. Long-term depressant effects	Swallowed	Withdrawal symptoms with frequent, prolonged use	Gastritis, vomiting, anorexia. Blackouts with heavy use.
Marijuana	Relaxation, depressant. May have mild hallucinogenic effects	Smoked, swallowed	Referred to as "gateway" drug, may lead to use of other products. Tolerance with regular use	Chronic users develop apathy, decreased motivation, flat affect, global cognitive impairment (memory, problem-solving), chronic cough
Cocaine	Stimulant, produces euphoria, increased physical activity, may lead to aggression, paranoia	Smoked, snorted, sniffed	Highly addictive, tolerance develops	Hypertensive crisis, coronary artery vasospasm, arrhythmias may occur
Methamphet-amine	Stimulant, similar to cocaine	Snorted, smoked, ingested	Withdrawal symptoms with cessation	Similar to cocaine, tachycardia
Hallucinogens (LSD, PCP, MDMA, "Ecstasy")	Visual, auditory hallucinations, altered mood and dream-like state	Ingested	MDMA commonly abused at "raves" to produce euphoria	Hallucinations may occur weeks after use. Renal damage may occur with Ecstasy.
Inhalants (glue, paint thinner, gasoline, freon)	Euphoria, dream-like state, often with hallucinations. Some products may have aphrodisiac properties	Directly inhaled or inhaled by huffing (putting a substance-soaked cloth in a bag and inhaling)	Commonly used by younger teens because of easy access	Most are CNS toxins, possible permanent sequelae such as peripheral neuropathy, ataxia, cognitive loss, language difficulty, loss of coordination. Lung, kidney damage may occur.

CONTINUED

TABLE 18–7 CONTINUED
EFFECTS OF DRUG ABUSE

NAME OF DRUG	EFFECT	METHOD OF USE	CHARACTER-ISTICS	EFFECTS ON USER
Heroin	Sedation, soothing and numbing effect with euphoria	Snorted, sniffed, subcutaneous (skin popping), and IV use	Sniffing most common method of use with adolescents	Chronic symptoms include constipation, chronic pruritus, bronchospasm
Prescription medications (opioids, ben-zodiazepine, stimulants	Concurrent with drug of use	Ingested	Often manifests as patients presenting with pain complaints	Necessary to treat patient for pain; however, recognize addiction can present this way

Physical Exam

▶ Stimulants

  » Anxiety, agitation, panic, restlessness, irritability, aggression

  » Mood swings, grandiose, elated mood, hallucinations

  » Tachycardia, arrhythmias, chest pain, hypertension; hypothermia, hyperthermia

  » Abdominal pain, nausea, vomiting, insomnia, mydriasis

  » Hypersexuality, frequent urination

▶ Depressants

  » Dysphoria, depressed affect, apathy, psychomotor retardation, slurred speech, drowsiness

  » Diaphoresis, hypotension, miosis, rhinorrhea, sneezing, headache, nausea, vomiting

  » Myalgia, muscle pain, ataxia, tremors, impaired coordination, impotence

  » Mood swings, aggression, combativeness, lack of impulse control, disinhibition

  » Impaired attention, memory, and judgment; hallucinations; paranoia

▶ Hallucinogens

  » Mydriasis, nystagmus, tachycardia, hypertension, ataxia, tremors

  » Severe anxiety, panic, mood swings, aggression, hallucinations, paranoia, flashbacks

  » Impaired concentration, memory, judgment, ability to make decisions

▶ Cannabis

  » Paranoia, confusion, hallucinations, distortion of time and spatial orientation

▶ Inhalants and solvents

  » Odor on breath, ataxia, slurred speech, euphoria, agitation, tachycardia, arrhythmias

  » Delirium, confusion, stupor, hallucinations, organic brain damage

Diagnostic Studies

▶ Urine and serum toxicology screens

▶ CBC; chemistry profiles; liver, kidney, cardiac, thyroid functions to rule out other disorders

▶ VDRL, HIV because of high rate of STDs and bloodborne disease in this population

▶ CT, MRI scans, X-rays as indicated by history and physical to rule out other conditions

Differential Diagnosis

▶ Polysubstance abuse

▶ Psychiatric disorders

▶ Hypothyroidism, hyperthyroidism

▶ Hypoglycemia, hyperglycemia

▶ Head trauma

▶ Stroke, dementia, delirium, seizure disorder

Management

▶ Treatment and management depend on patient motivation, characteristics, and ability to engage in a therapeutic relationship. Nonjudgmental support by provider facilitates recovery.

▶ Before treatment, identify type and amount of substance ingested and route taken.

▶ Minimization and denial are hallmark characteristics and interfere with recovery.

Nonpharmacologic Treatment

▶ Multiple treatment modalities and interventions

  » Behavioral therapy

  » 12-step programs (Narcotics Anonymous, Cocaine Anonymous, Marijuana Anonymous)

  » Long-term residential treatment programs

Pharmacologic Treatment

▶ Methadone hydrochloride, levo-alpha-cetyl methanol (LAAM) used to treat heroin addiction, to block effects of heroin and yield stable, noneuphoric state free from drug craving

▶ Buprenorphine (Buprenex), a controlled narcotic similar to morphine with longer duration of action and no physical dependence upon withdrawal

▶ Stimulant abuse

  » Diazepam (Valium) 5–10 mg q3h; drug of choice for cocaine toxicity

  » Monitor cardiac rate and rhythm

▶ Depressant abuse

  » Phenobarbital for withdrawal

  » Haloperidol (Haldol) commonly used to treat assaultive and psychotic behaviors

How Long to Treat

▶ Varies according to individual response

▶ Substance abuse commonly occurs with psychiatric disorders, requiring treatment of other disorder.

▶ Prognosis and recovery are highly dependent on personal motivation and social support.

▶ Residential treatment needs to exceed 90 days to be effective.

▶ Methadone maintenance is 12 months minimum.

▶ Opiate treatment is a minimum of 2 years.

Special Considerations

▶ Legal issues are common with substance abuse disorders.

▶ Abuse of substances during pregnancy increases the risk of spontaneous abortion, premature birth, preeclampsia and eclampsia, low birth weight, and birth defects.

▶ DSM-IV criteria apply to adult population and may not be applicable to adolescents and children.

When to Consult, Refer, Hospitalize

▶ The role of the primary care provider is diagnosis, referral to substance abuse specialist, and co-management of medical consequences.

▶ Hospitalize for severe intoxication and medical compromise.

Follow-up

▶ Frequency dictated by substance abuse specialist

Expected Course

▶ Substance abuse is a chronic disorder characterized by periods of relapse and remission.

▶ Outcomes are contingent on adequate length of time in treatment and support systems.

Complications

▶ Long-term use results in significant changes in brain function, as well as severe impairment in social, vocational, and interpersonal relations.

▶ High-risk behavior places substance abusers at risk for infections such as HIV, STDs, and hepatitis.

▶ Poor nutritional status, dental problems, poor personal hygiene

DOMESTIC VIOLENCE AND ABUSE

DOMESTIC VIOLENCE

Description

▶ Physical, emotional, economic, or sexual pain and injury inflicted deliberately upon a partner or family member with the express goal of controlling, manipulating, or intimidating that person within the relationship

Etiology

▶ Genetic predisposition toward aggression

▶ Personality disorders (antisocial disorder, narcissistic disorder, borderline personality disorder)

▶ Environmental stressors; comorbid medical disease (depression, mania, schizophrenia)

▶ Low self-esteem; exposure to violence at an early developmental age

Incidence and Demographics

▶ Domestic violence is the leading cause of injury to women ages 15–44.

▶ 1 in 4 pregnant women has a history of domestic violence.

▶ 22%–35% of all women seen in emergency rooms suffer injuries as a result of domestic violence.

▶ 50% of homeless women are victims of domestic violence.

▶ Women who leave their abusers are at 75% greater risk of being murdered than those who stay.

▶ Profile of known, reported abusers: Male under age 25, lower socioeconomic status, inner-city resident.

▶ Male victims are underreported.

Risk Factors

▶ Female gender

▶ Physical, emotional, financial dependence

▶ Poverty, housing problems, lack of education, lack of vocational skills

▶ Divorced and single-parent families

▶ Psychiatric diagnosis

▶ Alcohol and substance abuse

▶ Pregnancy or other physical and emotional disabilities

▶ Family or personal history of physical or sexual abuse; long-term exposure to violence

▶ Social isolation, lack of support systems

Prevention and Screening

▶ Public education and awareness campaigns

▶ Educated primary care providers

▶ Provide community resources, support

▶ Community emergency shelters, hotlines, and safe houses

▶ Organizations such as the National Coalition Against Domestic Violence

Assessment

History

▶ Interview patient alone.

▶ Include questions concerning domestic violence in medical history.

▶ Appropriate documentation

  ▸ Trouble expressing anger

  ▸ Passive role in the relationship

Physical Exam

▶ Withdrawn, fearful, evasive

▶ Poor personal hygiene, neglect; bruises, burns, fractures, injuries to abdomen, breasts, torso, pelvic region; injuries inconsistent with explanation offered

▶ Significant delay between time of injury and treatment

▶ Substance abuse; depression, anxiety; suicidal or homicidal ideation; somatization of symptoms

Diagnostic Studies

▶ As injuries warrant:

  ▸ X-ray

  ▸ CT, MRI

  ▸ CBC, chemistry profiles, electrolytes, STD testing, VDRL, HIV

Differential Diagnosis

▶ Accidental injuries

▶ Depression or anxiety

▶ Hypochondriasis

▶ Substance abuse

▶ Borderline personality disorder

Management

Nonpharmacologic Treatment

▶ Establish safe, supportive environment, including counseling to develop a safety plan.

▶ Develop plan of action regarding safety and escape.

▶ Provide information on community resources, shelters, and hotlines.

▶ Cognitive–behavioral therapy

Pharmacologic Treatment

▶ Varies according to individual injuries

▶ Antidepressants

▶ Anti-anxiety agents

Special Considerations

▶ Victims of domestic violence have greater incidence of substance abuse.

▶ Persons with a history of being a victim of domestic violence are more likely to commit violent acts.

▶ People who are feeling trapped or hopeless have a greater incidence of suicidal ideation and depression.

▶ It is mandatory by law to report all acts of violence or abuse against children or elderly; check state laws for reporting domestic violence.

When to Consult, Refer, Hospitalize

▶ Refer all cases to a mental health specialist for counseling.

▶ Refer patients with injuries to an emergency department.

Follow-up

▶ Long-term with mental health specialist often needed, or return to therapy at later time

ELDER AND DISABLED ADULT ABUSE AND NEGLECT

Description

▶ Emotional or physical injury deliberately inflicted upon an older or disabled adult partner or family member with the goal of control and intimidation by a person who has control or a position of trust. Goal is manipulation, intimidation, or control of the dependent individual.

Etiology

▶ Physical, emotional, sexual, and financial dependency due to disability or age; unreasonable physical restraint; deprivation of food, water, shelter, or medical treatment; and physical abandonment

▶ Limited economic and financial resources

Incidence and Demographics

▶ More than 2 million adults > 60 years of age are abused annually.

▶ Adults > 84 are more likely to be abused.

▶ Women are more likely to be victimized than men.

▶ There is a greater incidence of abuse by family members than paid providers.

▶ More than 50% of victims are cognitively impaired.

Risk Factors

▶ Over age 84

▶ Social isolation, lack of support

▶ Cognitively impaired

▶ Physical, financial dependency

Prevention and Screening

- ▶ Public education and awareness
- ▶ Social programs such as Adult Protective Services
- ▶ Caregiver support and respite
- ▶ Assess caregivers for depression.

Assessment

History

- ▶ Interview patient alone.
- ▶ Mental status exam
- ▶ Determine primary caregivers, living arrangements, legal custodian, and power of attorney.
- ▶ History of medical treatment, accidents, fractures, physical injuries, traumas, overdose of medications
- ▶ Determine environmental, psychosocial, and financial stressors.

Physical Exam

- ▶ Monitor nutritional status for dehydration, malnutrition.
- ▶ Lacerations, bruises, wounds, burns, fractures
- ▶ Poor skin and personal hygiene
- ▶ Evidence of sexual abuse: Pain or soreness in anal-genital area, venereal diseases, vaginal or rectal bruises or bleeding.
- ▶ Fearful, evasive, guarded, depressed

Other

- ▶ Unusual or inappropriate activity in bank accounts
- ▶ Numerous unpaid bills
- ▶ Lack of amenities
- ▶ Missing belongings
- ▶ Missed medical appointments

Diagnostic Studies

- ▶ Specific to presenting symptomology
- ▶ Signs of poor nutritional status

Differential Diagnosis

- ▶ Accidental injury
- ▶ Depression
- ▶ Self-neglect due to cognitive status or physical impairment

Management

Nonpharmacologic Treatment

▶ Goal is to maintain independence of the patient and caregiver. If patient needs care beyond ability of caregiver, consider institutionalization, homecare services, respite for caregiver, adult daycare program, etc.

▶ Potential removal from the home for care and safety

▶ Monitor nutritional status and vital signs, cognitive status, medical status as symptomology presents.

▶ Counseling for the perpetrator and the abused may be indicated; consider need for psychiatric or alcohol abuse treatment.

Pharmacologic Treatment

▶ Antidepressants may be indicated.

Special Considerations

▶ It is mandatory by law to report all elder and disabled adult abuse and neglect to Adult Protective Services.

When to Consult, Refer, Hospitalize

▶ Hospitalization or institutionalization when in the best interest of the patient

Follow-up

▶ Routine medical follow-up for signs of further abuse

Complications

▶ Wide variety of medical and emotional consequences is possible.

CHILD ABUSE AND NEGLECT

Description

▶ Physical or emotional pain and injury inflicted deliberately upon a child or failure to provide a child with adequate food, clothing, shelter, supervision, or care

▶ Includes physical abuse; sexual assault; unreasonable physical restraint; deprivation of food, water, shelter or medical treatment; emotional deprivation; and physical abandonment

Etiology

▶ No single set of factors produces abusive or neglectful individuals

▶ Often abuser was a victim of abuse

Incidence and Demographics

▶ 2.5 million cases are reported each year in the U.S.

Risk Factors

▶ History of abuse in family is common.

▶ Nonbiologic primary caregiver, live-in girlfriend or boyfriend of child's parent

▶ Increased family stress and social isolation are linked to abuse.

▶ Low socioeconomic level and financial stress are correlated with increased rates of neglect and abuse.

▶ Some psychiatric conditions in parents or guardians are associated with abuse and neglect.

▶ Alcohol and drug abuse are related to high rates of neglect and abuse.

▶ Characteristics of the child, including dependency, being a fussy baby, slow growth, developmental delay, disability, and male gender, increase rates of abuse and neglect.

Prevention and Screening

▶ Public education and awareness

▶ Government social programs such as Child Protective Services

Assessment

History

▶ Interview child and parents separately. Start with open-ended questions.

▶ Interview by professionals with specialized training in the history process is preferred.

▶ If physical injury is present, ask specific questions eliciting detailed answers, including when and how it occurred.

▶ Inconsistencies, contradictions, and failure to adequately explain should arouse suspicion of abuse.

▶ Take a complete social history, including information about parents, caretakers, and family functioning; determine environmental, psychosocial, or financial stressors.

▶ Explore child's past and present history of medical treatment, including accidents, fractures, physical injuries, traumas, ingestions, and illnesses.

▶ Explore child's developmental and behavioral history, including the perinatal period, labor and delivery, neonatal period, feeding difficulties, sleeping problems, toilet training, encopresis, or enuresis.

Physical Exam

▶ Measure height and weight, using growth chart and comparing findings to norms and child's own growth curve; note nutritional status and hydration.

▶ Findings on physical exam suggestive of abuse include:

  » Bruising: In unexpected areas (abdomen, lower back, inner thighs, neck, around the mouth, pinna, inner aspects of arms — as child raises arms to protect face), in infants < 6 months of age; multiple bruises in various stages

» Marks with characteristic shapes: Belt buckles, looped cords, palm of hand, human bite marks, marks around the wrists or ankles may indicate tying the child down

» Burns: Cigarette marks, specific objects (curling iron), immersion burn from hot bathtub (discrete water level marks are around buttocks and feet and hands). Scalds from tap water are the most common type of intentional burn.

» Hair: Patchy areas of alopecia from pulling out hair

» Mouth: Torn frenula, petechial lesions, lacerations or bruising to the palate

» Neurologic signs (signs of increased intracranial pressure [ICP] from bleeding into the head): Bulging anterior fontanel, palpable split in suture lines, increasing head circumference, papilledema, behavior changes or decreased level of consciousness, vomiting. Most subdural hematomas are due to abuse. Head trauma accounts for approximately 50% of deaths due to physical abuse.

» Eyes (fundus): Retinal hemorrhages (from shaking), papilledema (from increased ICP)

» Abdomen: Vomiting, abdominal distention, tenderness, decreased or absent bowel sounds may indicate trauma; bruising on the abdomen may not always be present. Abdominal trauma is the second leading cause of death from physical abuse.

» Genitalia and buttocks: Most sexual abuse leaves no visible scars; injuries that occur heal quickly. In girls: Unusually enlarged hymenal opening (requires expert evaluation because of wide range of normal in sizes and shapes), extensive vaginal adhesions, purulent vaginal discharge. In boys: Penile or scrotal injuries are uncommon; most findings are in the rectal area and may include abrasions, perirectal skin tags outside the midline (develop as small areas of bleeding heal), hemorrhoids (normally very uncommon in children), poor rectal tone (dilation > 15 mm), penile erection during entire exam in prepubertal boys (may be a normal variant). In both sexes: Any sexually transmitted skin lesions such as warts are highly suggestive of abuse.

Diagnostic Studies

▶ Bony injuries are most common in children < 3 years.

▶ Fractures highly suggestive of abuse include metaphyseal (or buckle handle fracture), rib, scapular, vertebral, spiral fractures of the humerus or femur in the young infant, fractures of the hands or feet in children < 2 years of age.

▶ Metaphyseal injuries are fractures through newly forming bone that occur when limbs are forcefully moved (usually rotated), such as commonly seen in the distal humerus and femur or proximal tibia. They are highly suggestive of abuse. Changes may not be seen on X-ray for days to weeks.

▶ Skull fractures suggestive of abuse are wide (> 3 mm), complex (branching, involvement of suture lines), occurring outside the parietal area, or multiple. Simple skull fractures may or may not be associated with abuse. Falls of less than 2½ feet do not usually result in skull fractures.

▶ Multiple fractures in various stages of healing are almost pathognomonic of abuse once osteogenesis imperfecta is ruled out.

▶ Fractures not highly suggestive of abuse are those of the distal radius and ulna (from falling on outstretched hands), simple linear fracture of a long bone, mid-clavicular fractures, and nondisplaced spiral fracture of the tibia in a toddler.

▶ Blunt trauma to a bone can cause subperiosteal hemorrhage, with subsequent periosteal thickening and elevation visible on X-ray.

▶ Full skeletal surveys are recommended in children < 3 years of age who are suspected of being abused.

▶ New, nondisplaced fractures may not be evident on X-ray for 1–2 weeks and a repeat X-ray or a bone scan is recommended.

▶ Sexual abuse requires a specialized exam and collection of laboratory and forensic evidence.

Differential Diagnosis

▶ Unintended injury

▶ Poverty resulting in poor hygiene, poor clothing, or poor nutrition

▶ Osteogenesis imperfecta

Management

▶ Suspicion of neglect or abuse mandates reporting to local (or state, depending on region) child protection authority. Consider reporting to local law enforcement authority.

▶ Inform parent or guardian that you are required by law to report suspected abuse.

Special Considerations

▶ The child protection agency is responsible for investigating the case and assisting the family and child to obtain access support services.

▶ Documentation is critical and should be done carefully; it may become part of a court case.

When to Consult, Refer, Hospitalize

▶ If injuries are severe or involve suspected sexual abuse, child should be referred to the hospital for evaluation and treatment by child abuse team.

Follow-up

▶ The FNP has the responsibility to follow up closely and advocate for safety and medical well-being of the child.

Complications

▶ Victims are at risk for depression; other psychological, educational, and behavioral problems; and repeating the cycle of violence.

SEXUAL ASSAULT AND ABUSE

Description
▶ Any sexual act or penetration committed through coercion or physical force, including rape, incest, sodomy, oral and anal acts, or use of hands or a foreign object

Etiology
▶ Character disorders

▶ Behavioral: Act of violence is reinforcing; once done, likely to do again

▶ Social: Exposure to violence in culture, media, and home

Incidence and Demographics
▶ Women have a greater incidence of being assaulted; men are more frequently perpetrators.

▶ The most common form of abuse is by persons the victim knows: fathers, stepfathers, uncles, older siblings, and dates.

▶ Incestuous behavior is reported more frequently among families of low socioeconomic status.

▶ Alcohol is involved in 34% of all rapes.

▶ Only 1 out of 4 rapes is reported.

Risk Factors

In the Abuser
▶ Substance abuse disorders, psychiatric disorders

▶ Divorce, pregnancy

▶ Family or personal history of physical or sexual abuse

▶ Long-term exposure to violence

▶ Lower socioeconomic status

▶ Social isolation, lack of support systems

▶ Factors such as unemployment, financial difficulty, housing problems, overcrowding

In the Abused
▶ Vulnerable, dependent, young

▶ Opportunity for abuser to be alone with them

Prevention and Screening
▶ Public education and awareness campaigns

▶ Providing community resources, support

▶ Community emergency shelters, hotlines, and safe houses

▶ Organizations such as the National Coalition Against Domestic Violence

▶ Assertiveness and self-defense training

Assessment

▶ The FNP is required to know and follow specific rape evaluation protocols regarding history, physical, and collection of specimens, or information and findings may not be admissible in court.

▶ If not educated in rape evaluation, refer to a specially trained provider.

History

▶ Social history, living environment, relationships

▶ Inclusion of questions concerning domestic violence in medical history

▶ Interview patient alone when possible.

Physical Exam

▶ Withdrawn, frightened appearance; depressive symptoms

▶ Dislocations and fractures

▶ Unexplained bruises, abrasions, cuts, laceration, burns, soft tissue swellings, hematomas

▶ Sexually transmitted diseases, genital rash, discharge

▶ Rectal tissue swelling, discharge

Diagnostic Studies

▶ Forensic specimens and extensive STD testing per protocol, including HIV screening

▶ Pregnancy test now and at later time for female victims past puberty

▶ X-rays, CT scans, MRI as indicated

Differential Diagnosis

▶ Consenting sex among adults

▶ Accidental injury to pelvic and groin area

▶ Posttraumatic stress disorder

Management

▶ Ensure safety, well-being, confidentiality

▶ Accurate documentation

▶ Be aware of depressive symptoms and potential for suicide.

Nonpharmacologic Treatment

▶ Cognitive–behavioral therapy

▶ Psychoanalysis

▶ Support groups and community resources

▶ Legal intervention

Pharmacologic Treatment

▶ Emergency contraception for postpubertal females (rule out pregnancy with urine or serum hCG first)

　▹ Emergency contraceptive tablet *or*

　▹ Norgestrel 0.3 mg and ethinyl estradiol 0.03 mg (Lo/Ovral) or other 30 mcg pill: 4 tablets within 72 hours of incident with 4 tablets 12 hours later

　▹ Levonorgestrel 0.25 mg and ethinyl estradiol 0.05 mg (Preven): 2 tablets within 72 hours of incident then 2 tablets 12 hours later

　▹ Antiemetic may be necessary with emergency contraception.

How Long to Treat

▶ Varies with individual medical and emotional needs

Special Considerations

▶ People with other mental disorders at higher risk of abusing others

▶ Nature of relationship between abuser and the individual affects recovery

▶ Persons with developmental delays at risk of being abused

When to Consult, Refer, Hospitalize

▶ All injuries and all cases of recent rape should be referred to an emergency department (with rape protocol).

▶ Refer all those with recent or past sexual abuse to mental health professional with experience in sexual abuse for treatment of psychosocial issues and possible posttraumatic stress disorder.

Follow-up

▶ Depends on individual coping strategies and support system

Complications

▶ Posttraumatic stress disorder, injuries to external genitalia, STIs, pregnancy

EATING DISORDERS

Description

▶ Disorders that are characterized by severe disturbances in eating behavior. The two major types are anorexia nervosa and bulimia nervosa. Binge eating also is a disorder that exists by itself (without purging).

ANOREXIA NERVOSA

Description

▶ Eating behavior characterized by refusal to maintain a normal body weight (and body weight is < 85% of expected), severe restriction of caloric intake, intense fear of gaining weight and a severely distorted perception of one's body, and absence of menses in women; weight loss to > 15% below expected weight for height

▶ Types: Restricting, binge eating and purging

Etiology

▶ Biological

　▹ Genetic vulnerability and predisposition, neurotransmitter abnormalities

▶ Psychodynamic

　▹ Reaction to the demand of adolescence; perfectionist personality with obsessive, rigid characteristics

　▹ Lacking self-confidence; close, troubled relations with parents; influence of family dynamics; parents may be overbearing or demanding; father may be distant while mother is overprotective and intrusive

▶ Sociocultural

　▹ Peer pressure to be thin; media and cultural emphasis on thinness, youth, body image

▶ Pathophysiology of starvation: Lack of energy and nutrients causes fat and protein store breakdown

Incidence and Demographics

▶ Approximately 90% of patients are female

▶ 85% of cases have onset at 14–18 years of age

▶ Maximum frequency of occurrence is age 17–18

▶ Mortality rates are 5%–18%, making it the psychiatric disorder with highest rate of fatalities

▶ Associated with depression in 65% of cases, social phobia in 34%, obsessive-compulsive disorder in 26%

Risk Factors

▶ Family histories of mood disorders, alcoholism, or eating disorders

▶ Perfectionistic, compulsive, high expectations of self

▶ Caucasian, middle-class females; adolescence

▶ Dancers, athletes, gymnasts

Prevention and Screening

▶ Public education and awareness

▶ Early intervention

Assessment

History

▶ Weight history, onset of weight loss

▶ Symptoms such as constipation, cold hands and feet, fatigue

▶ Dietary habits, patterns of eating, food rituals, weight loss, binge eating or purging

▶ Menstrual history: Amenorrhea

▶ Perception of body weight and shape, fears of gaining weight

▶ Exercise history, frequency and duration — may be excessive

▶ Use of medication for weight control

▶ Psychiatric history, including comorbidity and previous eating disorders

▶ Family history of eating or psychiatric disorders

▶ Previous psychiatric treatments

Physical Exam

▶ Weigh patient without clothes. Weight is often 15% below ideal body weight with significantly low BMI.

▶ Amenorrhea, lanugo, delayed growth and sexual maturation

▶ Altered vital signs: Hypothermia, hypotension, bradycardia

▶ Muscular atrophy, ridges in fingernails, erosion of enamel of teeth from stomach acid

Diagnostic Studies

▶ A multitude of endocrine and medical problems can occur secondary to the starvation that occurs with this disorder. There are no definite laboratory tests to diagnosis anorexia.

▶ ECG (look for flattening or inversion of T waves, ST-segment depression, lengthening of QT interval), CBC (anemia, leukopenia), chemistry panel with electrolytes (low potassium level), LH and FSH diminished, TSH, T3, T4, glucose levels

Differential Diagnosis

▶ Bulimia nervosa

▶ Mood disorders

▶ Substance abuse

▶ Medical disorders such as cancer, diabetes mellitus, Crohn's disease, endocrine disorders

Management

▶ First consideration in treatment is to restore the patient's nutritional state.

Nonpharmacologic Treatment

▶ Nutritional and medical management

  ▹ Establish appropriate eating habits.

  ▹ Rehydrate and correct electrolyte balance.

    ▹ Restore weight; stop exercising.

▶ Psychotherapy

  ▹ Cognitive–behavioral therapy is treatment of choice

  ▹ Individual and family therapy

  ▹ Nutritional and dietary education and weekly monitoring

Pharmacologic Treatment

▶ SSRI antidepressants are the most commonly used and may or may not be helpful in treating anorexia, but may be used in prevention of relapse of symptoms after weight is restored.

▶ Other antidepressants, such as TCAs or amitriptyline (Elavil), antipsychotics (olanzapine [Zyprexa]), mood stabilizers, and appetite stimulants (cyproheptadine [Periactin]), have also been tried.

How Long to Treat

▶ Varies according to individual characteristics, severity of symptoms and motivation

▶ Inpatient stays may last 4–8 weeks, followed by day treatment program of 4–6 weeks

Special Considerations

▶ Denial is a classic characteristic of this disorder.

▶ Patients with eating disorders resist medical treatment.

▶ Symptoms of bulimia occur in 30%–50% of anorectic persons.

▶ In a pregnant patient, poor nutritional status may endanger fetus and status of the pregnancy.

When to Consult, Refer, Hospitalize

▶ A psychiatric consult should always be obtained.

▶ Mandatory hospitalization should occur when the risk of death from complications of malnutrition is likely.

▶ Required when total body weight is 30% below expected

Follow-up

▶ The role of the primary care provider is to monitor the medical component, including weekly weight and nutritional status, periodic lab tests, and collaboration with involved professionals.

Expected Course

▶ Varies widely

▶ 10-year outcome: ½ markedly improved, ¼ recovered completely

▶ Short-term response to hospitalization is good, but relapse is common.

▶ Food rituals, low self-esteem, and distorted body image commonly persist after treatment.

▶ Indicators of a favorable outcome are decreased denial, admission of hunger, and improved self-esteem and perceptions of body image and self.

Complications

▶ Cardiac arrhythmias if purging, heart failure, convulsions, osteoporosis, infertility, death

BULIMIA NERVOSA

Description

▶ Recurrent episodes of overeating followed by purging behavior (episodes occur at least twice a week for 3 months). Feeling of self-worth unduly influenced by weight.

   ▹ Eating a larger amount of food than most in a discrete time period

   ▹ Sense of lack of control over eating during episode

▶ Recurrent compensatory behavior to prevent weight gain with use of laxative, diuretic, enema, induced vomiting (purging type); or fasting or excessive exercise (nonpurging type)

Etiology

▶ Neurotransmitter abnormalities: Poor serotonergic function; depression

▶ Poor impulse control disorder; high prevalence of alcoholism and drug abuse in this population

▶ Genetic predisposition

▶ Social, cultural, and peer pressure to be thin

▶ Demands of adolescence

▶ Family dynamics, particularly family disorganization and lack of interest

Incidence and Demographics

▶ More common in females than in males

▶ More common than anorexia, but may occur with it

▶ Occurs in late adolescence

Risk Factors

▶ Approximately 90%–95% are female; adolescents and young adults; family history of obesity, family conflict

▶ Poor impulse control, low self-esteem; high expectations of self-performance

▶ Normal weight or overweight; history of dieting, obesity, fluctuating weight

▶ Substance abuse, mood disorders

Prevention and Screening

▶ Public education and awareness

▶ Early intervention

Assessment

History

▶ Onset of symptoms such as constipation, muscle cramps; menstrual history

▶ Dietary habits, patterns of eating, food rituals, and purging behaviors

▶ Use of medication, especially for weight control; use of laxatives

▶ Weight history, exercise history

▶ Psychiatric history, body perception

Physical Exam

▶ Complete physical exam to rule out medical causes

▶ Weight measurement without clothes (weight fluctuations — typically remain within 20% of normal)

▶ Dental carries, dental erosions, gum disease, parotid swelling

▶ Abdominal distress (from putting pressure on the abdomen to vomit), esophagitis, irritation of the pharynx

▶ Ridges in fingernails, calluses or abrasions on knuckles (Russell's sign)

Diagnostic Studies

▶ CBC, chemistry panel with electrolytes (low potassium), ECG, TSH, T3, T4

▶ Amylase levels elevated with vomiting, return to normal in 72 hours after vomiting stops

Differential Diagnosis

▶ Anorexia nervosa

▶ Gastrointestinal disorders

▶ Endocrine disorders

▶ Neurologic disorders

▶ Mood disorders

▶ Anxiety disorders

▶ Personality disorders

Management

Nonpharmacologic Treatment

▶ Cognitive-behavioral therapy, including individual and family therapy

▶ Nutrition counseling: Goal is to restore appropriate eating patterns

▶ Community support groups and resources

Pharmacologic Treatment

▶ Antidepressant medications — SSRIs and TCAs — are considered effective in reducing binge eating and purging behaviors. Use doses given in the treatment of depressive disorders.

▶ Avoid MAO inhibitors due to potential for severe food interactions and hypertensive crisis.

▶ Medication is used as adjunct therapy, combined with psychological and nutritional counseling.

How Long to Treat

▶ Duration varies; often months to years

Special Considerations

▶ Patients will try to hide behaviors associated with the disorder; family may see patient make frequent trips to bathroom after eating, excessive exercise, up during night binging

When to Consult, Refer, Hospitalize

▶ Refer every case to a mental health professional who is an eating disorder specialist.

▶ Treatment may be managed on an outpatient basis in consultation with a nutritionist and psychotherapist.

▶ Hospitalization is indicated when outpatient treatment is unsuccessful, or if cardiac complications, hemodynamic instability, or hypovolemia present.

Follow-up

▶ Role of primary care provider is to monitor medical aspects, including nutritional status (weekly weight) and periodic lab testing, and coordinate care with other involved professionals

Expected Course

▶ Frequent relapses

▶ Better prognosis than anorexia

▶ Prognosis depends on severity, electrolyte imbalances, and other medical complications

Complications

▶ Chronic induced emesis results in volume depletion, renal compensation, cardiac arrhythmia, esophagitis, dental decay

OTHER DISORDERS

ATTENTION-DEFICIT HYPERACTIVITY DISORDER (ADHD)

Description

- ▶ A neurobiological disorder affecting attention, impulse control, and level of activity
- ▶ One of the most common psychiatric disorders of childhood and adolescence; also recognized in adults
- ▶ Main behavioral aspects: Inattentiveness, impulsivity, and hyperactivity, more frequent and severe than what would be expected for child's developmental level. Symptoms vary from person to person and may include:
  - ▹ Easily distracted
  - ▹ Daydreams
  - ▹ Appears to be in another world
  - ▹ Fidgety, restless
  - ▹ Inappropriate or excessive activity
  - ▹ Seems to be "driven by a motor," always on the go
  - ▹ Talks constantly
  - ▹ Interrupts others
  - ▹ Has difficulty getting along with others
  - ▹ Forgetful: Fails to turn in work or complete assignments ("forgets")
  - ▹ Poor sustained attention
  - ▹ Poor self-esteem
- ▶ Symptoms may vary with the type of setting. Often minimized in highly supervised situations, one-on-one encounters, and when an activity is new or enjoyable. Symptoms may worsen when the activity is nonpreferred, difficult, or unstructured.
- ▶ Age of onset of symptoms is usually before age 7 (diagnosis may be made later).
- ▶ **Subtypes** (DSM-IV-TR)
  - ▹ Attention-Deficit Hyperactivity Disorder, Combined Type
  - ▹ Attention-Deficit Hyperactivity Disorder, Predominantly Inattentive Type
  - ▹ Attention-Deficit Hyperactivity Disorder, Predominantly Hyperactive-Impulsive Type

Etiology

- ▶ No single known cause; may be multiple etiologies. Possible causes:
  - ▹ Genetic factors: Up to 50% of children may have inherited this disorder
  - ▹ Adoption: Adopted children five times more likely to have ADHD than nonadopted children; may be related to poor prenatal care, malnutrition, or lack of stimulation
  - ▹ Neurochemical differences: Possible dopamine or norepinephrine deficiencies

- Brain structure differences: Possible frontal lobe and striatum alterations
- Pregnancy and delivery complication
- Prenatal substance abuse
- Low birth weight
- Traumatic brain injury

Incidence and Demographics

▶ Approximately 3%–7% of all school-age children have ADHD.

▶ Ratio of boys to girls with ADHD approximately 3:1; however, girls may be underdiagnosed because, although they are inattentive, their behavior tends to be less aggressive than that of boys.

▶ Most common psychiatric disorder in school-age children; less recognized in adults

▶ One of the most common referrals for mental healthcare providers

Risk Factors

▶ See Etiology.

Prevention and Screening

▶ Public education and awareness

▶ Early screening and evaluation

▶ Patient and family education

Assessment

History

▶ Specific symptoms, age of onset (< 7 years), duration of symptoms (> 6 months), presence in more than one setting

▶ Has a negative impact on child's quality of life

▶ Central nervous system insult or injury such as fetal alcohol syndrome, prematurity, CNS infection or injury, lead poisoning, neurodegenerative disorders and seizures

▶ Family or child history of medical conditions such as anemia, thyroid dysfunction, fragile X syndrome

▶ Interpersonal dynamics:interactions between the child and each family member and peer relationships

▶ Past or present stressors such as divorce or loss of a parent

▶ School history: Grades (past and present), school problems, absenteeism

▶ Family history of psychiatric illnesses, ADHD, or "school problems" (diagnosed or undiagnosed)

▶ History should be obtained from multiple sources, including parents, child, teachers, or other persons involved with the child such as mental healthcare providers.

Physical Exam

▶ Usually no findings on physical exam. There may be an increased incidence of neurologic "soft signs," which can aid with diagnosis.

▶ Perform a complete physical exam to rule out possible medical etiologies.

▶ Obtain vision and hearing tests

Diagnostic Studies

▶ No laboratory tests diagnose ADHD.

▶ Parent and teacher rating scales, such as Connor's, Vanderbilt, Achenbach, and Barkley's, should be used in addition to the clinical history.

▶ Psychological, educational, and language evaluations may be performed if learning disabilities are suspected. Psychoeducational testing may be obtained through the child's school or a psychologist.

▶ If indicated, obtain a CBC, lead level, and thyroid studies.

▶ EEGs may be obtained to rule out seizure disorders; MRIs are only indicated for children with neurologic findings.

Differential Diagnosis

▶ Anxiety

▶ Depression

▶ Learning disabilities

▶ Pervasive developmental disorder

▶ Substance abuse

▶ Medical disorders—absence seizures, hypothyroidism, anemia, lead poisoning

▶ Hearing and vision impairment

▶ Disorganized and chaotic family

Possible Comorbid or Coexisting Conditions

▶ Depression

▶ Dysthymia

▶ Learning disabilities

▶ Oppositional defiant disorder

▶ Conduct disorder

▶ Bipolar disorder

▶ Tourette's syndrome

▶ Drug or alcohol abuse

▶ Adjustment disorder

▶ Posttraumatic stress disorder (PTSD)

Management

Nonpharmacologic Treatment

▶ Education of child and family

  ▹ Assess their understanding of ADHD and provide information as needed.

  ▹ Discuss the treatment plan with the child and family, including behavioral and educational plans and medication use.

  ▹ Often one of the parents has symptoms and may need support and assistance. Adults often have history of problems in school and jobs, and require assistance with organization, social skills.

▶ Social skills training

   » Children with ADHD often have problems with peer relationships, due to their inability to read social cues and impulsive, hyperactive, or aggressive behaviors; tend to be immature

   » Training facilitates the child in recognizing problem areas in relationships and teaches strategies to help improve social skills.

▶ Psychotherapy

   » Often helpful in understanding ADHD and its impact on the child and family

   » May include cognitive–behavioral therapy (CBT) for the child and family, and group therapy

   » Behavioral and educational interventions (see Table 18–8)

TABLE 18–8
SELECTED BEHAVIORAL AND EDUCATIONAL INTERVENTIONS FOR CHILDREN WITH ADHD

BEHAVIORAL INTERVENTIONS AT HOME	ACCOMMODATIVE INTERVENTIONS AT SCHOOL
Establish a list of appropriate behaviors (a targeted small number but consistently reinforced)	Assess for possible learning disorders
Provide a structured environment (predictable routines)	Tutoring
	Untimed testing
Give only 1–3 shortly stated instructions at a time	Preferential seating in the class room
Use chart for reminders	Note-taking services
Use timers or bells for transitions	Modified textbooks
Reward positive behaviors	Tailoring of homework assignments
Ignore minor misbehaviors or give nonverbal cues	Organizational aids
Consistently discipline targeted behaviors	Use visual cues
	Use peer helper

Pharmacologic Treatment

▶ Approximately 80% of children with ADHD respond positively to medication; adults may also respond (see Table 18–9).

▶ Some positive effects of medication include improvement in attention, concentration and academic achievement; decrease in hyperactive, disruptive, and aggressive behaviors and emotional lability (emotional ups and downs).

▶ Psychostimulants are the first-line choice for the treatment of ADHD.

▶ Side effects of the psychostimulants include

   » Decreased appetite, insomnia, headache, stomachache, irritability, dysphoria

   » Rebound effect (increased hyperactive or impulsive behavior or marked irritability as medication wears off)

   » Most side effects dissipate after several days; however, if they persist, medication change should be considered.

   » Less common side effects seen, particularly with methylphenidate, are tics in susceptible children (5%–10%) and possible growth suppression at high doses.

▸ Nonstimulant medication may be used to treat ADHD if the child does not respond to or tolerate stimulants. These may include clonidine (Catapres), imipramine (Tofranil), venlafaxine (Effexor), or bupropion (Wellbutrin).

▸ Unlike psychostimulants, nonstimulants may not treat all behaviors associated with ADHD. A combination of stimulants and nonstimulants may be needed.

TABLE 18-9
PHARMACOLOGIC MANAGEMENT OF ADHD

MEDICATION	DAILY DOSE RANGE	MAXIMUM DOSE
Methylphenidate HCl		
Ritalin, Ritalin LA, Ritalin SR	5–60 mg	60 mg
Metadate CD, Metadate ER	10–60 mg	60 mg
Concerta	18–54 mg	54 mg
Dextroamphetamine Sulfate (Dexedrine, Dexedrine Spansule)	5–30 mg	40 mg
Dextroamphetamine/amphetamine (Adderall, Adderall XR)	5–30 mg	40 mg 30 mg (XR)
Dexmethylphenidate HCl (Focalin)	2.5–10 mg	20 mg
Atomoxetine HCl (Strattera)	10–60 mg	100 mg
Pemoline (Cylert) (Not used as first-line therapy due to liver toxicity)	18.75–75 mg	112.5 mg

How Long to Treat

▶ The child may continue on medication throughout adulthood; however, as the child matures, he or she may learn compensatory mechanisms, which decreases the need for medication.

Special Considerations

▶ The diagnosis of ADHD before the age of 4 years should be done cautiously.

▶ Females may often be underdiagnosed, particularly if child is inattentive but does not exhibit impulsive or hyperactive behavior.

▶ Adolescents typically are not hyperactive, but restless.

▶ Hyperactive children often exhibit quiet behavior while in an office setting.

▶ If hyperactive behavior appears suddenly, this is often due to a stressor in the child's life, not ADHD.

▶ Inattention or lack of motivation may be easily confused with ADHD and needs to be examined further.

▶ Children with ADHD are at an increased risk for developing other conditions, such as substance abuse, depression, conduct and anxiety disorders, and driving violations.

When to Consult, Refer, Hospitalize

▶ If the child has an atypical ADHD presentation or has a complicated comorbid condition

▶ When the child does not respond to treatment

▶ If the child exhibits severe antisocial or aggressive behavior

▶ If the child is threatening or attempting suicide

Follow-up

▶ Medications should be monitored closely to determine effectiveness and possible side effects.

▶ Behavioral rating scales are useful to establish the effectiveness of medication during school.

▶ Initially frequent telephone follow-up with an office visit 1 month after starting medication

▶ Frequent follow-up when titrating medication dosage and every 3–6 months when stabilized

▶ Monitor height, weight, and blood pressure at every visit.

▶ Provide close monitoring of the child's functioning in school and at home, and make appropriate adjustments and recommendations as needed.

AUTISM SPECTRUM DISORDERS (ASD)

Description

▶ A group of neurodevelopmental disorders characterized by impairments in 3 major domains: socialization, communication, and behavior

▶ The DSM-IV categorizes these disorders under pervasive developmental disorders and includes autistic disorder, Asperger syndrome, and pervasive developmental disorder — not otherwise specified (PDD-NOS).

Etiology

▶ No single known etiology; multiple genetic and environmental factors suspected to play a role

Incidence and Demographics

▶ Five times more common in males than females

▶ Prevalence increased since 1970s, particularly since late 1990s, partially due to changes in case definition and increased awareness

▶ Estimated prevalence ranges from 1 in 88 to 1 in 500 children, depending on study methodology and area

Risk Factors

► Genetic (multigenomic) factors lead to altered brain development, resulting in neurobehavioral phenotype.

► Little evidence to link any single environmental factor to autism

► Overwhelming majority of evidence does not support an association between immunizations and autism.

Prevention and Screening

► Commonly recognized symptoms of autism most often recognized in second year of life

► Screening not diagnostic, but helps determine whether additional diagnostic evaluation by a specialist is warranted

► Developmental-behavioral assessments should be done for all infants and young children routinely; an autism specific screening tool should be used in children with delayed language or communication milestones, regression in milestones, a sibling with autism, parents who raise concern, and all ages 18 to 24 months.

Assessment

History

► Impaired social interaction, including a baby who resists cuddling, avoids eye contact, or fails to spread arms in anticipation of being picked up

► Failure to develop peer relationships, prefers solitary play, older children lack understanding of social conventions or needs of others

► Use valid screening tools such as CHAT, ITC, ASSQ

► Assess for comorbid conditions, including seizure disorders, lead poisoning, genetic disorders, mental health disorders, sleep problems, gastrointestinal problems, nutrition problems, delays in acquisition of self-help skills.

Physical Exam

► Refer for a comprehensive diagnostic evaluation by a team that has expertise in the diagnosis and management of ASD.

► Complete a developmental and neurologic exam.

► Evaluate for medical causes (uncommon).

Diagnostic Studies

► Genetic testing

► Metabolic testing

► Neuroimaging not recommended

Differential Diagnosis

► Phenylketonuria

► Rett syndrome

► Fetal alcohol syndrome

► 15q chromosome disorders

► Tuberous sclerosis complex

► Smith-Lemli-Opitz syndrome

► Fragile X

► Other chromosomal disorders

Management

Nonpharmacologic Treatment

▶ Main role of the primary care provider is to coordinate referrals to specialists for evaluation and management; routine health maintenance; and provision of support, guidance, and advocacy.

▶ Parental education

▶ Early intensive behavioral and educational interventions that target the core symptoms are key.

Pharmacologic Treatment

▶ Medications may be helpful for management of symptoms such as hyperactivity, aggression, anxiety, obsessive–compulsive behaviors, depressive symptoms, and sleep dysfunction.

▶ Psychopharmacologic interventions do not treat the underlying symptoms, but can improve the child's functioning and ability to participate in behavioral interventions.

How Long to Treat

▶ Individualized; management goal is to maximize functioning, improve quality of life, and move child toward independence

When to Consult, Refer, or Hospitalize

▶ All suspected cases should be referred to a specialized team for comprehensive evaluation and management.

Follow-up

▶ Close monitoring of support and treatment for child and family as needed

Expected Course

▶ Outcome is variable and difficult to predict. Some children will retain diagnosis despite improvement and others with milder symptoms may no longer meet diagnostic criteria for autism, yet still have delays or other mental health disorders.

▶ Early identification and early intervention are associated with better outcomes.

CONDUCT DISORDER

Description

▶ Persistent antisocial behavior, violating others' rights and inconsistent with societal norms. Conduct disordered individuals exhibit at least one of these symptom clusters:

  ▹ Aggressive, bullying behavior toward people or animals

  ▹ Vandalism, fire-setting, and property destruction

  ▹ Lying, "conning," or theft

» Serious violation of rules (truancy) or running away from home overnight

» No sign of remorse for misconduct

Etiology

▶ No single known etiology; multiple genetic and environmental factors suspected to play a role.

▶ Parental inconsistency, chaotic home environment, harsh and punitive parenting

▶ Parental depression, parental antisocial personality disorder

▶ Children who lack permanent family or father

▶ Children with ADHD and oppositional defiance disorder

▶ New evidence suggests neurotransmitters such as serotonin, and abnormalities in catecholaminergic and peptidergic systems, are linked to aggressive conduct disorder.

Incidence and Demographics

▶ Occurs in 1%–10% of children, more common in boys

▶ As many as 50% of patients < 18 years seen in outpatient psychiatric care have a conduct disorder.

▶ Prevalence in U.S. is increasing; boys < 18 years have 6%–16% prevalence, girls have 2%–9% prevalence

Risk Factors

▶ Dysfunctional family

▶ Socioeconomically deprived

▶ Family history of antisocial personality

▶ Substance abuse

▶ Learning disorders or ADHD

Prevention and Screening

▶ Early management of associated disorders decreases the likelihood that antisocial behaviors will develop.

» Parent education about child development and parenting techniques

» Social skills training

Assessment

History

▶ Specific behaviors of the patient and effects on self and others

▶ Comorbid conditions such as depression, anxiety, substance abuse, learning disabilities, ADHD

▶ Academic history, past and present

▶ Family history of sociopathic or psychiatric illnesses

▶ Family functioning

▶ CNS insults or injuries, disorders, or symptoms

Physical Exam

▶ Evaluate for trauma or abuse

▶ Evaluate for medical causes (uncommon)

Diagnostic Studies

▶ Neuropsychiatric assessment

▶ Psychoeducational testing to rule out learning disabilities

Differential Diagnosis

▶ Oppositional defiant disorder

▶ Depression

▶ ADHD

▶ Specific developmental disorders

▶ Substance abuse

▶ Bipolar disorder

▶ Psychotic disorders

▶ Dissociative disorder

▶ PTSD

Management

Nonpharmacologic Treatment

▶ Psychotherapy and anger management; individual and family therapy

▶ Parent training

▶ Treat comorbid conditions if present (depression, personality disorders, anxiety).

Pharmacologic Treatment

▶ Medications helpful for management of aggressive and antisocial behavior include lithium, risparidone (Risperdal), olanzapine (Zyprexa); atypical antipsychotics (diminish aggression); stimulants (with co-existing ADHD); clonidine (Catapres), and SSRIs (with coexisting depression or anxiety).

How Long to Treat

▶ Variable

Special Considerations

▶ Early age of onset and higher number of behaviors correlate with poorer prognosis.

▶ Medication and patient management should be by a psychiatrist who specializes in this area.

When to Consult, Refer, or Hospitalize

▶ All cases should be referred to a mental health professional.

▶ Emergency referral or hospitalization for aggressive, threatening behavior that jeopardizes safety of others or patient; homicidal or suicidal ideation

Follow-up

▶ Close monitoring of medications and support for child and family as needed

Expected Course

▶ Course is variable and dependent on multiple factors, including patient's receptivity to treatment, stability of family, and access to resources; early intervention has a more favorable outcome.

Complications

▶ Treatment failure may result in criminalization and placement in a correctional facility.

INSOMNIA

Description

▶ *Chronic insomnia*

　　» Difficulty initiating or maintaining sleep of a restorative nature that lasts for at least 1 month and causes significant distress or social, educational, or occupational impairment

▶ *Transient insomnia*

　　» Lasts only a few days and is induced by substances, medications, jet lag, medical illness, stressful events

Etiology

▶ Normal sleep has two basic phases: REM (time of physical and mental activation) and NREM (deep rest), which cycle in 90 minutes and repeat 4–5 times a night; with insomnia, the typical pattern is lost due to:

　　» Substance or medication effects

　　» Situational stressors

　　» Medical disorders

　　» Sleep apnea conditions

　　» Disturbance in circadian rhythms from jet lag, shift work

　　» Psychiatric disorders such as anxiety, major depressive disorders

　　» Primary sleep disorders with unknown etiology

Incidence and Demographics

▶ It is estimated that close to 60% of the population has suffered from insomnia at some time.

▶ Most common and widely recognized sleep disorder

▶ More prevalent with increasing age

▶ More common in women than men

Risk Factors

▶ Older adults

▶ Persons under severe situational stress, such as divorce, job loss, financial distress

▶ Occupations that require shift work, frequent travel through time zones

▶ Alcohol and substance abuse

Prevention and Screening

▶ Regular bedtime routines

▶ Normalized work hours

▶ Reduced daily stress, avoidance of stimulants late in the day

Assessment

History

▶ Inquire about onset, frequency, and duration of insomnia.

▶ Elicit present and past history of sleep patterns, routines, and naps.

▶ Inquire about patterns of use of caffeine, nicotine, alcohol, or substances.

▶ Review current medications, including OTC and herbal products.

▶ Obtain psychiatric and medical history.

Physical Exam

▶ Physical exam should be tailored to the presenting symptomology because primary insomnia is an illness of exclusion of other underlying medical conditions.

Diagnostic Studies

▶ CBC, chemistry profile, electrolytes, ECG

▶ EEG if warranted by abnormal exam or associated symptoms

Differential Diagnosis

- ▶ Alcohol or substance abuse
- ▶ Medication side effects
- ▶ Acute reaction to stressful life events

Psychiatric Disorders

- ▶ Anxiety disorder
- ▶ Major depressive disorder
- ▶ Grief reactions
- ▶ Bipolar disorder

Medical Conditions

- ▶ Cardiac disease
- ▶ Gastrointestinal disease
- ▶ Respiratory problems
- ▶ COPD
- ▶ Sleep apnea
- ▶ CNS lesions
- ▶ Endocrine disorders

Management

Nonpharmacologic Treatment

- ▶ Primary treatment consists of treating underlying cause.
- ▶ Eliminate or restrict use of caffeine, nicotine, and other CNS stimulants; alcohol may cause rebound stimulation.
- ▶ Establish routine:
  - ▹ Maintain a consistent bed time.
  - ▹ Only go to bed when tired.
  - ▹ Do not use the bedroom for any activity other than sleeping and sex.
  - ▹ Rise from bed at the same time every day, regardless of hours slept.
  - ▹ Do not nap during the day.
  - ▹ Provide patient with literature and community resources.

Pharmacologic Treatment

- ▶ Medications commonly prescribed for the treatment of insomnia include benzodiazepines, zolpidem (Ambien), and trazodone (Desyrel). Most medications (see Table 18–10) have some adverse effects, such as hangover, loss of effectiveness (tolerance), dependence, or constipation. Trazodone has TCA adverse reactions. Benzodiazepines are addictive; zolpidem may cause psychological dependence.
- ▶ Melatonin is not FDA-approved, but has shown some effectiveness in self-treatment of insomnia.

How Long to Treat

- ▶ Nonbenzodiazepines: Prescribe for short term (1 month), except rozerem which can be used long-term.
- ▶ Benzodiazepines: Prescribe for 7–10 days.
- ▶ Use lowest effective dose and discontinue gradually.
- ▶ Rebound insomnia may occur when medications discontinued.
- ▶ Be aware of potential for drug tolerance, dependence, and withdrawal with benzodiazepines.

TABLE 18–10
INSOMNIA MEDICATIONS

MEDICATION	DOSE
Nonbenzodiazepines	
Zolpidem (Ambien)	10 mg h.s.
Zaleplon (Sonata)	10–20 mg h.s.
Trazodone (Desyrel)	25–100 mg h.s.
Ramelteon (Rozerem)	8 mg h.s.
Benzodiazepines	
Triazolam (Halcion)	0.125–0.25 mg h.s.
Temazepam (Restoril)	15–30 mg h.s.
Flurazepam (Dalmane)	15–30 mg h.s.
Estazolam (ProSom)	1–2 mg h.s.
Quazepam (Doral)	15–30 mg h.s.

Special Considerations

▶ Do not prescribe for pregnant or lactating women or people with sleep apnea or renal or hepatic disease.

▶ Dose in older adults is usually lower and short-acting agents are generally safer.

▶ Benzodiazepines have a potential for abuse; do not prescribe if patient has history of substance abuse or mental illness.

When to Consult, Refer, Hospitalize

▶ Refer to mental health specialist when symptoms are secondary to anxiety disorder or mood disorder.

▶ When symptoms continue for longer than 1 month, refer to a sleep disorder specialist, neurologist, psychiatrist, or other qualified mental health practitioner.

Follow-up

▶ Weekly monitoring of effectiveness of treatment, compliance, and potential abuse

Expected Course

▶ Most cases of primary insomnia will resolve with short-term management.

Complications

▶ Medication dependence

CASE STUDIES

Case 1. A 7-year-old male child is brought in by his mother because he is having difficulty in school. The mother has brought a note from the school nurse and teacher. The child makes careless mistakes in schoolwork, is unable to sustain attention to tasks, does not listen, and does not follow through on assignments or finish schoolwork. He is constantly on the move, interrupts, cannot wait his turn, blurts out answers, and talks in class. He has lost his backpack twice and has difficulty remaining in his seat on the school bus.

PMH: Fracture left tibia at age 5 years due to bike accident, 7 stitches for laceration to forehead due to a fall from tree-climbing at age 6 years. No serious illnesses, no hospitalizations.

> ▶ What additional history would you ask for?
> ▶ What do you think is happening?
> ▶ What diagnostic tests would you offer?
> ▶ What is your treatment plan?

Case 2. An 18-year-old female, on break from her first semester at college, presents to you with her mother. The chief complaint is amenorrhea, fatigue, and weight loss. The mother blames the weight loss and fatigue on the poor quality of college food, dorm life, and being away from home.

HPI: It is revealed that the patient is a dance major with daily dance classes at the university and evening dance classes at a private studio. She has always been a competitive student and graduated from high school with a grade point average of 4.0. During her senior year, she was the school social activities director, and participated in extracurricular activities and volunteer work. Although the patient is new to college life, she is already involved in dance performances and volunteer work, has joined the poetry club, and is co-editor of its publication.

> ▶ What additional history would you ask for?

Exam: BP is 110/70, respiratory rate 18 and regular, heart rate 80 and regular, skin is dry, weight just at the 30th percentile with low BMI, negative for syncope or orthostatic hypotension, negative for parotid enlargement, negative for oral lesions or dental caries, alert with intact cranial nerves, good muscle strength and coordination. Normal pubic hair development and small breasts. Fingernails dry and brittle, no ridges, skin over knuckles intact and normal.

> ▶ What do you think is happening?
> ▶ What diagnostic tests would you offer?
> ▶ What is your treatment plan?

Case 3. A 70-year-old male presents to you reporting several incidents of shortness of breath and a choking sensation, accompanied by dizziness, diaphoresis, and feelings of doom and loss of control. These "spells" have occurred 4 times in the past 4 weeks and start without warning. He denies seizure disorder and has not experienced loss of consciousness. Two days ago, he went to the hospital emergency room because he thought he was having a heart attack. He was told it was not a heart attack and to see his regular provider.

> ▶ What additional history would you ask for?

Exam: Patient appears calm, alert, oriented, and concerned. Physical exam is unremarkable with normal vital signs.

> ▶ What do you think is happening?
> ▶ What diagnostic tests would you offer?
> ▶ What is your treatment plan?

REFERENCES

American Academy of Pediatrics. (2013). *Child abuse and neglect.* Retrieved from www.aap.org/en-us/advocacy-and-policy/aap-health-initiatives/Medical-Home-for-Children-and-Adolescents-Exposed-to-Violence/Pages/Child-Abuse-and-Neglect.aspx

American Psychiatric Association. (2000). *Diagnostic and statistical manual of mental disorders* (4th ed., text rev.). Washington, DC: American Psychiatric Association.

American Psychiatric Association. (2006). Practice guideline for the treatment of patients with major depressive disorder (3rd ed.). Retrieved from http://psychiatryonline.org/guidelines.aspx

American Psychiatric Association. (2010). Practice guideline for the treatment of major depressive disorder (3rd ed.). *American Journal of Psychiatry, 167,* 10(supplement).

American Psychiatric Association. (2011). *Guideline watch: Practice guideline for the treatment of patients with eating disorders* (3rd ed.). Retrieved from http://psychiatryonline.org/content.aspx?bookid=28&sectionid=39113853

Anton, R. F., O'Malley, S. S., Ciraulo, D. A., Cisler, R. A., Donovan, D. M., Couper, D., ... Zweben, A. (2006). Combined pharmacotherapies and behavioral interventions for alcohol dependence: the COMBINE study: A randomized controlled study. *JAMA, 295*(17), 2003–2017.

Arcangelo, V. P., & Peterson, A. M. (2011). *Pharmacotherapeutics for advanced practice.* Philadelphia: Lippencott Williams & Wilkins.

Brickner, M. (2007). Elder abuse detection and intervention: A collaborative approach. *Care Management Journals 8*(4), 219–223.

Bush, B., Shaw, S., Cleary, P., Delbanco, T. L., & Aronson, M. D. (1987). Screening for alcohol abuse using the CAGE questionnaire. *American Journal of Medicine, 82,* 231–235.

Centers for Disease Control and Prevention. (2006). Mental health in the United States: Parental report of diagnosed autism in children aged 4–17 years — United States, 2003–2004. *MMWR: Morbidity and Mortality Weekly Report, 55*(17), 481.

Centers for Disease Control and Prevention. (2011). Vital signs: Current cigarette smoking among adults aged ≥ 18 years — United States, 2005–2010. *MMWR: Morbidity and Mortality Weekly Report, 60*(33), 1207–1212.

Centers for Disease Control and Prevention. (2012). Prevalence of autism spectrum disorders — Autism and Developmental Disabilities Monitoring Network, 14 sites, United States. *Morbidity and Mortality Weekly Report Surveillance Summary, 61*(3), 1.

Council on Children with Disabilities. (2006). Section on Developmental Behavioral Pediatrics, Bright Futures Steering Committee, Medical Home Initiatives for Children with Special Needs Project Advisory Committee. *Pediatrics, 118* (1), 405.

Eisendrath, S. J., & Lichtmacher, J. E. (2013). Psychiatric disorders. In M. A. Papadakis, S. J. McPhee, & L. M. Tierney (Eds.), *Current medical diagnosis & treatment* (52nd ed., pp. 847–948). Norwalk, CT: Appleton & Lange.

Fombonne, E. (2009). Epidemiology of pervasive developmental disorders. *Pediatric Research, 65*(6), 591.

Gardener, H., Spiegelman, D., & Buka, S. L. (2011). Perinatal and neonatal risk factors for autism: A comprehensive meta-analysis. *Pediatrics, 128*(2), 344.

Getahun D., Jacobsen, S. J., Fassett, M. J., Chen, W., Demissie, K., & Rhoads, G. G. (2013). Recent trends in childhood attention deficit/hyperactivity disorder. *JAMA Pediatrics, 167*(3).

Goroll, A. H., & Mulley, A. G. (2009). *Primary care medicine* (6th ed.). Philadelphia: Lippincott Williams & Wilkins.

Griffith, H. W., & Dambro, M. R. (2012). *The 5-minute consult.* Malvern, PA: Lea & Febinger.

Hay, W. W., Levin, M. J., Deterding, R. R., Abzug, M. J., & Sondheimer, J. M. (2012). *Current pediatric diagnosis & treatment.* New York: McGraw-Hill.

Kroenke, K., Spitzer, R. L., & Williams, J. B. (2001). The PHQ-9: Validity of a brief depression severity measure. *Journal of General Internal Medicine, 16*(9), 606.

Maglione, M. A., Gans, D., Das, L., Timbie, J., Kasari, C., Technical Expert Panel, & HRSA Autism Intervention Research—Behavioral (AIR-B) Network. (2012). *Pediatrics, 130*(Suppl 2): S169.

Monod, S. (2013). Promoting good clinical care to prevent elder abuse. *JAMA Internal Medicine, 173*(7), 289–290.

Myers, S. M. (2009). Management of autism spectrum disorders in primary care. *Pediatric Annals, 38*(1), 42.

Myers, S. M., Johnson, C. P., & American Academy of Pediatrics Council on Children with Disabilities. (2007). Management of children with autism spectrum disorders. *Pediatrics, 120*(5), 1162.

Papadakis, M. A., McPhee, S. J., & Tierney, L. M. (2013). *Current medical diagnosis & treatment* (52nd ed.). Norwalk, CT: Appleton & Lange.

Ramsey, J., Carter, Y., Davidson, L., Dunne, D., Eldridge, S., Feder, G. ... Warburton, A. (2009). Advocacy interventions to reduce or eliminate violence and promote the physical and psychosocial well-being of women who experience intimate partner abuse. *Cochrane Database of Systematic Reviews*, Jul 8;(3):CD005043.

Rhodes, K. V., & Levinson, W. (2003). Interventions for intimate partner violence against women: Clinical applications. *Journal of the American Medical Association, 289*, 601–605.

Rubinsky, A. D., Kivlahan, D. R., Volk, R. J., Maynard, C., & Bradley, K. A. (2010). Estimating risk of alcohol dependence using alcohol screening scores. *Drug Alcohol Dependence, 108*(1–2), 29.

Stead, L. F., & Lancaster, T. (2012). Combined pharmacotherapy and behavioral interventions for smoking cessation. *Cochrane Database of Systematic Reviews* 10:CD008286.

U.S. Senate Special Committee on Aging. (2011). *Justice for all: Ending elder abuse, neglect and financial exploitation* [Kindle Edition].

Websites With Important Information:

Centers for Disease Control and Prevention: www.cdc.gov

National Institutes of Health: www.nih.gov

National Institutes of Mental Health: www.nimh.nih.gov

Case Studies Discussion

CHAPTER 2: IMPORTANT FACTORS INFLUENCING THE NURSE PRACTITIONER ROLE

Case 1. Joan

1. Is Joan legally authorized to provide care to prenatal women? To children?

   If her certification has been maintained as a family nurse practitioner, she is legally authorized to provide care.

2. Should she accept this assignment? Why or why not?

   She is legally authorized and she can accept this assignment because adequate supervision will be provided to her during this training period.

3. What standards of care should she follow in providing care to prenatal patients?

   Standards of care are developed by professional organizations such as the American Nurses Association, which has created the *Standards for Advanced Practice Nursing,* **and the American Association of Colleges of Nursing and the National Organization of Nurse Practitioner Faculties (NONPF), which have created population-focused** *Nurse Practitioner Primary Care Competencies.* **The NP should use established guidelines and standards of practice that guide safe and appropriate care for prenatal patients.**

Case 2. Lee Ann

1. What are the legal issues presented in this case?

   The main legal issue is the provision of care to minors without the consent of parent or legal guardian. This patient is a minor and does not have a life-threatening illness. Thus, the patient should return with her mother/guardian for treatment or the NP

should contact the mother by phone to receive authorization for care before initiating any interventions. Informed consent is necessary to provide care.

2. What ethical principles will guide you in making a decision regarding this case?

You will involve Lee Ann in the decision-making process by asking whether she would like to call her mother and making a new appointment with her mother present. In this way, you are using the principle of beneficence — duty to help others — as well as compassion and caring. You also can speak with the mother and call the school nurse to clarify the need for Lee Ann's absence from school.

Case 3. Alice

1. What theoretical model will assist you in planning an intervention for Alice?

The developmental model proposes that families progress through developmental processes that are predictable. Because this is a non-traditional family, Alice may be experiencing some disappointment that she cannot enjoy just being a mother in the launching phase of family life, but instead must also assume the role of grandmother and caretaker for her daughter's child. In addition, the daughter's developmental stage of adolescent carries with it several developmental tasks that are not being met when caring for a child. Alice's daughter may be exhibiting conflict over not being able to finish high school and the need to care for her child rather than spend time with her peers. Conflict over development processes is apparent.

2. What additional information would you like to obtain?

What coping mechanisms and support systems does Alice have for handling stress? Who else would be considered part of the family — does Alice have a partner? What about the baby's father? What roles do other members of the family assume? What are the financial resources? What are the strengths of the family? Are there any safety issues for the baby, Alice, or her daughter? What is the developmental stage and anticipatory guidance needs of the adolescent daughter?

3. How can you best help her today?

Acknowledge the stress in Alice's life and treat her headaches. Ask about her willingness to engage a counselor for additional help for both her and her daughter, either alone or in family therapy. Identify and strengthen Alice's coping skills. Encourage Alice to see that she, her daughter, and the baby maintain regular health promotion visits. Consult with social services for a referral to a program for teenage mothers for Alice's daughter and needed resources for the baby.

CHAPTER 3: HEALTHCARE ISSUES

Case 1. Emily

1. What vaccines will Emily need today?

   DTaP, IPV, HBV, HIB, PCV, rotavirus

2. What developmental milestones would you assess for in a 2-month-old?

   Regards faces, eyes follow to midline, smiles, laughs, squeals, vocalizes, lifts head to 45° when prone, responds to bell, has equal movements.

3. There is no fluoride in the tap water; when should you start Emily on fluoride? How much will you give her per day?

   Begin at 6 months with 0.25 mg per day.

4. Emily's mother is thinking about discontinuing breastfeeding and starting infant formula. What information should you provide to her that might encourage her to continue to breastfeed?

   Breastmilk is nutritionally balanced, contains antibodies and macrophages, which are important to immunity and wound healing, and is free of bacteria. Allergic reactions are rare. Breastfeeding saves time and money.

Case 2. Travis

1. What vaccines will he need today?

   DtaP, IPV, MMR, hepatitis B, and varicella; depending on time of year, add influenza and give hepatitis A, if not given.

2. What safety issues will you discuss with Travis and his parents?

   Recreational sports protection gear (helmets, pads); swimming safety; automobile (street safety, seatbelts); knows his address, phone number, how to call 911; ipecac on hand for accidental poisoning; smoke alarms in the house; access/storage of guns in the home.

3. What will your assessment examination focus on?

   History, immunization status, vital signs, pubertal development, musculoskeletal and cardiopulmonary systems

4. What counseling does Josh need?

   Weight management (his BMI is 34.2), safety (seatbelts, recreational protective gear)

5. What immunizations might Josh need?

Hepatitis B (check that all 3 were given), varicella (if no history of vaccine or disease), Tdap and meningococcal MCV4 (if not given at 11–13 yrs), MMR (second shot, if not given previously), hepatitis A (if not given).

Case 3. Computer company health fair

1. What primary prevention topics will you address for parents of young children?

Nutrition, iron intake, fluoride, safety (car seats, falls, poisonings, drowning), immunizations, sunscreen, access/storage gun safety.

2. What secondary prevention topics will you address for adults ages 18–50?

Clinical breast exam, Pap smears, serum cholesterol

3. What secondary prevention topics will you address for adults 50 and older?

Clinical breast exam, mammography, Pap smears, testicular exam, digital rectal exam, PSA, fecal occult blood, flexible sigmoidoscopy, dental/oral screening, blood pressure, serum cholesterol, EKG, vision, hearing.

4. How would you educate the participants about stress management?

Large amounts of stress can lead to disease. Discuss stress management techniques (relaxation, imagery, time management). Seek out support. Recognize sources of stress for the geriatric clients—loss.

CHAPTER 4: INFECTIOUS DISEASES

Case 1. Male freshman

1. Should you be concerned about measles, mumps, rubella, polio, diphtheria, or pertussis since he does not know if his immunizations are up-to-date?

No, it is unlikely that he has missed these immunizations because they would have been required on entrance to college.

2. What other history is needed?

Health of his roommates, dormmates, and friends; any rash, specific joint pain, and swelling; how much weight has he lost; has he had any night sweats or cough; tick bite or outdoor exposure; and his sexual preference and partner history (how many, use of STI protection, any symptoms of STIs in partners), history and symptoms of STIs, any swollen glands, other associated symptoms

3. What is your differential diagnosis?

Rheumatic fever, mononucleosis (unlikely with no lymphadenopathy), Lyme disease (dependent on history of exposure), HIV primary infection (unlikely without additional symptoms), viral illness (unusual to last this long and be unaccompanied by rash)

4. What initial diagnostic and management plan is appropriate?

Aortic murmur is significant and rheumatic fever should be highly suspected. Immediate referral to cardiologist is essential with initiation of penicillin treatment. Initial diagnostic testing would include CBC, ESR, C-reactive protein, streptococcal antibody titer, and ECG.

Case 2. 6-year-old male

1. What are you looking for in a physical exam?

Fever, cervical lymphadenopathy, rash, skin desquamation in groin; eye, ear, nose, throat exam for signs of local infection; cardiac exam for signs of pericarditis, myocarditis; neurologic exam for signs of meningitis; abdominal exam for hepatosplenomegaly; musculoskeletal exam for arthritis; skin for rash

2. What do you suspect from this child's presentation?

Kawasaki disease

3. What is your management plan?

Immediate referral to pediatric cardiologist

Case 3. 14-month-old female

1. What other history is needed?

Her contact with other children and if any of them have been ill; does she seem to have a sore throat; how is she eating, sleeping; activity level

2. What screening tests need to be done?

If sore throat is present, a throat swab and a CBC with differential will rule out group A β-hemolytic streptococcal infection.

3. What is the likely diagnosis and what management is appropriate?

Given the history of high fevers that relented on the onset of rash on day 4, is likely to be roseola. Expected PE findings would be a blanching erythematous maculopapular rash and may have adenopathy. Rule out otitis media. Continue supportive management.

CHAPTER 5: COMMON PROBLEMS OF THE SKIN

Case 1. 15 year-old male

1. What pertinent history is it important to obtain?

   Any fever, systemic symptoms, any bites or other forms of exposure? Is there a history of irritant dermatitis or other rashes? What types of allergies does the patient have — environmental, food, seasonal, and/or drug? Did he walk in tall bushes/grass/swim in lake or pool?

2. What is the most likely diagnosis based on this history?

   Contact dermatitis, due to a plant such as poison ivy

3. What would you expect to find on PE?

   Eruptions along areas of skin exposure on arms and legs, possibly linear. Papules, dry scaling, and erythema. May see scratch marks. Later weeping and excoriation.

4. Is he contagious?

   No, contact dermatitis is not contagious unless clothing or other items are contaminated with the oil from the plant. All clothing or shoes with oil from the plant have the potential to cause irritation again until oil is removed.

5. How would you treat this patient?

   Identification and removal of offending agent; relief of symptoms with colloidal oatmeal, astringent, topical corticosteroids (do not use over large areas or if infected), oral steroids if a large area is involved, antihistamines, antibiotics (for cellulitis or impetigo only).

Case 2. A 26-year-old White male

1. What pertinent history is it important to ask?

   Has he used any new products? Allergies? Medications? Previous episodes of same? Any itching, scaling, flaking? Any associated symptoms of disease?

2. You note discrete, scattered, or confluent patches. Wood's lamp exam reveals faint yellow-green scales. What is the most likely diagnosis?

   Tinea versicolor

3. What laboratory tests would you order to confirm the diagnosis?

   KOH and microscope visualization

4. How would you treat this patient?

   Topical selenium sulfide 2.5% shampoo to skin for 30 minutes the wash off for tinea versicolor; repeat 2 weeks later

Case 3. 5-year-old girl

1. What pertinent history is it important to ask?

   How long have the lesions been there? Fever? Remedies tried so far? Crowded living conditions? In day care? Any contacts with similar? Vaccines current?

2. What is the most likely diagnosis given this presentation?

   Impetigo

3. What would you look for on PE?

   Possible poor hygiene evident in child's grooming; breakdown and secondary infection (impetiginizing) of neglected skin lesions; honey-colored fluid oozing from open lesions and others with crusted covering; may see bullous (large vesicle or bullae containing clear yellow fluid on erythematous base); ecthyma (ulceration with thick adherent crust); possible tenderness; possible regional lymphadenopathy

4. Is she contagious?

   Yes

5. What laboratory tests would you order?

   Diagnosis is primarily clinical; cultures may be warranted if diagnosis is in doubt or if the lesions fail to respond to an appropriate course of antibiotics; possible Gram stain; cultures demonstrate *S. aureus*, group A streptococci, possible methicillin resistant *S. aureus*; if recurrent, serology for anti-DNAse beta to look for prior strep infection.

6. How would you treat this patient?

   Wash area with soap to remove crusts prior to applying topical antibiotic penicillin for streptococci, Dicloxacillin (for staphylococcus); erythromycin may be used if allergic to penicillin; topical mupirocin for small lesions.

CHAPTER 6:
EYE, EAR, NOSE AND THROAT DISORDERS

Case 1: 16-year-old female

1. What additional history do you need?

    Details on history of frequent head colds (review the symptoms and signs, number of episodes in past few years, how treated, whether the episodes resolved). Any change in environment (dusty or damp, pets)? Has she ever had allergy tests or radiographic sinus imaging or endoscopy? Does she have asthma or allergic symptoms? Any symptoms/ signs of systemic disease (diabetes)? Any intranasal (or other) drug use? ETOH? OTC nasal decongestants? Does she use condoms? Assess her STI risk.

2. What are the risk factors for possible diagnoses?

    Cigarettes predispose to allergic rhinitis and sinusitis. Allergic rhinitis predisposes to sinusitis. Oral contraceptives may cause vasomotor rhinitis. Oral sex and new partner may cause gonococcal pharyngitis, risk for HIV, and immunosuppression

3. What diagnostic tests would you order?

    Probably none at this time unless the history and physical exam suggests HIV risk or other systemic disease (diabetes, anemia)

4. What is your differential diagnosis?

    Infectious rhinitis, probably viral; allergic rhinitis; acute bacterial sinusitis; vasomotor rhinitis

5. What treatment plan will you carry out?

    Patient/family education on various types of rhinitis/sinusitis and what treatment is appropriate in this case versus indiscriminate use of antibiotics; also prevention measures and maintenance care. Suggest saline lavage q.i.d., intranasal corticosteroid steroid spray, non-sedating antihistamine, OTC oral decongestants, infection prevention, and allergy control in her environment

Case 2. 22-year-old female college student

1. What are the most likely possibilities for a differential diagnosis?

    Peritonsillar abscess, streptococcal tonsillitis, infectious mononucleosis, antibiotic noncompliance, acute otitis media, antibiotic resistant infection

2. What information in the history is the most significant?

    Failure to improve on antibiotics; symptoms worse with ear pain, which may be referred from pharynx

3. What physical examination components are especially useful for this presentation?

Fever, erythematous posterior pharynx with exudative tonsil, trismus, palatal bulge, tender lymphadenopathy, negative ear findings

4. Are the findings from the history and physical adequate to make the diagnosis and what diagnostic studies will rule in or out any of the possibilities?

The history and physical are very revealing for peritonsillar abscess; however, CBC with differential, mono screen test, quick streptococcal screen, throat culture, and possibly blood cultures will help define her diagnosis.

5 What treatment plan will you carry out?

Start parenteral antibiotics (ceftriaxone is a good choice) and consult with ENT specialist for urgent evaluation and possible admission. If urgent referral to ENT is not possible, make arrangements for her to be evaluated at the nearest emergency department for evaluation and treatment.

Case 3. 6-year-old boy presents with severe right ear pain.

1. What additional history is important?

Any recent URI? Cigarette smoke exposure? Is the child in day care? Any siblings? Recent swimming? Has he ever had otitis externa or TM rupture? Has he ever put anything in his ear?

2. What is the differential diagnosis?

Acute otitis media with perforation, acute otitis externa, foreign body

3. What historical and physical exam features support the differential?

The external auditory canal is without erythema or edema, no tragal tenderness, so otitis externa is ruled out; the red, bulging TM with a perforation and acute illness supports acute otitis media; the whitish crust in the ear canal is from the perforation of the tympanic membrane with extrusion of exudate.

4. What are the risk factors for otitis media?

Male, day care, Eustachian tube dysfunction, secondhand cigarette smoke exposure

5. How will you treat this child?

Amoxicillin 80–90 mg/kg/day in divided doses; or ofloxacin (Floxin) otic 5 gtts b.i.d.; acetaminophen or ibuprofen for pain and fever; follow up in 2 weeks but instructed to return if not improving in 48–72 hours

CHAPTER 7: RESPIRATORY DISORDERS

Case 1. 15-month-old female

1. What additional history would you like to obtain?

   Frequency of the colds (a child normally will have 7–9 colds a year, particularly if he or she attends day care or has older siblings), onset, description of cough; sleep, activity, appetite, vomiting, change in stools; immunization status, particularly for Haemophilus and pneumococcal; history of respiratory disease, GERD, feeding problems; family history of asthma, allergies, cystic fibrosis; social factors such as siblings, day care, smokers in the home, foreign-born

2. What are the possible diagnoses?

   Bronchiolitis because of low-grade fever, URI symptoms, tachypnea, retractions, wheezing, rhonchi; croup because of barky cough, concurrent URI; viral pneumonia because of fever, cough, URI symptoms; cystic fibrosis because of frequent reoccurrence, cough, would have foul-smelling stools

3. What diagnostic tests would you initially order?

   Pulse oximetry to help determine degree of respiratory distress; CXR to determine infection, congenital anomaly; CBC with differential to determine infection; sweat test to rule out cystic fibrosis

4. Your working diagnosis is bronchiolitis. What is your treatment plan?

   Encourage parent to offer lots of clear liquids; acetaminophen as needed for fever; educate parents on signs and symptoms of respiratory distress and to return immediately or go to ER if present. Trial of bronchodilator in office, if significant reduction is wheezing, give Rx to use at home: albuterol 5 mg/mL 0.1–0.15 mg/kg in 2 cc of saline q4–6h if no nebulizer available for home use, oral Alupent 2 mg/5 mL 0.1 mg–0.15 mg/kg q4–6h. Follow up the next day.

5. On follow-up your patient is doing much better, but the results of the sweat test have returned positive. What is your course of action now?

   The child most likely has cystic fibrosis. Referral to a specialist is indicated.

Case 2. 76-year-old male

1. What additional history would you like to obtain?

   Living situation; any known exposures to others with pneumonia, flu, TB? Any recent travel? Does cough get worse at night or with exercise? Any history of asthma, wheezing? When the cough is productive, what does it look like — color, consistency, any blood? Any URI symptoms? Any symptoms of indigestion? Hx of allergies, clear nasal discharge, postnasal drip? Any night sweats?

2. What are the most likely differential diagnoses?

   Postnasal drip, most common cause of chronic cough; COPD; lung cancer; TB; CHF; anginal equivalent; GERD; psychogenic cause (recent loss of wife)

3. What diagnostic tests would you order?

   CXR—rule out COPD, lung cancer, TB; CBC—infection, cancer; PPD—TB; pulmonary function tests—COPD; upper GI if above negative—rule out GERD; bronchoscopy, based on results of other tests

4. If the PPD is negative, would you do anything further?

   Consider repeating the PPD in 1–3 weeks because of booster effect

5. What would you do for this patient on this visit?

   Discuss possibility of grief reaction to loss of wife, depression; assess eating habits, humidification, cough suppressant at night; consider nasal antihistamines or nasal steroids; suggest avoiding oral decongestants due to slight elevation in BP and potential for urinary retention in a man this age; update immunizations, pneumovax, flu (depending on season) and tetanus

Case 3. 35-year-old married Hispanic female

1. What are your working differential diagnoses?

   URI, bronchitis, viral pneumonia, TB, occupational exposure

2. What diagnostic tests would you order?

   PPD because of immigrant status, cough, low-grade fever. Other diagnostic tests are not indicated at this time. This patient has no signs of respiratory distress, bacterial pneumonia, or sinusitis.

3. What would you do for this patient at this visit?

   Nonpharmacologic: Increase fluids, rest, humidification, avoidance of secondhand smoke

   Pharmacologic: Antipyretic as needed, cough suppressant at night if having difficulty sleeping due to cough, bronchodilator inhaler

   Follow-up: 48–72 hr to read PPD and see if symptoms have improved

4. On return visit, the PPD is positive at 10 mm. She tells you her symptoms are not improved and her fever has been 101° F, but responds well to Tylenol. What is your differential diagnosis now?

   TB; bronchitis with secondary bacterial infection

5. What diagnostic tests would you order?

   CXR; CBC with differential, sputum cultures

6. What would you do regarding the other family members?

Have all family members get a PPD; discuss communicability of illness

7. The CBC with differential results are WBC 12,000, segmented 50%, lymphs 48%; CXR shows increased hilar markings. Would you order an antibiotic? If so, which and why?

Yes. Because this is a previously healthy patient with no recent antibiotic use, you would select a broad spectrum antibiotic that would cover for most of the causative organisms of secondary bacterial infection, which are *S. pneumoniae, Haemophilus, Chlamydia, Mycoplasma,* **and** *Moraxella.* **You would choose a macrolide (Azithromycin, Clarithromycin, and Erythromycin) or Doxycycline. Alternatively, you could also use a beta-lactam such as Augmentin, Ceftin or Vantin. Although the CXR was suggestive of pneumonia and not TB, her positive PPD warrants prophylaxis with INH and a referral to a pulmonologist. She will require baseline ALT and AST and benefit from some pyridoxine (vitamin B$_6$) to prevent neuropathy.**

CHAPTER 8: CARDIOVASCULAR DISORDERS

Case 1. Lori

1. What additional history would you ask regarding her cardiovascular status?

Personal and family history of CHD, DM, hyperlipidemia; any previous lipid evaluation; history of activity/exercise; comprehensive health maintenance history; previous attempt of smoking/alcohol cessation; history of psychosocial stressors; any comorbid disease; abdominal pain; rheumatic disorders; medication history including OTCs, pregnancies

2. Would you order any diagnostic test on this patient?

Baseline ECG; fasting lipid profile (total cholesterol, triglycerides, HDL, LDL, VLDL, risk ratio); apolipoprotein b; comprehensive metabolic panel, U/A, TSH, free T4; possibly CXR, CBC with differential, CMP

3. If your suspicions are correct, what actions would be required?

Step 2 diet and exercise program; referral to nutritionist for diet counseling; tobacco and alcohol cessation program; counseling for stress reduction

4. When Lori returns to the clinic 6 months later with total cholesterol 252, HDL 30, and LDL 170, how will you intervene?

Reinforce Step 2 diet and exercise. Start on a statin such as atorvastatin (Lipitor) 10 mg/day; plan on monitoring hepatic function panel every 4–6 weeks after starting therapy × 3 months and again with any dose

5. What complications can occur with this problem and the treatment regimens?

   Hyperlipidemia: CAD progression, stroke, peripheral vascular disease. Drug treatment: pancreatitis, rhabdomyolysis, hepatic dysfunction

Case 2. Baby Joe

1. Are there any other history questions you would like to ask?

   Weight history since birth; prenatal/delivery history; voiding/stooling history in past 24 hours; 24-hour intake history; feeding behavior, sleep pattern

2. What are your differential diagnoses?

   Patent ductus arteriosus, atriovenous malformations, venous hum, ventricular septal defect with aortic regurgitation, pulmonary atresia, persistent truncus arteriosus, aortopulmonary septal defect, peripheral pulmonary stenosis, total anomalous venous connection, tetralogy of Fallot.

3. What is your management plan?

   Refer child to emergency room for admission and evaluation with cardiologist.

Case 3. Mr. Jones

1. What additional history would you ask?

   Characteristics of cough and sputum; need for additional pillows to sleep — orthopnea; fever; detailed history on comorbid diseases.

2. What diagnostic studies would you order?

   CXR, ECG, echocardiogram, electrolytes, U/A, pulse oximetry, cardiac enzymes, BUN, arterial blood gases.

3. What is your differential diagnosis?

   CHF, renal disease, COPD, nephrotic syndrome, cirrhosis, pulmonary emboli, MI, pneumonia, asthma, chronic venous insufficiency.

4. What is your management plan?

   Give O_2 and consult with physician to plan hospital admission to stabilize; identify and treat underlying disease. At follow-up, educate about sodium and fluid restriction, control leg edema with elastic pressure stockings and elevation of legs, record daily weights; multiple medications needed to treat — diuretics, ACE, beta blocker, glycoside, vasodilators, and anticoagulants.

CHAPTER 9: GASTROINTESTINAL DISORDERS

Case 1. 6-week-old infant

1. What other history would you ask?

    Any choking during feeding (congenital anomalies), any bile or blood in regurgitation (obstruction), fevers URI sx (infection), other illnesses. Are developmental milestones appropriate (smiling, lifting head when prone; neurologic disorders), stooling pattern, irritability, consolability (intussusception, Hirschsprung's disease), any projectile vomiting (pyloric stenosis), feeding position and post feeding position. Family history of food allergies (food intolerances/allergies), sleeping pattern.

2. What laboratory tests would you order?

    CBC, to look for infection, anemia; electrolytes, to evaluate hydration status; U/A, to look for UTI, hydration status

3. What other studies would you order

    CXR, to look for congenital anomalies, lung status, cardiac enlargement

4. What is the most probable diagnosis and what treatment would you provide?

    If all studies are normal would consider change in formula to Nutramigen for possible allergy. Upright with feeding and post feeding. Review burping techniques and frequency during feedings. Close follow-up and if not resolving referral to pediatric gastroenterologist.

Case 2. 18-year-old female

1. What other history questions would you ask this patient?

    Stool pattern > 3/day or < 3/week, straining or feeling of incomplete evacuation, mucus in stools, feeling abdominal distention (IBS) any blood in stools, nocturnal diarrhea (UC), fever, anorexia, weight loss (UC), LMP, birth control, hx of STIs (PID, ectopic pregnancy), any association with certain foods (lactose intolerance), UTI sx, family hx of bowel disease, nausea, vomiting, low fiber diet (diverticulosis)

2. What laboratory tests would you order?

    CBC: infection, anemia, blood loss; ESR: inflammatory process; hCG: pregnancy; stool for WBCs, culture, O & P: infectious etiology; Albumin: malabsorption, chronic disease

3. What other studies would you consider?

    Abdominal US: ectopic, ovarian abscess; sigmoidoscopy: UC; colonoscopy: Crohn's disease

4. What is the likely diagnosis if laboratory tests are normal and what treatment would you provide?

   If all laboratory tests are normal, the most likely diagnosis is IBS. Have patient keep a diary of food intake and symptoms, avoid foods that increase symptoms, trial for two weeks of a lactose-free diet, increase fiber. Antidiarrheal or anticholinergic as needed. Close follow-up, if unresponsive refer for further evaluation.

Case 3. A family of three

1. What other questions would you ask this family?

   » **Frequency of vomiting, color of vomitus, waking at night to vomit**

   » **Frequency of diarrhea, description of stools, blood, mucus**

   » **Fever, lethargy, urine output, crying with tears**

   » **Recent travel, camping, day care**

   » **Any common food source that all members have eaten**

2. What laboratory tests would you order?

   » **CBC with diff-infection, parasites**

   » **U/A- hydration status**

   » **Stool for WBC, culture, O&P**

3. Are any other diagnostic studies warranted at this time?

   No

4. What is the likely diagnosis and what treatment would you provide?

   » **Acute gastroenteritis**

   » **While awaiting lab results, maintain and improve hydration status**

   » **Give oral replacement therapy (ORT) at 50 mL/kg over a 4-hour period, start with sips and gradually increase if no vomiting occurs. If vomiting occurs, either wait an hour and retry or give an antiemetic, then try to rehydrate again with ORT. Once child is rehydrated (crying with tears, alert, good urine output, thirsty), resume regular diet.**

CHAPTER 10: RENAL DISORDERS

Case 1. 49-year-old woman

1. What additional history will you need?

   Characteristics and duration of pain, presence of abdominal or chest pain, other gastrointestinal symptoms, fever, gross hematuria, current symptoms of UTI. PMH of kidney stones or urologic structural abnormalities, any new sexual partners.

2. What are the differential diagnoses?

Pyelonephritis, back strain, urolithiasis, nephrolithiasis MI, gallbladder disease, other gastrointestinal problem. Because of the patient's history of frequent UTIs during her reproductive years, current dysuria and urinary frequency plus the CVA tenderness on exam, pyelonephritis is first in the differential.

3. What diagnostic studies will you consider?

Urinalysis, CBC with differential; BUN, creatinine

4. What treatment will you consider?

Strain urine; save any retrieved stones for laboratory analysis. Increase fluid intake to maintain urinary output at 2–3 L /day, increase fiber in diet; decrease animal fat in diet. Pain management with NSAIDs and opioids as required; antiemetics as needed. Return if inadequate pain relief from NSAIDs, severity of pain increases, urine output decreases despite increasing fluids, or unable to keep fluids down.

Further work-up will be required only if she does not improve or she has a recurrent symptoms.

Case 2. 25-year-old female

1. What are the differential diagnoses?

Cystitis, vaginitis, female urethral syndrome, interstitial cystitis, meatal stenosis

2. What diagnostic studies will you order?

Clean catch urinalysis; urine culture not necessary because she is afebrile and it is not a recurrent infection. Physical exam confirmed cystitis as the top differential.

3. What risk factors can you identify?

Female, diaphragm use, recently married.

4. What treatment measures will you prescribe?

Hygiene measures, hydration, voiding after coitus. Trimethoprim/sulfamethoxazole (Bactrim) DS b.i.d., or ciprofloxacin (Cipro) 500 b.i.d. for 3 days. Phenazopyridine (Pyridium), 200 mg t.i.d. for no more than 2 days for pain relief.

5. What follow-up is necessary?

No follow-up necessary, expect resolution of symptoms in 72 hours, return as needed

6. What will you do if this patient follows up 2 weeks later with another UTI?

Obtain culture and sensitivity and retreat as indicated. Trial of cranberry juice or cranberry tablets. Review hygiene, use of diaphragm, and voiding after coitus. Consider post-coital antibiotic prophylaxis or alternate method of birth control.

Case 3. 10-year-old boy

1. What additional history would you like?

   What the family thinks about his bedwetting. What he thinks. Family history of bedwetting. Day time incontinence pattern, constipation, food allergies, stress issues, sleep pattern — snoring?

2. What are the differential diagnoses?

   Primary nocturnal enuresis (PNE), UTI, diabetes, sleep disorder

3. What diagnostic studies will you order?

   Urinalysis, HgbA1C if diabetes is suspected ,

4. What treatment would you consider?

   Discuss with patient and parents the causes of PNE, i.e., primarily an arousal disorder. Reinforce to the family that bedwetting is nobody's fault, is a common problem and generally resolves on its own over time. However, he has had some changes in his daily routine that may be also causing him to wet the bed more frequently. Describe motivational and conditioning exercises as well as use of alarms and pharmacologic agents. Start by having parents restrict fluids 2 hours before bedtime and begin bladder exercises. Keep a motivational chart that has rewards for every morning his bed is dry. Have patient return in 2 weeks for follow-up. Consider addition of either DDVAP or an alarm at that time.

CHAPTER 11: FEMALE REPRODUCTIVE SYSTEM DISORDERS

Case 1. 39-year-old sexually active woman

1. What might you find on examination of vaginal fluid if this woman has bacterial vaginosis?

   Thin, homogenous, white-gray discharge; pH > 4.5; clue cells visible on microscopic exam; positive KOH whiff test

2. Should her partner be evaluated and treated?

   No, treatment of men has not shown to alter relapse/reinfection rate in female partners.

3. What is the standard treatment for non-pregnant women?

   Metronidazole 500 mg p.o. b.i.d. for 7 days or metronidazole gel 0.75% intravaginally b.i.d. for 5 days

45. What does the patient need to know regarding use of this medication?

Patient is to avoid alcohol for 48 hours prior to initiating medication treatment, while taking the medication, and for 48 hours after taking the last dose due to the Antabuse effect of this drug.

Case 2. Jane S.

1. What further history do you need from Jane?

Age at menarche, LMP, menstrual history, gynecologic history, obstetrical history, PMH, medications, social history

2. What will you include in her physical assessment?

Height, weight, blood pressure, complete physical exam, breast exam, pelvic exam including bimanual exam for fundal height, fetal heart rate depending upon weeks of pregnancy

3. What screening tests will you order?

Urine screen for protein and glucose followed by urinalysis and urine culture; CBC, blood type, Rh and antibody screen; RPR; rubella titer; hepatitis screen; Pap smear; STI screening if indicated

4. What prenatal education will she need?

Include plan for smoking cessation. Nutrition, exercise, changes during pregnancy, prenatal vitamin and folic acid supplementation, smoking cessation through behavior modification techniques, usual schedule of prenatal visits

Case 3. 52-year-old woman

1. What additional history would you like before advising her on treatment?

Obstetrical and gynecologic history; complete medical history for history of breast cancer or breast mass, thromboembolic disease, gallbladder disease, hypertension, cardiovascular disease, hyperlipidemia, liver tumor, migraines; osteoporosis risk factors; method of contraception, chance of pregnancy

2. What laboratory tests will you do to confirm menopause?

No tests are essential; by history she is perimenopausal. TSH not necessary unless having additional symptoms of hyperthyroidism; LH, FSH, and estradiol will fluctuate. Significant FSH and LH elevations may not be seen until 1 year after cessation of menses.

3. What information will you review about hormonal treatment in menopause?

Hormone replacement now reserved for short-term use in patients with severe symptoms. Long-term use is not cardioprotective and may increase risk for stroke,

MI, breast cancer, and perhaps dementia. Advise herbal preparations or symptomatic treatment rather than HRT at this time.

4. What other recommendations should the FNP provide?

Calcium intake of 1,200–1,500 mg/day; vitamin D 400–800 IU/day; exercise and weight management; vaginal lubrication for intercourse if dryness occurs, Kegel exercises to prevent urinary incontinence, check active ingredient and dosage of herbal product to determine its value (Black Cohosh, soy in large amount, flaxseeds may be helpful).

CHAPTER 12: MALE REPRODUCTIVE SYSTEM DISORDERS

Case 1. 17-year-old male

1. How can you elicit more information from this patient?

Ask his mother to step out of the room during the examination and continue to question him in a matter-of-fact, nonjudgmental manner. Tell him you review this information with all adolescents and adults. Tell him what the differential diagnosis is because it is important to treat the right cause. Assure him that confidentiality is always respected in adolescents seeking treatment for STIs.

2. What additional information would you like?

Other symptoms such as fever, urinary complaints, urethral discharge; history of STIs and current sexual practices; description of the injury

3. Can testicular torsion be ruled out?

Yes, patient has a positive Prehn's sign, no nausea or vomiting.

4. What is the most likely diagnosis?

Epididymitis

5. Is diagnostic testing necessary to initiate treatment?

No. Test for gonorrhea and chlamydia, but empirically initiate treatment with ceftriaxone and doxycycline. Also consider testing for syphilis and HIV.

6. What additional intervention is needed?

Advise bedrest and scrotal elevation until fever and pain subside. Avoid sexual activity and pelvic strain until infection completely resolved. Refer if no improvement in 3 days. Teach safe sex practices, use of condoms, notify partners within past 30 days, and advise need for STI evaluation and treatment prior to resuming intercourse.

Case 2. 1-week-old, full-term male infant

1. What additional history would you like?

   Has the baby been circumcised? How have the parents been caring for the uncircumcised penis? Was the foreskin retracted?

2. What is the differential diagnosis?

   Balanitis, phimosis

3. How would you treat this patient?

   Replace foreskin to non-retracted position if possible. If unable, obtain emergency urologic consult.

4. What follow up is necessary?

   Attention to penis during well-child visits.

5. What infant care teaching do parents need?

   Care of uncircumcised penis

Case 3. 67-year-old retired postal worker

1. What additional history would you like?

   Any irritative symptoms; sexual activity; medications, including over-the-counter antihistamines and decongestants, saw palmetto, or other herbal products; family history of prostate cancer; date and results of last digital rectal exam (DRE), date and results of last prostate-specific antigen (PSA), if done in past.

2. What diagnostic tests would you perform?

   Urinalysis, serum BUN, creatinine, and prostate-specific antigen (PSA). Note: Prostate-specific antigen (PSA) may be helpful to distinguish cause (BPH or prostate cancer) of large gland; use of this test is controversial if patient is asymptomatic and results are 4–10 ng/mL. Results > 10 ng/mL may be associated with cancer, but not necessarily correlated. PSA increases as gland enlarges, but do not assume increases are due only to gland enlargement. Acute urinary retention, prostatitis, urinary tract instrumentation, or prostatic infarction may elevate the PSA.

3. What does the clinician need to know regarding the indicated diagnostic test necessary for this patient?

   The PSA needs to be drawn *before* the digital rectal exam (DRE) being performed because increased levels may be noted 1–24 hours post-DRE; therefore, avoid lab work during this time period.

4. Can you make a diagnosis?

   Should you refer this patient? Diagnosis of BPH based on clinical findings can be made and treatment could be instituted with medications. Refer if AUA score > 8, unresponsive to medication, suspicious for malignancy, or complications with medications.

5. What is your treatment plan?

   Treat with an alpha-adrenergic blocker (terazosin or doxazosin) for both BPH and HTN. Increase dose gradually over 1 month and monitor BP until therapeutic effect is reached in 4–6 weeks. Avoid bladder irritants, decrease fluid in the evening. Once medication therapy is initiated, encourage patient to keep a log noting urinary symptoms in relation to medication dosage, and bring log to each follow-up visit for evaluation.

6. What follow up and screening recommendations would you give this patient?

   DRE annually; baseline ECG, serum cholesterol, annual fecal occult blood testing and sigmoidoscopy every 3–5 years (see Chapter 3, Adult Screening Guidelines); BP check-ups every 3–6 months when stable (see Hypertension, Chapter 8).

CHAPTER 13: SEXUALLY TRANSMITTED INFECTIONS

Case 1. 23-year-old sexually active male

1. What additional information will help you evaluate this patient?

   Presence and characteristics of penile discharge, number of sexual partners, history of STIs

2. What is the differential diagnosis?

   Gonococcal urethritis, NGU, HIV

3. Should any diagnostic tests be done?

   Tests for gonorrhea and *Chlamydia* **using one of the following: Gram stain (gonorrhea only), culture using special media for each, DNA probe, nucleic acid amplification test on first-void urine**

4. What are your treatment considerations?

   Consider empiric therapy for both gonorrhea and *Chlamydia,* **notify partner(s) of need for evaluation and treatment, abstain from intercourse until treatment complete (7 days), report to public health after confirmation of gonorrhea or** *Chlamydia,* **no follow-up necessary if resolves, refer for persistent or recurrent urethritis, condom use, HIV screening**

Case 2. 17-year-old female

1. What additional information should you obtain?

   History of STIs, current symptoms of STIs, signs and symptoms of primary HIV infection (fever, adenopathy, pharyngitis, rash, myalgias, diarrhea, headache, nausea and vomiting, thrush)

2. What screening tests should be done?

   Pap smear; gonorrhea and *Chlamydia* tests; vaginal microscopy for trichomoniasis, bacterial vaginosis, and candidiasis; syphilis serology; HIV testing; pregnancy test

3. What treatment should be considered today?

   Rule out pregnancy before treatment of HPV and other infections.

4. What education and prevention topics should be discussed with this patient?

   HIV risk factors; perinatal transmission of HIV; how to change unsafe sexual behavior; additional birth control measures; annual screening for cervical cancer, gonorrhea, *Chlamydia,* condom use

CHAPTER 14: MUSCULOSKELETAL DISORDERS

Case 1. 12-year-old White male

1. What other history would you like?

   Recent illness, description of pain, associated symptoms

2. What type of examination should be done?

   Observe gait, assess for muscle atrophy and tenderness, assess for limited ROM. Exam reveals patient has local tenderness over hip with decreased flexion, abduction, and internal rotation.

3. What diagnostic tests should be ordered?

   AP and lateral of hip/frog-leg X-ray

4. What is the diagnosis and plan for management?

   Slipped capital femoral epiphysis; refer to orthopedic surgeon immediately for evaluation.

Case 2. 34-year-old man

1. What other history would you like?

   Able to lift objects, even cup or liquid; able to squeeze a hard ball; has this problem occurred before. Any fever, rash, or other recent illnesses? Any history of Lyme disease, recent tick bites? Any prior history of similar symptoms? Any treatment at home (rest, ice, compression, medications, topical preparations)?

2. What should be done on physical exam?

   Inspect for edema, redness, palpate joint for crepitus, fluctuancy. Assess for muscle atrophy and limited ROM.

3. What diagnostic tests should be ordered?

   None indicated.

4. What is the diagnosis and plan for management?

   Epicondylitis. Nonpharmacologic treatment will consist of RICE protocol, avoid aggravating activities, and oral NSAIDs. Symptoms should resolve in 3 months with conservative treatment.

Case 3. 15-year-old girl

1. What other history would you like?

   Precipitating factors, description of pain, any redness or swelling, associated symptoms, alleviating factors

2. What type of examination should be done?

   Vital signs, inspection for redness and swelling; palpation for warmth, tenderness, effusion; assess for swelling at tibial tubercle, ROM, ligament stability

3. What diagnostic tests should be ordered?

   None indicated unless symptoms do not improve

4. What is the diagnosis and plan for management?

   Osgood Schlatter's disease. Avoid activities that cause pain, ice for 20 minutes after exercise, quad strengthening exercises, NSAID if necessary

CHAPTER 15: NEUROLOGIC DISORDERS

Case 1. 49-year-old Black female

1. What other history is needed?

   Family history of headache, including migraine. Are patient's symptoms becoming progressive? History of head injury? Does she have headache with exertion, (straining, sexual activity, or coughing)? Any change in mental state, focal neurologic deficits, or fever?

2. What type of physical exam would you do?

   Screening neurologic exam including funduscopic, cranial nerves, motor exam, gait and coordination, reflexes (would be normal in primary headache syndrome). Focused general exam to include vital signs, HEENT, and other systems as the history suggests to rule out secondary headache. Heart and lung exam routine for woman this age

3. What screening tests would you do?

   CBC if chronic anemia or infection is suspected. Consider CT due to new-onset headache lasting more than a few weeks. Do immediate CT if headache with exertion, staining, sexual activity, or coughing; or on exam there is change in mental state, focal neurologic deficits, or fever. Other diagnostic testing as directed by history and physical exam to rule out infectious, metabolic or autoimmune process

4. What is the most likely diagnosis?

   Migraine headache

5. How would you manage this patient?

   The patient has started with analgesics, Excedrin, which did not work. Can try NSAID, but avoid opioids to prevent rebound headache. Move on to 5-HT agonists if nonnarcotic analgesics ineffective. Sumatriptan (Imitrex)—oral: 25 mg taken as soon as possible at onset, 25–100 mg every 2 hours up to 300 mg in 24 hours. Injection: 6 mg SC adults. Perform first injection in office. Intranasal: single dose of 5, 10, or 20 mg administered in one nostril, may repeat once after 2 hours, not to exceed 40 mg in 24 hours. See her back at weekly to monthly intervals until headaches under control. Consider prophylactic treatment for attacks occurring more than twice a month, or impairing daily function, or medications contraindicated due to hypertension or cardiovascular disease.

Case 2. 3-year-old Asian male

1. What other history do you want to obtain?

   How long has he been febrile? (Febrile seizure usually occurs within the first 24 hours of fever.) Any symptoms of URI, otitis, tonsillitis? Is there a family history of febrile

seizures? Or other risk factors for febrile seizures such as neonatal discharge ≥ 28 days; delayed development; day care attendance; very high fever? Complete description of the seizure, duration, recovery, motor involvement, etc. Any history of recent illness or exposure to illness, onset of headaches, vomiting or unusual symptoms? Recent trauma; lead, toxin, or medication exposure? Prenatal/perinatal history, including developmental history.

2. What physical examination would you perform?

   Complete physical exam. Identify underlying illness requiring treatment; look for signs of physical abuse. Complete neurologic exam, including level of consciousness, presence of meningismus, or a tense bulging fontanel; obtain head circumference. Look for neurocutaneous skin lesions.

3. What further diagnostic tests would you want to order?

   Probably none: lumbar puncture would have been done in ER if any clinical suspicion of meningitis or for children under age 18 months with first seizure; MRI would be done for child with focal seizures. Consider serum lead and routine lab studies only if no source of fever can be elicited on physical examination.

4. How will you initially manage this patient?

   Because febrile seizures are very frightening to the parents, parental reassurance and education are vitally important, as is an active search for the underlying cause of the fever and appropriate treatment with each incidence. Vigorous control of fevers by antipyretics and sponging with tepid water. Acetaminophen 10–15 mg/kg per dose either orally or per rectum. Ibuprofen 10 mg/kg per dose orally.

Case 3. 78-year-old male

1. What other history is important?

   Onset, duration, and progression of symptoms most important in determining etiology and management. Resolution of symptoms in minutes to hours is suggestive of a TIA. Detailed description of symptoms or deficits including visual changes, aphasia, motor weakness, paresthesias may give clue to location of lesion. Review of systems: for associated seizure, loss of consciousness, syncope, vertigo, vomiting, chest pain. Past medical history: cardiac disease; peripheral vascular disease; diabetes; IV drug abuse; and previous neurologic conditions such as seizure, head trauma, dementia, brain tumors. Review all medications including home remedies and supplements, particularly those that can alter level of consciousness or cause bleeding.

2. What systems will you examine?

   Complete neurologic exam for any neurologic deficits (no lasting deficits with TIA). Cardiovascular exam for hypertension, atrial fibrillation, heart murmurs, carotid bruits, abdominal bruits.

3. What is the most likely diagnosis?

   TIA; also has significant risk factors for cardiovascular and cerebrovascular disease.

4. What is your plan?

   Consult with primary care physician or refer to neurologist immediately for work-up that will include CT scan; consider obtaining CBC, ESR, baseline coagulation studies, chemistry panel, lipid profile, RPR, ECG, and chest X-ray in meantime. Provide initial education to patient and family about need for immediate response for subsequent episodes, which could be stroke. Also provide initial education about risk factors — smoking, hypertension, hyperlipidemia — that will need to be modified. Prescribe aspirin 325 mg daily to be started immediately, until more definitive management is begun.

CHAPTER 16: HEMATOLOGIC DISORDERS

Case 1. L.O.

1. What additional history would you like?

   Diet recall, any pica, family history of anemia, any gastrointestinal ailments

2. What type of anemia is most likely in this case?

   Iron deficiency anemia

3. What is the most likely cause of L.O.'s anemia?

   Inadequate dietary intake of iron due to intake of cow's milk before 12 months of age and onset of rapid growth

4. What corrective actions might you recommend at this time?

   Parental education about appropriate diet for age, referral to nutritional assistance program if needed, consider vitamin with iron supplement, follow up in 1 month and then monitor at well child exams

Case 2. B.C.

1. What type of physical exam would you do?

   General appearance, presence of cyanosis or pallor, vital signs, thyroid exam, neurologic exam, breath sounds, cardiac auscultation, abdominal exam, pelvic exam, rectal exam for occult blood.

2. At this point what might you include in your differential diagnosis?

   Anemia due to blood loss, hypothyroidism, fatigue due to depression (related to caregiver burden)

3. What diagnostic studies would you order?

   CBC, TSH, chemistry panel; consider lipid panel, ECG

4. What would your recommendations be for B.C. at this point?

   Iron supplementation to treat iron deficiency anemia due to heavy periods. Consider additional laboratory studies such as serum iron, ferritin, TIBC. Work up or referral for menorrhagia. Offer support for caregiver burden. Follow up monthly until corrected.

Case 3. B.W.

1. What would you include in your differential diagnosis at this time?

   Dementia due to Alzheimer's disease or multi-infarct dementia; reversible causes of dementia such as vitamin B_{12} deficiency; depression; occult malignancy; sensory deficits.

2. What diagnostic studies would you order at this time?

   CBC, chemistry panel, TSH, B_{12} and folate levels, RPR and PSA, fecal occult blood tests (FOBT) × 3.

3. B.W. comes to see you 1 week later and has the following laboratory results: Hgb: 9 g; Hct: 27.2%; MCV: 72; reported as hypochromic; all other parameters are WNL. He has lost two more pounds despite the fact that his daughter has been cooking for him and encouraging him to eat. His FOBT are all positive. What type of anemia does this man most likely have and what would be the next step in your diagnostic work-up of this gentleman?

   Iron deficiency anemia, probably due to blood loss. You urgently refer him to a surgeon or gastrointestinal specialist for colonoscopy, and order iron replacement therapy. You caution him to gradually increase the iron pills to three a day between meals and increase fluids and fiber to prevent constipation.

CHAPTER 17: ENDOCRINE DISORDERS

Case 1. 52-year-old Hispanic female

1. What additional history would you ask?

   Allergies, sleeping pattern, appetite/weight change, level of activity/exercise, 24-hour diet recall, social history including ETOH and cigarette use, family history of DM, thyroid disorders, hypertension, cardiovascular disease. ROS questions should include a statement about how the patient feels in general, changes in skin integrity, nails or hair, visual changes, problems with breathing, chest pain/palpitations, urinary symptoms such as incontinence, urgency, burning; vaginal dryness, frequent yeast infections, bowel habit changes such as constipation, diarrhea, bloating, frequent hunger or thirst.

2. What diagnostic tests would you order?

Complete metabolic panel to check glucose level, renal and hepatic function due to the history of hypertension and exam findings; complete blood count to rule out anemia or other blood dyscrasias due to complaint of fatigue; thyroid panel to rule out hypothyroidism due to increased risk of age and gender and the complaint of fatigue and weight increase; lipid profile for risk of lipid abnormalities with the history of hypertension, obesity and age; urinalysis to rule out infection as a result of the history of frequency; may consider ECG and CXR as baseline studies.

3. If your suspicions were correct, what actions would be required?

Order fasting blood glucose on a separate day to confirm the diagnosis

4. What is your treatment plan and follow-up?

If her blood glucose was > 250 mg/dL and < 400 mg/dL, this would require immediate treatment with oral medications. If her blood glucose was < 250 mg/dL, diet and exercise would be the initial therapy. Nonpharmacologic therapy to include patient education: basic pathophysiology, cause, general management, and long-term complications of type 2 diabetes, lifestyle modifications including diet and exercise counseling and plan, foot care, medic alert bracelet, self-glucose monitoring and log; pharmacotherapy would include initial monotherapy. The medication will be adjusted based on home glucose monitoring in 1 week. Referral to a diabetes educator and dietitian should be considered.

Case 2. A mother with her 7-year-old daughter

1. What additional history would you ask?

Family history, medication use or medications in the home, history of chronic disease, onset of menses, recent increase in rate of growth, changes in behavior or mood, illness or head trauma

2. What diagnostic tests would you order?

Consider hormone and GnRH testing, thyroid function test. May consider bone age, MRI of pituitary gland, and CT of adrenal glands

3. What is your next course of action?

Refer to a pediatric endocrinologist for management if precocity is confirmed.

Case 3. Black parents and their 11-year-old son

1. What additional history would you ask?

Incidence of fatigue, abdominal pain, nausea, vomiting or diarrhea, headaches, medication use or drug ingestion; changes in behavior of school performance

2. What are your differential diagnoses?

   DM type 1, urinary tract infection, hypercalcemia, sepsis, acute abdomen, salicylate intoxication

3. What diagnostic tests would you order?

   Blood glucose (by monitor) and urine dip for glucose, ketones, and signs of infection; urgent comprehensive metabolic panel

4. Your lab results return with a glucose of 420 mg/dL (fasting) and urine dip positive for ketones and glucose. What is your next course of action?

   Consult with pediatrician or endocrinologist for hospitalization and management; educate parents on cause/course of illness and need for hospitalization

CHAPTER 18: PSYCHIATRIC AND MENTAL HEALTH DISORDERS

Case 1. 7-year-old male

1. What additional history would you ask?

   Family history, prenatal history, developmental history, history of neurologic compromise or head trauma, behavioral history, academic history, history of ear infections, vision or hearing problems, any comorbid conditions such as depression or anxiety. Any siblings or family members with ADHD, learning disabilities, or attending/attended special education programs. Onset of symptoms, duration, environmental influences or changes (including possible exposure to deer tick/Lyme disease), stressors or precipitators. Ask about symptoms to determine inattentiveness, hyperactivity, impulsivity per DSM-IV criteria. Explore parenting skills, discipline techniques, possibility of abuse or neglect.

2. What do you think is happening?

   Probable attention-deficit hyperactivity disorder (ADHD)

3. What diagnostic tests would you offer?

   Blood tests are not routinely done. Sometimes a CBC, TSH, or serum lead may be done if there is anything in the history or physical to suggest these. ADHD rating scales may be used by the teacher and parents. Vision and hearing screening should be done to rule out deficits in these areas. ADHD is a clinical diagnosis made by history, clinical observation, and neuropsychological testing.

4. What is your treatment plan?

   Refer to a pediatric neurologist or psychiatrist for pharmacologic management. Psychostimulant medication has been helpful and the medication most frequently used is methylphenidate (Ritalin). Offer information, counseling, resources, and support to parents. Behavior modification programs and social skills training are frequently helpful. With parental consent, communicate with school officials and advocate for child's appropriate educational placement and accommodations as needed.

Case 2. 18-year-old female

1. What additional history would you ask?

   Onset of symptoms, weight history, dietary history with patterns of eating and caloric intake, identify any food rituals, binging, or purging. Menstrual history, age of menarche, and date of LMP, sexual history, exercise history, psychiatric history including history of eating disorders and previous treatments, family history of psychiatric or eating disorders, use of medication for weight control, history of substance abuse, history of abuse or neglect, perception of body. Identify presence of other physical symptoms such as bowel habits, cold hands or feet, fatigue, signs of sexual maturation, patterns of hair growth, skin changes or acne, temperature tolerance, ridges in fingernails, parotid hypertrophy, calluses on fingers, dental erosion. Determine medical history and recent illnesses.

2. What do you think is happening?

   Possible eating disorder—anorexia nervosa, restrictive type. Rule out medical disorders such as thyroid disease, diabetes, pregnancy, CNS lesion or malignancy, or a communicable disease such as acquired immunodeficiency.

3. What diagnostic tests would you offer?

   Start with CBC, chemistry panel with electrolytes and FBS, LH, FSH, hCG, thyroid panel (TSH, T3, T4), electrocardiogram. Other tests based on history and physical findings.

4. What is your treatment plan?

   Psychiatric referral or consultation with a specialist in eating disorders. Make sure patient is hydrated and in stable condition. Primary care provider may monitor medical status in collaboration with specialist.

Case 3. 70-year-old male

1. What additional history would you ask?

   Ask about onset, duration, and severity of symptoms and to what extent daily functioning is impaired. Identify any precipitating events or recent life changes. Obtain complete medication history, caffeine intake, alcohol or drug use, prescription, OTC medication, and alternative medication or treatments, including herbal supplements. Obtain complete past medical history, any current medical problems, psychiatric history, social history, and family medical and psychiatric history.

2. What do you think is happening?

   Panic attacks.

3. What diagnostic tests would you offer?

   Diagnostic labs depend on physical findings. Consider chest X-ray and electrocardiogram due to symptoms and age; consider chemistry panel, TSH, and CBC to rule out other medical conditions; Hamilton Anxiety Scale, or similar rating tool .

4. What is your treatment plan?

   Referral for cognitive behavioral therapy. Pharmacologic treatment with SSRI. With the elderly, "go low, start slow". Dose is generally half the usual starting dose and increased slowly.

Review Questions

1. A 6-month-old infant is brought to the clinic for a well-child visit. The developmental assessment should include evaluation of the infant's ability to:
   a. Pick up small objects with the thumb and forefinger.
   b. Say "no-no" and "bye-bye."
   c. Sit up, with and without support.
   d. Pull-up to a standing position.

2. A 15-year-old female comes in for routine treatment of acne vulgaris. She has been using benzoyl peroxide facial scrubs with no improvement. Numerous open and closed comedones are seen on exam, as well as numerous papules and a few pustules. No cysts or scarring are noted. The preferred treatment regimen would be:
   a. Isotretinoin (Accutane) in the morning and minocycline hydrochloride (Minocin) 100 mg b.i.d.
   b. Erythromycin 1% gel (E-Mycin) gel in the morning and 0.025% tretinoin (Retin-A) cream at bedtime
   c. Tretinoin (Retin-A) 1% cream at bedtime
   d. Oral erythromycin 250 mg t.i.d.

3. A 21-year-old female is having a very severe asthma exacerbation. Which of these physical findings may be *absent* during an asthma attack?
   a. Tachypnea
   b. Wheezing
   c. Prolonged expiration
   d. Tachycardia

4. The differential diagnosis of gastroesophageal reflux (GERD) in an infant (> 2 months old) would include all of the following *except:*
   a. Overfeeding
   b. Hirschsprung's disease
   c. Urinary tract infection
   d. Gastroenteritis

5. A 62-year-old nulliparous diabetic female presents with complaint of watery vaginal discharge without itching or irritation. You notice no discharge, erythema, or lesions on pelvic exam. Your initial work-up should include all *except:*

    a. Microscopy with KOH for fungal elements and spores

    b. CA 125

    c. Pap smear and transvaginal ultrasound

    d. Microscopy for clue cells

6. You suspect that a 27-year-old woman with profuse, yellow vaginal discharge has trichomoniasis. Besides visualizing characteristic trichomonads on microscopy, what other findings would support your diagnosis?

    a. Clue cells and fishy odor

    b. Hyphae

    c. Pruritus and cervical motion tenderness

    d. Vaginal pH > 4.5

7. An older patient is taking carbidopa-levodopa (Sinemet) for Parkinson's disease. He develops depression. Which of the following medications to treat depression would be *contraindicated* for this patient?

    a. Monoamine oxidase inhibitor (MAOI)

    b. Serotonin selective reuptake inhibitor (SSRI)

    c. Tricyclic antidepressant

    d. Lithium

8. The preferred medication regimen for treating newly diagnosed hypothyroidism in older clients who have heart disease is:

    a. 100 mg of propylthiouracil, followed by an increase in dosage every 2–3 weeks

    b. 150 mg of propylthiouracil, followed by an increase in dosage every 4–6 weeks

    c. 0.025 to 0.05 mg of levothyroxine sodium (Synthroid), followed by an increase in dosage every 4–6 weeks

    d. 0.1 mg of levothyroxine sodium (Synthroid), followed by an increase in dosage every 4–6 weeks

9. Joanne is planning to go for an interview for a job with a physician practice that has not hired NPs previously. Joanne is asked, "How can we bill for the services you provide?" Joanne should explain:

    a. In most states, NPs take direct payment from patients, so the patients will pay her.

    b. Medicaid is the only insurance plan that does not reimburse FNPs.

    c. Medicare will reimburse for Joan's services at 85% of the customary physician rate.

    d. Reimbursement is available from Medicare at the full physician rate, even if the MD is not in the office.

10. A mother brings her 2-year-old child in for a sick visit. The child's face looks as though it has been slapped. What is the most likely cause?

    a. High fever

    b. Varicella

    c. Fifth's disease

    d. Roseola

11. A 10-year-old boy complains of a sore throat, fever, and fatigue for 2 days. Findings include pharyngitis, anterior cervical adenopathy, and an oral temperature of 101.6° F (38.6° C). Which of the following tests should be ordered at this time?

    a. Antistreptolysin O titer

    b. Cytomegalovirus titer

    c. Culture for streptococcal infection

    d. Monospot and complete blood count

12. A client who is starting warfarin sodium (Coumadin) therapy should be counseled to *avoid*:

    a. Alcohol, salicylates, and large amounts of green leafy vegetables

    b. Alcohol, antacids, and large amounts of yellow vegetables

    c. Anything containing acetaminophen

    d. Participation in contact sports

13. Initial symptoms of acute glomerulonephritis most commonly seen by the clinician include:

    a. Generalized edema and anorexia

    b. Periorbital edema and hematuria

    c. Fever and hypotension

    d. Flank pain and pyuria

14. A 22-year-old male with history of undescended testicles presents for his first adult health maintenance examination. You will make all of these recommendations *except*:

    a. Self testicular exam and annual clinical exam to detect testicular cancer

    b. DRE and PSA level every 3–5 years for early detection of prostate cancer

    c. Use of condoms if sexually active, to prevent unintended pregnancy and sexually transmitted infection

    d. BP check every 2 years to detect hypertension

15. An overweight adolescent boy complains of pain in his hip that radiates to the medial aspect of his knee. He denies trauma and has not had a fever. You note upon exam that he is walking with a limp. The most likely diagnosis is:

    a. Transient toxic synovitis

    b. Slipped capital femoral epiphysis

    c. Avulsion fracture of the tibial tuberosity

    d. Legg-Calvé-Perthes

16. Factors that may precipitate a sickle cell crisis include which of the following?

    a. Increased environmental humidity

    b. Over-hydration

    c. Exposure to extreme cold or heat

    d. Lack of activity and exertion

17. In addition to features of depression, bipolar disorder is characterized by:

    a. Excessive worry and feelings of apprehension

    b. Refusal to maintain normal body weight, due to intense fear of gaining weight

    c. Grandiose or delusional thinking

    d. Increased sleep

18. At what Tanner stage is a 10-year-old female with pubic hair mainly around the labia and breast budding?

    a. Stage 1
    b. Stage 2
    c. Stage 3
    d. Stage 4

19. A mother reports that her 14-year-old child has developed generalized itching and hives after being stung by a bee. Further assessment for more serious signs indicating the need for emergency intervention would be:

    a. Fluid oozing from lesions
    b. Pain, erythema, and honey-colored crusting of lesions
    c. Angioedema, shortness of breath, and wheezing
    d. Tachycardia

20. A 68-year-old man with chronic obstructive pulmonary disease (COPD) has continuous symptoms with FEV_1 at 60% normal. Which medications should be considered for initial treatment?

    a. Steroids
    b. Theophylline
    c. Antibiotics
    d. An anticholinergic

21. A 1-year-old presents for a well-child exam and you notice that the child has fallen off the growth curve for height and weight; otherwise, the P.E. is normal. You begin a work-up for FTT. What diagnostic tests would you initially order?

    a. CBC, CT of abdomen
    b. CBC, U/A, electrolytes
    c. CBC, TSH, abdominal flat plate
    d. CBC, HIV, U/A

22. Latoya, 22, presents for her annual Pap smear and mentions that she has had a yellowish, irritating vaginal discharge with dysuria and dyspareunia for 7–10 days. If she is a reliable patient, what is generally recommended in regard to her Pap smear when an infection is present?

    a. Obtain Pap smear; infectious process will not interfere with accuracy of cervical cytology results.
    b. Assess and treat for infectious process first and defer Pap smear for 3–6 months.
    c. Treat infectious process and refer for colposcopy to assess for cervical pathology.
    d. Obtain Pap smear and cultures for sexually transmitted infections; await results before treating.

23. A patient with a positive DNA probe test for chlamydia has no medication allergies, is on no medications, and had an LMP 3 weeks ago. You will treat her with:

    a. Azithromycin 1 g p.o. in a single dose
    b. Bactrim DS bid for 14 days

    c. Nothing until pregnancy can be ruled out

    d. Metronidazole gel 0.75% intravaginally b.i.d. for 5 days

24. How often should blood levels of anticonvulsant medications be routinely checked for a patient with a clinically controlled seizure disorder?

    a. Every 3 months

    b. Annually

    c. When adjusting dosage and there has been a change in seizure frequency

    d. If neurologic sequelae appear, such as intention, facial tics, or slurred speech

25. Which of the following statements indicates a client's understanding of what should be done to care for the client's diabetes mellitus when he or she is ill?

    a. "I should take my usual dose of insulin."

    b. "I should avoid eating sweets, especially when I'm sick."

    c. "I should check for ketones if my blood sugar is over 150."

    d. "I should alter my regular insulin, but take my usual NPH insulin."

26. Which of the following statements about Duvall's theory of the stages in family development is true?

    a. The stages cannot overlap.

    b. The stages are based on the age and school placement of the firstborn child.

    c. There are four stages.

    d. Marriage is strongest during the fourth stage.

27. The family nurse practitioner has just diagnosed a 27-year-old with Lyme disease. What is the appropriate management?

    a. Bactrim 400 mg b.i.d. for 14–21 days

    b. Amoxicillin 100 mg t.i.d. for 10 days

    c. Doxycycline 100 mg b.i.d. for 14–21 days

    d. Keflex 500 mg q.i.d. for 14 days

28. Acute otitis media can be distinguished from otitis media with effusion by:

    a. Hearing loss with ear popping and crackling

    b. Otalgia and decreased mobility of tympanic membrane

    c. Temporomandibular joint pain

    d. Eustachian tube obstruction

29. A new 58-year-old patient has a blood pressure reading of 162/90 mm Hg. The family nurse practitioner should:

    a. Tell the patient she has hypertension and begin treatment today.

    b. Have the client return for a total of 3 successive blood pressure checks and discuss therapeutic life style changes.

    c. Initiate treatment with 25 mg of hydrochlorothiazide daily.

    d. Plan to recheck the client in 3 months.

30. A patient complains of burning during urination, frequency, and urgency. The patient's history reveals that she has recently become sexually active and is on oral contraceptives. A urine dipstick reveals leukocyte esterase and nitrite. The best course of action is to perform a pelvic exam and obtain vaginal cultures to rule out vaginitis and cervicitis followed by:

   a. Placing the patient on amoxicillin 250 mg 4 times a day for 14 days

   b. Placing the patient on nitrofurantoin (Macrodantin) 100 mg 4 times a day for 5 days

   c. Placing the patient on trimethoprim-sulfamethoxazole (Bactrim DS) 160/800 mg every 12 hours for 3 days

   d. Obtain urine culture and sensitivity results before placing the patient on antibiotic therapy

31. Your evaluation of a 6-year-old male with an asymptomatic, firm, pear-shaped sac behind the testicle would include:

   a. Fluid aspiration for culture and sensitivity

   b. Transillumination

   c. Doppler ultrasound

   d. If on right side, immediate referral

32. You examine a patient you suspect has a meniscus injury. To assess for this injury, you examine the patient supine and the knee fully flexed. The tibia is externally rotated and mild varus or valgus stress is placed on the knee. This test is called:

   a. Lachman's test

   b. McMurray's

   c. Anterior drawer

   d. Thompson test

33. P.I. presents to clinic requesting a pregnancy test. The test is positive. In addition to referral for obstetrical care, what dietary supplements might you recommend at this time?

   a. None; patient is healthy and does not need supplements

   b. Prenatal vitamin with folic acid

   c. Vitamin C

   d. Vitamin E

34. A 12-year-old boy is brought in by his parents for increasing behavior problems in school and in the neighborhood. Which of the following descriptions would prompt your referral for a possible conduct disorder?

   a. Disregards the rights of others

   b. Shows remorse for misconduct

   c. Easily distracted, forgetful, does not complete tasks

   d. Mood swings, agitation, restlessness

35. A 22-year-old female presents to your office with a complaint of sudden onset of shortness of breath. Her history reveals she is sexually active and takes oral contraceptives. She has just returned from a trip to Australia and tells you she slept and watched movies for the whole 22-hour flight. You are immediately concerned that this patient may have:

   a. Hepatitis

   b. Pulmonary embolis

   c. Migraine headaches

   d. Urinary tract infection

36. You diagnosed pityriasis rosea in a 12-year-old female who came to you presenting with a maculopapular scaling rash for 2 days. Upon history, her mother revealed that the patient had a large, single, bright-red patch that preceded this rash eruption by about 2 weeks. Typical additional symptoms include which of the following?

    a. Fever of 102° F for more than 72 hours
    b. Fever for 24 hours before rash, followed by rhinorrhea and cough
    c. Non-pruritic rash, clear runny nose and cough
    d. Absence of fever, pruritis confined to trunk and upper extremities

37. You order a PPD on a 7-year-old who has a parent with suspected TB. The PPD result is 7 mm in duration. Your treatment plan is:

    a. Counsel family about TB and repeat PPD in 3 months.
    b. Order a chest x-ray (CXR) and begin medication if CXR is suggestive of pulmonary disease.
    c. Order a chest x-ray (CXR) and refer patient to begin treatment with INH.
    d. Begin INH.

38. A 70-year-old man presents with anemia, recent weight loss, and heme-positive stools. He has no GI complaints. The diagnosis until proven otherwise is:

    a. Ulcerative colitis
    b. Peptic ulcer disease
    c. Hemorrhoids
    d. Colon cancer

39. All of the following are symptoms of premenstrual syndrome *except*:

    a. Difficulty concentrating
    b. Psychotic episodes
    c. Fatigue, lethargic
    d. Irritability

40. You are working in a college health clinic that offers free HIV testing. A student has had unprotected intercourse with a new partner. You advise:

    a. Screening for Chlamydia and gonorrhea, and provide syphilis prophylaxis treatment
    b. Review history, STI screening, HIV testing, provide hepatitis B vaccination series
    c. Use of condoms for 3 months, then return for HIV testing
    d. Qualitative viral RNA level to assess for HIV

41. A 12-year-old male with a recent history of otitis media presents with 1 day of acute right facial weakness, including flattening of the forehead furrows, inability to completely close the ipsilateral eye, flattening of the nasolabial fold, and drooping of the mouth. What is the most likely diagnosis?

    a. Bell's palsy
    b. Acoustic neuroma
    c. Recurrence of otitis
    d. Trigeminal palsy

42. The family nurse practitioner sees an active 11-year-old girl who has type I diabetes. The child plays softball and basketball, and swims on the school team. The FNP tells the child and her mother that:

    a. Insulin dosing and eating patterns should not be changed during periods of frequent exercise.

    b. Nocturnal hypoglycemia may occur on significantly active days.

    c. Type I diabetic patients should avoid strenuous physical activity.

    d. Nocturnal hyperglycemia may occur on weekends.

43. The family nurse practitioner should:

    a. Rely on tradition, intuition, and personal preference to deal with clinical problems

    b. Accept and use clinical practice guidelines, regardless of the source of the recommendations

    c. Understand that cultural influences rarely influence health behaviors

    d. Use evidence-based practices and critically evaluate and participate in outcome studies

44. A 34-year-old male presents for your care with what appears to be obvious oral candidiasis. You treat him with nystatin oral suspension 500,000 units swish-and-swallow 3–5 times/day for 10 days. His infection clears, but he returns with the same symptoms in 1 month. Which of the following would *not* be part of your evaluation for this patient?

    a. Diabetes mellitus

    b. HIV infection

    c. Malnutrition or substance abuse

    d. Multiple sclerosis

45. Which of the following helps you differentiate croup from bronchiolitis?

    a. Age

    b. Presence of fever

    c. Tachypnea

    d. Wheezing

46. During a clinic visit, a woman known to rely on advertising claims for a wide variety of alternative therapies tells the family nurse practitioner that her husband is limiting his daily fluid intake to one glass of liquid to keep from passing blood in his urine. Which of the following responses by the nurse practitioner would be most appropriate?

    a. "Your husband can become dehydrated with small amounts of fluid."

    b. "Your husband needs to be seen for a kidney evaluation as soon as possible."

    c. "Tell me how you think this is helping your husband."

    d. Nothing, because the family nurse practitioner does not see the woman's husband.

47. Initial treatment for lateral epicondylitis includes all of the following *except*:

    a. NSAIDs

    b. Tennis elbow band

    c. Cortisone injection

    d. Physical therapy

48. In a female with vitamin B$_{12}$ deficiency, you would expect which laboratory profile?
    a. Hgb 10.6, MCV < 80
    b. Hgb 10.6, MCV > 100
    c. CBC normal between episodes of hemolysis
    d. Decreased hgb and hct, normal MCV

49. A sexually active patient with multiple partners presents with fever, adenopathy, rash, myalgias, headache, pharyngitis, and hepatosplenomegaly. You suspect:
    a. Syphilis
    b. Primary herpes simplex, type 1 infection
    c. Disseminated gonorrhea
    d. Primary HIV infection

50. A G1 P1 mother of a 7-day-old presents with right breast pain and fever since night-time yesterday. She is breastfeeding but uses 2–3 ounces of formula at 1 to 2 nighttime feedings. On exam, you note that her nipples have small central fissures and the right breast has some redness in the lower outer quadrant. She has no allergies and her temperature is 100.5° F. The infant is gaining adequate weight. Which of the following statements is **false**?
    a. When indicated, one possible antibiotic choice is dicloxacillin (Dycill) 500 mg p.o. q.i.d. for at least 10 days.
    b. Breastfeeding should be continued and encouraged more frequently and exclusively, regardless of the usual antibiotic therapy.
    c. Using formula to replace a feeding is a possible etiology of mastitis.
    d. Sore nipples with skin breakdown are normal and no improvement of the latch is necessary.

51. Which of the following liver function tests would you expect to be elevated in the presence of bone disease?
    a. GGT (gamma-glutamyl trans peptidase)
    b. ALT (alanine aminotransferase)
    c. Amylase
    d. ALP (alkaline phosphatase)

52. Jane, a 35-year-old corporate lawyer, presents with a 3-month history of abdominal pain, bloating, a stool pattern that varies from constipation to frequent loose stools over the course of the week, and occasional blood on the toilet paper, especially on days when she strains to eliminate stool or has several diarrhea-type stools. What is your diagnosis?
    a. Crohn's disease
    b. Irritable bowel syndrome
    c. Acute gastroenteritis
    d. Ulcerative colitis

53. Medicare part A pays for which of the following services?
    a. Outpatient services
    b. Inpatient services
    c. Homecare services
    d. Prescription services

54. You discover the practice you have recently joined plans to bill your services as "incidental to." You are aware that:

   a. Payment would be at 85% of the physician fee.

   b. This type of billing can only be used in a rural setting.

   c. This type of billing can only be used in a hospital setting.

   d. This would be Medicare fraud, as you are the only provider in the office.

55. You have just graduated from your NP program and are investigating malpractice insurance. You are aware that there are several different types of coverage. You select a policy that covers any claim that results from an incident that occurs during the term of the policy, regardless of how long it takes before the claim is made. This is referred to as a:

   a. Claims made policy

   b. Tail policy

   c. Occurrence policy

   d. Nurse practitioner policy

56. The cost common prescription drug–herb interaction occurs with herbal preparations and:

   a. Antibiotics

   b. Ace inhibitors

   c. Warfarin

   d. Oral diabetes agents

57. Legislative authority for nurse practitioner practice is regulated by:

   a. The professional certifying organization, with a vote of the membership

   b. The board of medicine in each state jurisdiction, with consent of the board of nursing

   c. A legally designated authority that implements regulations such as state boards of nursing

   d. The federal government's Bureau of the Health Professions

58. A 65-year-old male presents with the following complaints for the past 6 months: difficulty starting/stopping stream of urine, hesitancy, dribbling, weakening force/size of stream, and sensation of full bladder after urinating. He reports his symptoms are worsening, causing him to wake up 2–3 times per night to urinate. Patient is afebrile. Digital rectal exam reveals: prostate gland is non-tender, firm, smooth, and rubbery. Symmetrical enlargement with obliteration of midline median sulcus is noted. These symptoms are consistent with which urologic condition?

   a. Prostate cancer

   b. Epididymitis

   c. Benign prostatic hyperplasia

   d. Acute bacterial prostatitis

59. Immediate referral for surgical intervention is required for which of the following urologic condition?

   a. Hydrocele

   b. Epididymo-orchitis

   c. Testicular torsion

   d. Varicocele

60. At 12 weeks postpartum, a 25-year-old woman who is caring for her newborn complains that she feels unbearably lonely and sad. She reports poor appetite and sleeplessness. She states she loves her baby, but questions her ability to be a "good mother." She should be treated for:
    a. Maternity blues
    b. Postpartum depression
    c. Postpartum psychosis
    d. Bipolar disorder

61. Of the following, the test of choice for screening pregnant women at 26 weeks for gestational diabetes is:
    a. 3-hour GTT following a 100 g glucose load
    b. Hemoglobin A1 C
    c. Random serum screen
    d. Serum screen after a 50 g glucose load

62. All of the following provide quick relief of after-birth uterine pain for a multiparous woman in the postpartum period *except*:
    a. Analgesia
    b. Empty bladder
    c. Prone position
    d. Suckling of the newborn

63. At 34 weeks' gestation, a woman presents to the clinic, stating: "I have bloody fluid leaking from my vagina today." She is not experiencing any other symptoms. Initial management would include all of the following *except*:
    a. Digital examination to determine cervical dilatation
    b. Speculum exam to view the cervix
    c. Microscopy exam to determine vaginal ferning
    d. Ultrasound determination of amniotic fluid volume

64. A woman who is Rh negative is given Rh-immune prophylaxis during this pregnancy. She should be advised that, for future pregnancies, she will:
    a. Be tested with each subsequent pregnancy
    b. Not need future testing
    c. Only be tested if this baby is Rh positive
    d. Only be tested if this baby is Rh negative

65. A 38-year-old Black woman presents for her first prenatal visit at 10 weeks. Her blood pressure is 144/98. A repeat BP is 146/100. She has trace amounts of protein in her urine and says her rings feel tight. Your initial clinical impression would be:
    a. Chronic hypertension
    b. Chronic hypertension with superimposed preeclampsia
    c. Preeclampsia
    d. Normotensive for the first trimester

66. You are prescribing ferrous sulfate for a patient with iron deficiency anemia. Which of the following is an appropriate patient instruction?

    a. Take the ferrous sulfate with other medications.

    b. Take the ferrous sulfate with meals.

    c. Take on an empty stomach.

    d. Do not take with vitamin C.

67. In evaluating a CBC, the earliest laboratory abnormality in iron deficiency anemia is:

    a. Low platelet count

    b. Low MCH

    c. Low hemoglobin level

    d. Increased RDW

68. Mr. C is a 77-year-old patient who presents for his annual checkup; PMH includes COPD, HTN, and anemia. You diagnose anemia of chronic disease. Anemia of chronic disease is which type of anemia?

    a. Macrocytic

    b. Microcytic

    c. Normocytic

    d. Pernicious

69. A common physical exam finding in patients with pernicious anemia includes:

    a. Bradycardia

    b. Decreased reflexes

    c. Retinal hemorrhages

    d. Beefy-red, shiny tongue

70. A 24-year-old woman of Asian descent presents for evaluation. She has no complaints. Her CC results are HgB: 9.1 g; hct: 28%; RBC: 6 million; MCV: 68 fl;RDW: 13%. The most likely diagnosis is:

    a. Vitamin B_{12} deficiency

    b. Alpha-thalassemia minor

    c. Anemia of chronic disease

    d. Fanconi anemia

71. Ms. C, a 24-year-old female, presents for her a checkup. She informs you she is trying to get pregnant. In discussing her reproductive health, you advise her to increase her intake of which of the following to minimize the risk of neural tube defects in the fetus?

    a. Niacin

    b. Iron

    c. Folic acid

    d. Vitamin C

72. The cause of pernicious anemia is:
    a. RBC enzyme deficiency
    b. Dietary deficiency of vitamin B_{12}
    c. A combination of micronutrient deficiencies caused by malabsorption
    d. Lack of production of intrinsic factor by the gastric mucosa

73. The expected change in visual fields in a patient with glaucoma is:
    a. Loss of central vision
    b. Enhanced peripheral vision
    c. Loss of peripheral vision
    d. Enhanced central vision

74. A 2-year-old girl is brought to the clinic by her grandmother for a runny nose with unilateral greenish drainage and a low-grade fever for 2 weeks with decreased appetite for the last week. Which physical finding would be particularly worrisome and indicate the need for further evaluation?
    a. Fussiness
    b. Unilateral nasal drainage
    c. Sporadic, loose cough
    d. Decreased appetite

75. To help differentiate an S3 from other heart sounds, the family nurse practitioner listens closely to identify its timing. At what point in the cardiac cycle does S3 occur?
    a. Early systole
    b. Late systole
    c. Early diastole
    d. Late diastole

Answers to the Review Questions

1. **Correct Answer: B.** Pincer grasp occurs at about 9 months; saying "no" and "bye-bye" occurs between 9 and 12 months, and pulling up to a standing position occurs between 8 and 12 months.

2. **Correct Answer: B.** Use of topical antibiotic due to pustules and tretinoin (Retin-A) as an effective comedolytic.

3. **Correct Answer: B.** Wheezing is absent when there is severe constriction of the bronchial tree.

4. **Correct Answer: B.** Hirschsprung's disease presents with constipation and abdominal distention rather than vomiting or spitting up.

5. **Correct Answer: C.** Pap smear may show AGCUS and ultrasound may show increased endometrial stripe, requiring referral for further endometrial cancer work-up.

6. **Correct Answer: D.** Vaginal pH > 4.5 indicate a trichomonas infection.

7. **Correct Answer: A.** Nonselective MAO inhibitors-A are contraindicated in combination with levodopa.

8. **Correct Answer: C.** Should have a lower starting dosage to avoid adverse effect of angina in a patient who has preexisting CAD.

9. **Correct Answer: C.** Provided that the FNP has her own Medicare provider number, Medicare will reimburse for Joan's services at 85% of the customary physician rate.

10. **Correct Answer: C.** Slapped cheek appearance with a sick appearing child is likely to be Fifth's disease.

11. **Correct Answer: C.** A culture for streptococcal infection can be used instead of or in combination with quick strep test.

12. **Correct Answer: A.** Due to increased risk of GI bleed and the large amounts of Vitamin K in the food, the client should avoid alcohol, salicytes, and large amounts of leafy green vegetables.

13. **Correct Answer: B.** Edema and gross hematuria are the major symptoms of post-streptococcal glomerulonephritis.

14. **Correct Answer: B.** DRE and PSA level testing every 3–5 years for early detection is not recommended at age 22.

15. **Correct Answer: B.** Slipped capital femoral epiphysis is most common in adolescents who are obese. It usually presents with a limp and knee pain referred from the hip.

16. **Correct Answer: C.** Exposure to extreme cold or heat is a risk factor for crisis.

17. **Correct Answer: C.** Grandiose or delusional thinking is part of the diagnostic description of bipolar disorder.

18. **Correct Answer: B.** A 10-year-old female with pubic hair mainly around the labia and breast budding is in Tanner stage 2.

19. **Correct Answer: C.** These are signs of anaphylaxis.

20. **Correct Answer: D.** An anticholinergic is in line with national guidelines.

21. **Correct Answer: B.** CBC, U/A, and electrolytes are the basics lab to order.

22. **Correct Answer: B.** Pap smear more likely to be accurate after inflammatory process has cleared.

23. **Correct Answer: A.** Azithromycin is first-line treatment and ensures compliance.

24. **Correct Answer: C.** Blood levels of anticonvulsant medications should be checked when adjusting dosage and when there has been a change in seizure frequency.

25. **Correct Answer A.** Insulin intake should be the same.

26. **Correct Answer: B.** In Duvall's theory of the stages in family development, the stages are based on the age and school placement of the firstborn child.

27. **Correct Answer: C.** Doxycycline is the drug of choice.

28. **Correct Answer: B.** Otalgia and decreased mobility of tympanic membrane occur in otitis media, not in otitis media with effusion.

29. **Correct Answer: B.** Exercise and reducing sodium and changing diet may help lower the blood pressure.

30. **Correct Answer: C.** A sexually transmitted infection may also present with dysuria, so this needs to be ruled out in newly sexually active client. Short course therapy with a sulfa drug or a fluoroquinolone has been shown to be safe and effective against the organisms most often responsible for uncomplicated UTI (e.g., *E. coli*.)

31. **Correct Answer: B.** There should be a red glow if hydrocele with shadow of testicle; smaller mass if spermatocele.

32. **Correct Answer: B.** The McMurray test is used to check for injury to the meniscus. The exam is as described.

33. **Correct Answer: B.** Begin prenatal vitamins with folic acid as early as possible during pregnancy; must have minimum of 400 mg of folic acid to help prevent neural tube defects.

34. **Correct Answer: A.** Disregarding the rights of other is a characteristic of conduct disorder.

35. **Correct Answer: B.** Patients on oral contraceptives with long periods of sitting such as airplane trips are at high risk for DVT and pulmonary embolism.

36. **Correct Answer: D.** Absence of fever, pruritis confined to trunk and upper extremities would be typical additional symptoms.

37. **Correct Answer: B.** Because child is a close contact of someone who may have TB, induration > 5 is considered positive PPD.

38. **Correct Answer: D.** Colon cancer often presents in elderly in late stage with only anemia, bowel changes, heme-positive stools, and possible weight loss.

39. **Correct Answer: B.** Psychotic episodes are not part of PMS.

40. **Correct Answer: B.** This woman is considered high risk because of new partner and should complete a full history, STI screening, HIV testing, and receive a hepatitis B vaccine.

41. **Correct Answer: A.** Bell's palsy affects the motor branch of the facial nerve, altering facial movements.

42. **Correct Answer: B.** Exercise requires additional energy, so diet and insulin doses should be adjusted accordingly; nocturnal hypoglycemia may occur on days the patient is very active.

43. **Correct Answer: D.** The nurse practitioner should use scientific resources, reliable sources for guidelines, and understand that culture influences health behaviors.

44. **Correct Answer: D.** Multiple sclerosis is not a risk factor for oral candidiasis.

45. **Correct Answer: A.** Croup affects children 7 months to 3 years; bronchiolitis is a disease of infants, newborns to 2 years, with peak incidence at 6 months. Both have little or no fever, cause tachypnea, and cause wheezing.

46. **Correct Answer: C.** This response validates that you understand what she believes but need to understand more why this makes sense to her. It opens communication that may lead to a therapeutic intervention.

47. **Correct Answer: C.** The initial treatment does *not* include using a cortisone injection in the area. This is considered a second line treatment.

48. **Correct Answer: B.** This is a macrocytic anemia, as in B_{12} deficiency.

49. **Correct Answer: D.** These symptoms generally indicate a primary HIV infection.

50. **Correct Answer: B.** Breastfeeding helps increase antibiotic dissemination.

51. **Correct Answer: D.** ALP (alkaline phosphatase) is found in liver, intestine, bone and placenta. It elevates in bone diseases such as bony metastasis and Paget's disease.

52. **Correct Answer: B.** These are classic presentations of irritable bowel syndrome.

53. **Correct Answer: B.** Medicare Part A pays for inpatient services.

54. **Correct Answer: D.** Incident to billing allows for 100% of the physician fee if all criteria are met. Location does not have an impact on "incident to" billing.

55. **Correct Answer: C.** An occurrence policy covers any claim that results from an incident that occurs during the term of the policy regardless of how long it takes before the claim is made.

56. **Correct Answer: C.** The most common prescription drug–herb interaction is between Warfarin and a variety of common herbal products, including garlic, ginkgo, and St. John's Wort.

57. **Correct Answer: C.** Authority for nurse practitioner (NP) practice is found in state legislative statutes and in rules and regulations.

58. **Correct Answer: C.** These symptoms and exam findings are consistent with benign prostatic hyperplasia.

59. **Correct Answer: C.** Testicular torsion requires surgical intervention within 4 hours of onset of pain and symptoms to preserve the testicle from necrosis.

60. **Correct Answer: B.** These symptoms are consistent with postpartum depression, which are prolonged, lasting greater than 6 weeks to 1 year.

61. **Correct Answer: D.** A serum screen after a 50 g glucose load is current standard diagnostic test for determining gestational diabetes.

62. **Correct Answer: D.** Suckling of the newborn would increase uterine pain as suckling stimulates the uterus to contract.

63. **Correct Answer: A.** Never insert fingers blindly into the vagina when a pregnant patient reports vaginal bleeding as this action could rupture membranes or perforate a potentially prolapsed placenta.

64. **Correct Answer: A.** Pregnant women need to be tested with each subsequent pregnancy.

65. **Correct Answer: A.** The patient presents with hypertension. It is too early to develop preeclampsia, and the blood pressure readings are not normotensive.

66. **Correct Answer: C.** Taking on an empty stomach will increase absorption.

67. **Correct Answer: D.** Increased RDW is the earliest laboratory finding.

68. **Correct Answer: C.** Anemia of chronic disease is a normocytic anemia.

69. **Correct Answer: D.** A beefy-red tongue is common in patients with pernicious anemia.

70. **Correct Answer: B.** Alpha-thalassemia minor is usually asymptomatic, with high prevalence in persons originating from Southeast Asia

71. **Correct Answer: C.** Folic acid helps prevent neural tube defects.

72. **Correct Answer: D.** Pernicious anemia is caused by a lack of production of intrinsic factor by the gastric mucosa.

73. **Correct Answer: C.** Loss of peripheral vision occurs with glaucoma.

74. **Correct Answer: B.** Any patient with unilateral nasal drainage should be evaluated for a foreign body in the nares, including tumors, as URI symptoms will produce bilateral nasal drainage.

75. **Correct Answer: D.** S4 is a low-pitched heart sound that occurs late in diastole, after S3 and immediately before S4.

Page numbers followed by *f* indicate figures; *t* tables; and *b* boxes.

A

Abnormal cervical cytology
 assessment of, 639–641
 etiology of, 636
 explanation of, 636
 follow-up for, 642
 incidence and demographics for, 636
 management of, 641
 prevention and screening for, 638
 recommendations for, 637–638
 risk factors for, 636–637
 special considerations for, 641–642
 when to consult, refer, or hospitalize for, 642
Abnormal liver function tests (LFTs)
 assessment of, 469–470
 etiology of, 467–469
 explanation of, 467
 follow-up for, 470
 management of, 470
 risk factors for, 469
 special considerations for, 470
 test interpretation, 471*t*
 when to consult, refer, or hospitalize for, 470
Abnormal uterine bleeding (AUB)
 assessment of, 613–614
 differential diagnosis of, 614
 etiology of, 613
 explanation of, 612–613
 follow-up for, 616
 incidence and demographics for, 613
 management of, 615–616
 risk factors for, 613
 special considerations for, 616
 when to consult, refer, or hospitalize for, 616
Abuse assessment, 86
Accreditation, 13
Acne
 hidradenitis suppurativa, 199–201
 rosacea, 197–199
 vulgaris and nodulocystic acne, 194–197
Acute abdominal pain
 assessment of, 480–482
 differential diagnosis of, 483
 explanation of, 480
 follow-up for, 484
 management of, 483
 special considerations for, 483
 when to consult, refer, or hospitalize for, 483

Acute bronchitis
 assessment of, 333–334
 differential diagnosis of, 334
 etiology of, 333
 explanation of, 332
 follow-up for, 336
 incidence and demographics for, 333
 management of, 335
 prevention and screening for, 333
 risk factors for, 333
 special considerations for, 335
 when to consult, refer, or hospitalize for, 336
Acute gastroenteritis, 484–486
Acute glomerulonephritis, 574–576
Acute pancreatitis, 517–519
Acute pyelonephritis, 559–561, 560*t*
Acute stress disorder (ASD), 985
Addison's disease, 932, 964–966
Addition. *See* Alcohol dependence; Substance abuse and dependence; Tobacco dependence
Adjustment disorder with depressed mood, 992, 994
Adolescent issues. *See also* Childhood issues
 nutrition and, 78–79
 pubertal changes, 66–67, 67*t*
 pubertal disorders, 972–980
 sports assessments, 75–76, 76*t*
Adrenal disorders
 Addison's disease, 964–966
 Adrenal insufficiency, 932, 964–966
 Cushing's syndrome, 961–964
Adrenal insufficiency, 932, 964–966
Adult issues. *See also* Geriatric issues
 health screening and supervision, 91–93*t*
 injury prevention in, 82, 83–86*t*
 nutrition and, 81–82
Adult onset diabetes. *See* Diabetes mellitus type 2
Advance directives, 15
Advanced Practice Registered Nurse (APRN) Compact, 11–12
Advertising, direct-to-consumer, 36
Agency for Health Care Research and Quality (AHRQ), 23
Agent-host relations, 56
Agent (organism) properties, 56
Age-related stresses, 59, 87
Aging, normal changes of, 94

AIDS. *See* HIV/AIDS; HIV exposure
Alcohol dependence
 assessment of, 1003–1004
 differential diagnosis of, 1004
 etiology of, 1001–1002
 explanation of, 1001
 follow-up for, 1005
 incidence and demographics for, 1002
 management of, 1004
 prevention and screening for, 1002, 1003*t*
 risk factors for, 1002
 special considerations for, 1005
 when to consult, refer, or hospitalize for, 1005
Allergy
 contact dermatitis, 183–186
 urticaria, 186–188
Alopecia areata, 240–242
Alternative medicine, 26–27
Alzheimer's disease/multi-infarct dementia, 853–857, 854*t*
Amenorrhea
 assessment of, 605–607
 differential diagnosis of, 607
 etiology of, 604
 explanation of, 603
 follow-up for, 608
 incidence and demographics for, 605
 management of, 607–608
 risk factors for, 605
 special considerations for, 608
 when to consult, refer, or hospitalize for, 608
American Academy of Family Physicians, 92
American Academy of Pediatrics, 75, 134
American Association of Colleges of Nursing (AACN), 22, 23
American Association of Sports Medicine Physicians, 75
American Cancer Society, 92, 637
American College of Nurse Practitioners (ACNP), 39
American College of Obstetricians and Gynecologists (ACOG), 92, 637
American Diabetes Association (ADA), 935
American Gasteroenterologic Association, 473, 496
American Heart Association, 382

About the Authors

Elizabeth Blunt, PhD, RN, FNP-BC, ANP-BC, has more than 30 years of nursing experience, with over 15 years' experience as a nurse practitioner, and has been teaching NP students since 1998. She teaches across the NP curriculum including physical assessment, leadership, and NP clinical courses and has been a directing NP programs for the last 10 years. She completed her PhD in 2004 with a focus on pharmaceutical company influence on NP prescribing. Dr. Blunt has multiple publications to her credit, including articles on the NP role in the emergency department, online learning, and development of NP skills labs. She presents at national and international conferences. Her clinical practice is in emergency department and outpatient practice settings.

Courtney Elizabeth Reinisch, DNP, MSN, FNP-BC, DCC, is a Clinical Assistant Professor of Nursing at Rutgers University College of Nursing, teaching in the graduate nurse practitioner program. She is a Hispanic, bilingual certified Family Nurse Practitioner since 1999. Presently, Dr. Reinisch maintains a clinical practice as an Emergency Department APRN. Her research and practice interest are in underserved communities and chronic disease prevention. She has worked with an urban charter school to promote exercise and nutrition knowledge in vulnerable youth. She also assisted in the opening of a family practice serving the community of LEAP Academy Charter School to provide primary care for the students and families in Camden, New Jersey. She received her BA in Biology-Psychology from Immaculata College, BSN and MSN from the University of Delaware, and her Doctor of Nursing Practice degree from Columbia University. Prior to joining Rutgers, Dr. Reinisch was an Assistant Clinical Professor of Nursing at Columbia University School of Nursing. Dr. Reinisch has presented and published numerous times, both nationally and internationally. She is an Executive Committee member of the American Board of Comprehensive Care. She was instrumental in achieving accreditation status for the certification examination administered by the American Board of Comprehensive Care.

Dawn Aubel, MS, MPH, FNP-BC, is a Family Nurse Practitioner in a corporate wellness center managing an onsite health center and global wellness programs. She is also an Adjunct Professor of Clinical Nursing at Columbia University School of Nursing. She received a BSN from the Medical College of Virginia, a Master's of Science — Family Nurse Practitioner from Columbia University School of Nursing, and a master's in public health from the Mailman School of Public Health at Columbia University. At present she is a doctoral student in the Nurse Executive program at Teacher's College, Columbia University. She is certified by the American Nurses Certification Center as a Family Nurse Practitioner. Ms. Aubel has extensive experience as a primary care provider, an advocate for cancer survivors, and as a health educator. She is a member of Sigma Theta Tau, the nursing honor society; the NYS Coalition of Nurse Practitioners; and the American Academy of Nurse Practitioners.

Dawn Bucher, DNP, FNP-BC, DCC, is a part-time Assistant Professor of Clinical Nursing at Columbia University, New York. She received her Doctorate of Nursing Practice degree from Columbia University in 2007 and is a diplomate in comprehensive care. Dr. Bucher practices as a family nurse practitioner providing care to underserved individuals, families, and communities in rural Minnesota, and Native American tribes in South Dakota and Arizona. Her focus is preventative care, family practice, with emphasis in internal medicine and chronic health conditions. Dr. Bucher has published many articles in peer-reviewed journals. She belongs to numerous professional organizations and was selected Distinguished Young Alumni award in 2008 from Columbia University School of Nursing and Alumni Association. She can be contacted at dr_bucher@yahoo.com.

Deborah Gilbert-Palmer, EdD, FNP-BC, received her associate degree in nursing in 1985 from the University of West Virginia. Her nursing career includes pediatric oncology nursing for 10 years at St. Jude Children's Research Hospital and Emergency Medicine at Leboneur Children's Hospital as well as the Elvis Presley Trauma Center in Memphis, Tennessee. In 1993, she completed her bachelor's degree in nursing at the University of Tennessee — Memphis and went on to complete a master's degree in nursing in the FNP Program at the University of Tennessee in 1995. She was credentialed as a Family Nurse Practitioner by the American Nurses Credentialing Center in 1995. She has practiced in primary care settings in rural Missouri and Arkansas for 18 years. In 2000, she accepted a tenured position as a FNP Program Faculty Member and has taught at the graduate level since that time. She is currently a Professor and Family Nurse Practitioner Program Faculty Member with Walden University. In 2001, she developed and implemented a program for the utilization of nurse practitioners as providers in the emergency room for White River Medical Center, Batesville, Arkansas. Deborah has received the Faculty Alumni Award from the University of Tennessee and Clinical Excellence Award from Sigma Theta Tau. She has presented at the international and national level and continues to maintain clinical practice in a private family practice clinic in rural Arkansas.

Julie A. Lindenberg, DNP, APRN, FNP-BC, DCC, is a certified family nurse practitioner. Her academic degrees include a bachelor of science in nursing from the University of Delaware and a master of science in nursing from The University of Texas Health Science Center (UTHSC) in Houston. She received her doctor of nursing practice degree from Columbia University, where she received the Macy Foundation scholarship. Dr. Lindenberg is an associate professor of clinical nursing at the UTHealth School of Nursing in Houston, where she has taught nurse practitioner students for more than 20 years. Her administrative roles there have included serving as director of the family nurse practitioner program and The University of Texas Health Services, a primary care and occupational health academic nursing center. Currently, she serves as the chief clinical officer (interim) at RediClinic, the largest independently owned retail health care operator in the United States, where she has clinical oversight for 60 nurse practitioners and physician assistants.

Barbara Rideout, MSN, ANP-BC, has more than 40 years' experience in nursing practice, leadership and education. She received her diploma from Sacred Heart Hospital in Allentown, PA; BSN from the University of Delaware; MSN in Nursing Education and post-master's in Nursing Administration from Villanova University; post-master's in Adult Primary Care NP from Temple University; and post-master's in Family NP from MCP–Hahnemann University. She has 16 years of NP experience, including acting as the Clinical Director in the development of two NP-managed health centers for underserved populations in North Philadelphia. She is currently employed in occupational medicine, and has published on ostomy and wound care topics, GI nursing topics, nurse managed health centers, and health assessment. Rideout's greatest personal achievement was to be selected as "Teacher of the Year" on three occasions by graduating nursing students at Temple University.

Colleen Stellabotte, RN, CCRN, MSN, FNP-BC, is an Adjunct Clinical Professor in the Family Nurse Practitioner Program at Villanova University. In addition, she is the lead NP for Mercy Philadelphia and Mercy Fitzgerald Emergency Medicine Departments, responsible for the operations of Fast Track. Ms. Stellabotte has presented numerous continuing education programs both locally and nationally. She belongs to numerous professional organizations.

Debra Shearer, EdD, MSN, FNP-BC, is the Director of the Doctor of Nursing Practice Program and Assistant Professor at Villanova University College of Nursing. Prior to her position at Villanova, Dr. Shearer served as Department Chair of the Nurse Practitioner Programs at Drexel University College of Nursing and Health Professions. She was the Chief Nurse Practitioner Officer and practiced as a family nurse practitioner at Drexel University's College of Medicine Convenient Care Center. In this position, Dr. Shearer held a faculty appointment in Drexel University's College of Medicine. Dr. Shearer currently practices at the Crozer Keystone Health System in the Occupational and Employee Health departments.

Barbara M. Siebert, DNP, CRNP, FNP-BC, CNE, is currently the Associate Director of Student Health Services at the University of the Sciences, Philadelphia, PA. In May 2012, she graduated from Duquesne University School of Nursing with a Doctorate in Nursing Practice. Her capstone research project was *The Academic Characteristics of Nursing Students with Undiagnosed Learning Disabilities: A Retrospective Case Study Analysis.* Dr. Siebert has more than 32 years of nursing education experience teaching nurse practitioner students in both women's health and family practice and undergraduate nursing students in a variety of nursing education settings. As an FNP, she has extensive clinical experience providing comprehensive primary care and family planning/gynecologic health care to adolescents as well as addressing primary care health issues affecting male and female adults across the life span. Dr. Siebert continues to provide health care to diverse and vulnerable patient populations in urban, suburban, and rural health care settings. She has practiced for more than 20 years at the Department of Adolescent Medicine at St. Christopher's Hospital for Children in Philadelphia, and currently maintains an additional practice in Addiction Medicine at the Livengrin Foundation, providing comprehensive health care to patients in the drug and alcohol recovery program.

Made in the USA
Charleston, SC
09 July 2014